The Echocardiography Companion

Tarak Rambhatla • Gila Perk

The Echocardiography Companion

Study Guide and Review

Springer

Tarak Rambhatla
Miami Cardiac and Vascular Institute
Baptist Health South Florida
Miami, FL
USA

Gila Perk
Icahn School of Medicine
at Mount Sinai
New York, NY
USA

ISBN 978-3-030-47040-1 ISBN 978-3-030-47041-8 (eBook)
https://doi.org/10.1007/978-3-030-47041-8

This Springer imprint is published by the registered company Springer Nature Switzerland AG
The registered company address is: Gewerbestrasse 11, 6330 Cham, Switzerland

Contents

1 Echo Physics

Learning Objectives

- Understand the principles of US image formation
- Learn basic terminology related to US physics and how they relate to image formation
- Review the various components of image resolution
- Recognize image artifacts and learn ways to avoid or minimize them

General Considerations

Basic process of US image formation (Fig. 1.1):

- US signal sent to tissue → US-tissue reflector interaction → Returned signal recorded.
- The returned signal is analyzed for:
  - Time for the signal to return → translated to distance to the reflector
  - Amplitude of the retuning signal → translated into brightness

This process can be broken down to the following components, each of which will be discussed in the following sections:

- The US transducer
- Ultrasound wave and pulses
- US-tissue interaction (specular and Doppler)
- Image formation
- Image resolution
- US artifacts

1.1 US Transducer

A transducer is a device that converts one form of energy into another. The basic components of a transducer include (Fig. 1.2):

1. Piezoelectric crystal (e.g. quartz, barium titanate)
   - Element that creates an US wave and reacts to US
     - Electric current applied to crystal → change in shape → US wave produced
     - US wave hits a crystal → deformation occurs → electrical impulse produced
   - The same crystal can serve both as a transmitter and receiver
   - The main frequency of the emitted US depends on the thickness of the crystal
   - However, every US pulse created by a crystal contains more than one frequency (termed the band width of the US beam created)

T. Rambhatla, G. Perk, *The Echocardiography Companion*,
https://doi.org/10.1007/978-3-030-47041-8_1

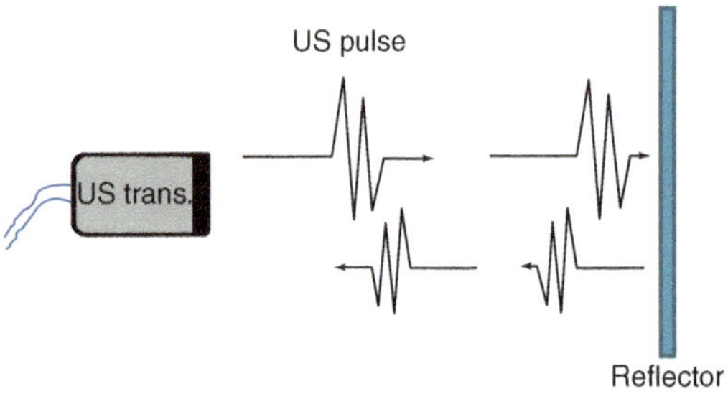

Fig. 1.1 **Image formation**. The basic sequence of events for image creation in echocardiography; an ultrasound pulse is generated by a transducer (US trans.) and sent to the body. The pulse propagates in the body until it encounters a reflector. A reflector is a boundary between two media that have different acoustic properties. The US pulse is then reflected back to the transducer

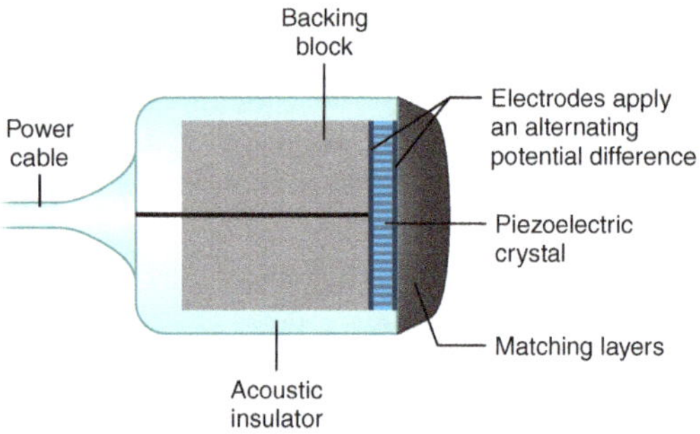

Fig. 1.2 **Basic components of the US transducer**. The important components that make an US transducer include the piezoelectric crystal, electrodes, matching layers, backing block and power cable. See text for detailed description

2. Electrodes (apply alternating electrical current)
3. Matching layers
   - Acoustic impedance matching between the body and the piezoelectric elements (to prevent reflection of the US wave immediately at the skin level)
   - The acoustic impedance of the matching layer is intermediate, between that of the crystal and biological tissue
4. Backing block
   - Absorbs the acoustic energy and shortens the ringing response of the piezoelectric material after electric current is applied to the crystal
   - Reduces spatial pulse length (see below) for improved resolution
5. Power cables

If one element is used, an "ice pick" view of the heart is obtained, at the site where the beam traverses the heart (Fig. 1.3).

The returned signal can be displayed as an amplitude graph (A mode) or as a dot with varying brightens which represents the amplitude of the returned signal (B mode)

When repeated sampling is done along one line and presented over time utilizing the brightness mode, the movement of structures in the line of imaging can be tracked over time (M mode)

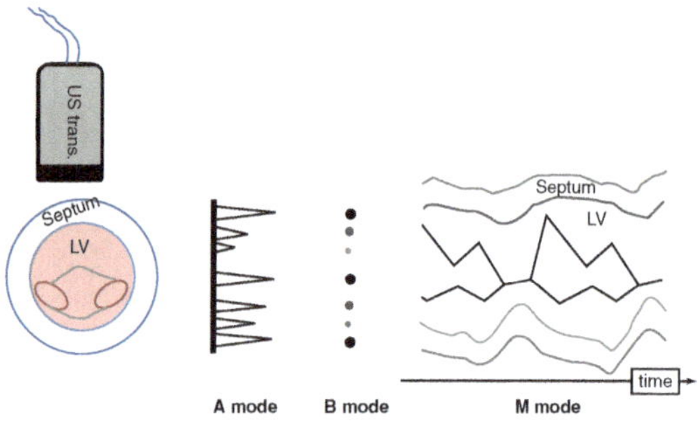

Fig. 1.3 **A, B, M Mode imaging**. When a single element is used for imaging, several forms of display are available. The returned signal can be displayed as an amplitude graph (A mode) or as a dot with varying brightness which represents the amplitude of the returned signal (B mode). When repeated sampling along one line is done and presented over time utilizing the brightness mode, the movement of structures in the line of imaging can be tracked over time (M mode)

For two dimensional imaging, several scan lines need to be combined into one image

- One element can be mechanically steered across an area; the returning signals are combined to form an image
- Alternatively, more than one element is used; an array of US crystals is used to create sector scanning
- For cardiac US, phased array transducers are used; in this configuration the various elements are activated with a time delay → a wave front that is the sum of the individual wavelets is created (Fig. 1.4)

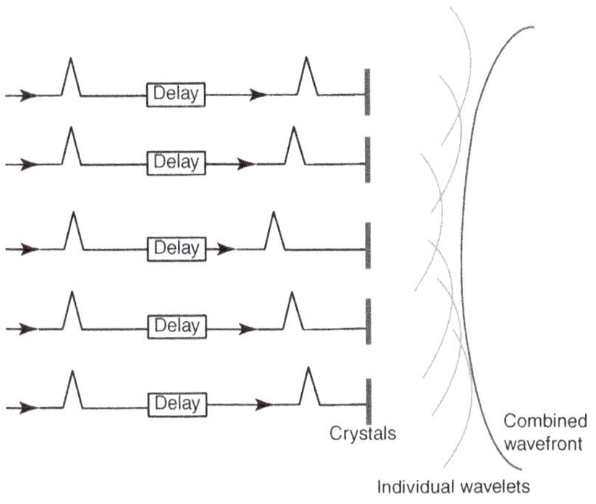

Fig. 1.4 **Phased array transducer**. When multiple elements are used, a 2D image can be obtained; an array of US crystals is used to create sector scanning. For cardiac US, phased array transducers are used; in this configuration the various elements are activated with a time delay creating a wave front that is the sum of the individual wavelets

- The wave front can be steered and focused towards the region of interest

1.2 US Wave and Pulses

US wave is a pattern of compression and refraction which propagates through a medium. It can be described by the following properties (Fig. 1.5):

- Period—the time it takes to complete one cycle
- Frequency—number of wave cycles in one second (f – measured in Hz: $\frac{cycles}{s}$)
- Wave length—distance from peak to peak of an ultrasound wave (λ)
- Propagation velocity—speed by which the US wave travels through biological tissues. US travels through different tissues at different speeds; propagation through lung (~700 m/s) is much slower as compared to propagation through bone (3000 m/s). Propagation velocity through soft tissue and blood is 1540 m/s (C – measured by $\frac{m}{s}$)
  – Frequency, wave length, and propagation velocity are related by:

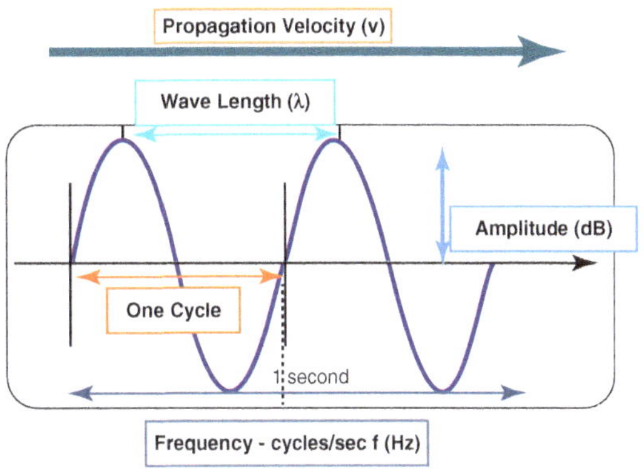

Fig. 1.5 **US wave characteristics**. US wave is a pattern of compression and refraction, which propagates through a medium. It can be described by the following properties: period, frequency, wavelength, propagation velocity, and amplitude. See text for detailed description

$$\lambda = \frac{c}{f}$$

  – For cardiac ultrasound:

$$\text{since } C = 1540\ \frac{m}{s}$$

$$\rightarrow \lambda = \frac{1540}{f(Hz)}\ (\text{m}) = \frac{1.54}{f(MHz)}\ (\text{mm})$$

- Amplitude—maximal displacement relative to the resting state; measures the energy of the US wave. Uses a logarithmic scale comparing the measured amplitude relative to a reference value and presented in Decibels (dB)
  – Related parameters:
    Power—energy per unit time
    Intensity—power per unit area
    Intensity diminishes with propagation distance

Echocardiography uses pulses of US: A short burst of US is sent from the transducer, followed by a "listening period" for the returning signal (Fig. 1.6)

- Pulse—few cycles of US
- Pulse repetition period—time from beginning of one pulse to the beginning of the next one
- Pulse repetition frequency (PRF)—number of pulses that are generated in one second (measured in Hz – $\frac{\#\,of\ pulses}{s}$)
- Pulse duration (PD)—the time it takes for one pulse to occur

  - Depends on the wave period and the number of cycles per pulse
  - Pulse duration decreases when the number of cycles decreases or when the wave frequency increases (wave period decreases)
- Spatial pulse length (SPL)—distance in space over which the pulse occurs
  - Measured in millimeters
  - Related to pulse duration: SPL = PD × C (propagation velocity)
- Listening period ("Dead time")—determines the depth of imaging
  - Longer "listening period" → deeper structures can be imaged; machine waits longer between pulses and records returning signals from structures that are further away

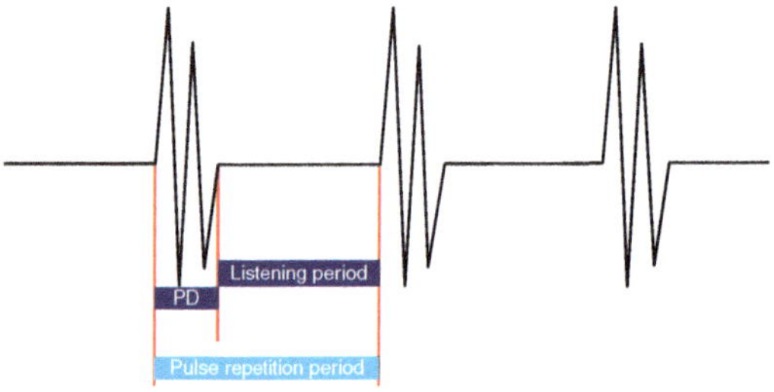

Fig. 1.6 **US pulses**. Echocardiography uses pulses of US: A short burst of US is sent from the transducer, followed by a "listening period" for the returning signal. Each pulse is made of a few cycles of US. Pulse repetition period—time from beginning of one pulse to the beginning of the next one. Pulse duration (PD)—the time it takes for one pulse to occur

  - When PRF is changed the listening period changes (→ depth of imaging changes)
- Duty factor—fraction of time the transducer is "on" (sending pulses)
- Duty factor = $\frac{\textit{Pulsed Duration}}{\textit{Pulse Repition Period}}$

1.3 US-Tissue Interaction

US image is formed after a wave interacts with biological tissue boundaries and a returning signal is detected by the transducer.

US travels through biological tissue/medium ("medium 1") until it encounters a boundary of a second medium ("medium 2") that has different acoustic properties. This tissue boundary serves as a "reflector."

Several interactions can occur between US waves and a reflector (Fig. 1.7):

- Reflection
  Return of the signal back through "medium 1" towards the US source
- Refraction
  Deflection of the sound wave from a straight path
- Propagation/attenuation

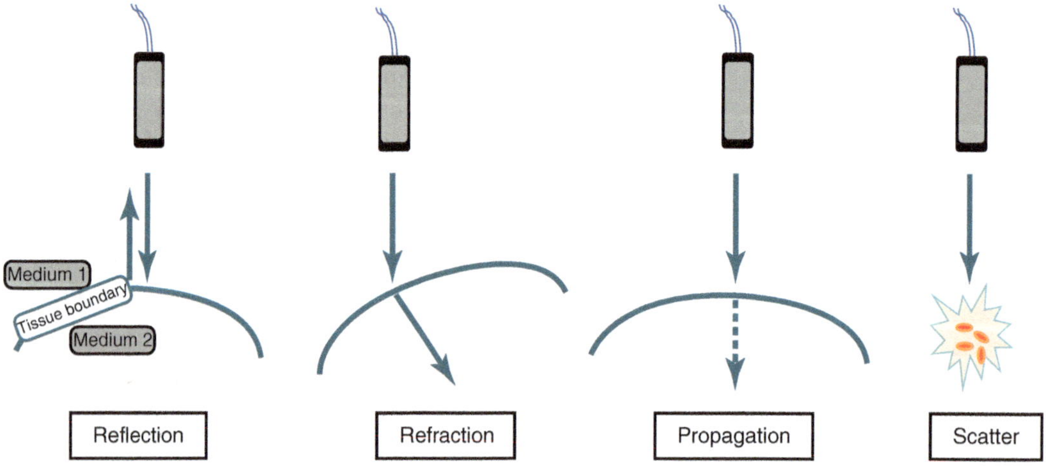

Fig. 1.7 **US-tissue interaction**. A tissue boundary ("reflector") is the border between two media that have different acoustic properties. When an US pulse hits a reflector, several interactions can take place: reflection—the pulse is reflected back towards the transducer, refraction—the pulse continues to propagate but at an angle relative to the original path, propagation—the pulse continues along the original path however at a lower energy (amplitude), scatter—dispersion of the US in multiple directions

Transmission of the sound wave through "medium 2" at lower amplitude than the original wave

- Scatter
  Dispersion of the reflected signals in all directions.
  - When a reflector size is small (relative to the wavelength) scattering (rather than reflection) occurs
  - Normally, the amplitude of the returning signal is much lower as compared to original wave's amplitude
  - Scatter can occur when US interacts with blood cells, heterogeneous medium, or irregular surfaces
  - This type of interaction is what allows imaging of the "texture" of the myocardium
    Note: scatter of US is relatively angle independent which helps image structures even if they are not perpendicular to the direction of the US beam

Factors that determine which interaction takes place include:

- Acoustic impedance difference between tissues
  Acoustic impedance is a tissue property that depends on tissue density and stiffness
- Angle of incidence
  Angle between US wave and reflector; Maximal reflection occurs with 90° angle of incidence (making it the best incident angle for two-dimensional imaging)
- Distance from the transducer
  The US wave loses energy ("attenuates") as it travels through tissues; the energy from the US wave is absorbed into the tissues
- Attenuation coefficient—loss of energy per distance per frequency
  In cardiac imaging 0.5 dB/cm/MHz
  Reflected signals from distant targets are lower in amplitude
- US wave frequency
  The frequency of the wave effects the penetration and attenuation; higher frequency results in more energy loss, meaning more attenuation (less penetration)

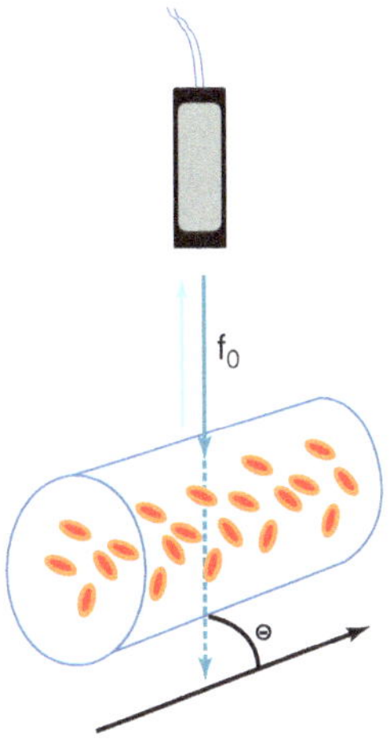

Fig. 1.8 **The Doppler principle**. When US interacts with a moving "target" (e.g. blood cells) the returned wave has a different frequency than the emitted wave (f_0). The difference in those frequencies (the emitted and the returned) is termed the "Doppler shift." The Doppler shift depends on the speed of the target and the angle between the US beam and the target's motion (angle Θ)

Doppler US is based on scatter interaction between US waves and red blood cells

- Since blood cells are a "moving target" the returned signal has a different frequency than the emitted signal, as stated by the Doppler principle (Fig. 1.8):
  - There is a change in frequency/wavelength of a wave, caused by motion
- The frequency change (shift) (Δf) depends on several factors, as given by the Doppler equation:

$$\Delta f = \frac{2 f_0 V}{C} \times Cos\Theta$$

- f_0—Emitted frequency, V—velocity of target, C—propagation velocity, Θ—angle of incidence
  - The Doppler shift is measured from the returning signal
  - The angle is assumed to be 0°
    Note: in clinical echocardiography, the US beam is aligned such that the angle of incidence is as close to 0 as possible; attempting to correct for other incident angle introduces too much error
  - The emitted frequency is known
- The equation can be re-written to solve for V:

$$V = \frac{\Delta f \, x C}{2 f_0}$$

The velocity of the target (blood flow) can thus be calculated

- Blood flow velocity is related to the pressure gradient driving the interrogated flow
  - The relationship is given by the Bernoulli equation, which has multiple components
  - In clinical echocardiography, the simplified Bernoulli equation is used:

$$\Delta P = 4\left(V_2^2 - V_1^2\right)$$

  - Most commonly the V_1 component (upstream velocity) can be ignored, such that:

$$\Delta P = 4V^2$$

Summary:

- Once blood flow velocity between two chambers is known (calculated by the Doppler equation utilizing scatter interaction between US wave and blood cells) the pressure gradient between the two chambers where this flow occurs can be calculated.
- See Chap. 7 for more details about hemodynamic assessment utilizing Doppler echocardiography
  Note: tissue velocity can also be calculated by Doppler based technique: scattered signals from the myocardium are analyzed for frequency shift allowing for myocardial tissue velocity to be calculated.

1.4 Image Formation

Image formation is based on two conversions:

- Pulse travel time—converted to distance
- Amplitude of the returning signal—converted to brightness

Range equation

- The time it takes for US pulse to go to and return from a reflector is measured (T)
- Propagation speed (velocity by which the pulse travels through soft tissues) is known (C)
- The distance (d) to the reflector is calculated by: d = ½ C × T (the ½ constant is used since the time measured is the time to the reflector and back)

Every returning signal is analyzed for

1. The distance it came from (by measuring the time it took the signal to go-and-return)
2. The amplitude of the signal

Based on the distance and the amplitude an image is created to represent the reflector that caused the signal to return

Modes of Imaging

1. A mode, B mode, M mode
   - One element is used to create an "ice pick" view of the heart at the site where the beam traverses the heart (Fig. 1.3)
2. 2D Imaging
   - Multiple elements are used (by the phased array transducer) creating multiple scan lines
   - A two dimensional sector-image of the heart is created
3. Doppler Echocardiography
   Types of Doppler US:
   - Spectral Doppler
     - Pulsed wave Doppler (PW)
     - Continuous wave Doppler (CW)
   - Color Doppler

1.4.1 PW Doppler

General principles

- Short intermittent bursts of US, each followed by fixed and brief period of "listening"
- Allows for recording of returning signals from a certain distance, thus measuring flow velocity at a known location

- However, since the rate of sampling is finite, there is a limit on the maximal frequency shift that can be accurately measured
- The length of the listening period determines the depth from which the Doppler signal is recorded; the length of the listening period is determined by the pulse repetition frequency

PRF and depth calculation:

- Go and return time—T
- $T = \frac{2D}{C}$
  D—distance to the reflector
  C—propagation speed of sound in soft tissue
- PRF—number of pulses per second, $PRF = \frac{1}{T}$
- $PRF = \frac{C}{2D} \rightarrow D = \frac{C}{2PRF}$

Nyquist Limit
The PRF also determines the maximal frequency shift that can be accurately resolved;

- In order to accurately discern the velocity and direction of the interrogated flow, the recorded frequency shift must be less than half the PRF

$$\Delta f_{max} = \frac{1}{2} \times PRF$$

- Higher frequency shifts will result in "aliasing" of the Doppler signal (meaning direction of the flow and velocity calculation would not be accurately discerned)
- As mentioned above, based on the Doppler principle:

$$V = \frac{\Delta f \times C}{2f_0}$$

- Utilizing the above equations:

$$V_{max} = \frac{C^2}{8Df_0}$$

- The maximum flow velocity that can be accurately resolved by PW Doppler is called the Nyquist limit
- Nyquist limit is inversely related to the distance to the flow being interrogated and the emitted frequency; far sampled flow (bigger D) → lower the Nyquist limit; high emitted frequency (bigger f_0) → lower Nyquist limit

1.4.2 CW Doppler

General principles

- Continuous transmission of ultrasound
- Continuous receiving of ultrasound signal
- Requires two separate elements—one acts as transmitter and one as receiver
- All reflected signals are sampled continuously
- Since there are no pulses:
  - No limit on maximal frequency shift (velocity) that can be measured
  - However, no range resolution available

Spectral Doppler Display (Fig. 1.9)
- Velocity—Y axis
- Time—X axis
- Flow towards the transducer—above baseline
- Flow away from the transducer—below baseline
- PW Doppler—thin envelope as only velocities from a certain location are displayed
- CW Doppler—full envelope; all velocities along the scan line are displayed

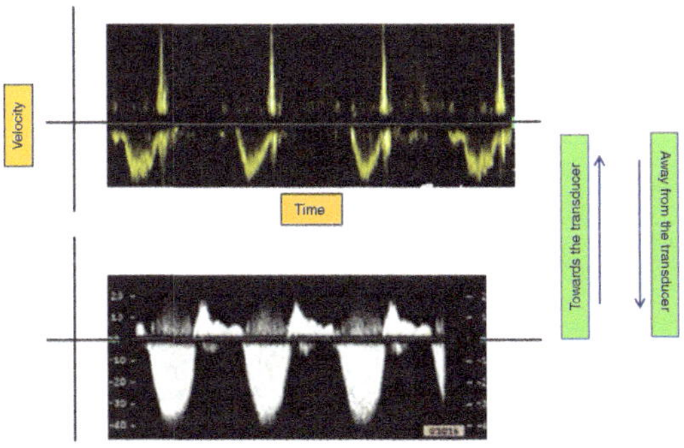

Fig. 1.9 Spectral Doppler display. By convention, velocity is displayed on the Y-axis and time on the X-axis. Velocity towards the transducer is displayed above the baseline; velocity away from the transducer, below

1.4.3 Color Doppler

- A form of pulsed wave Doppler—allows for some range resolution
- Multiple sample volumes along each scan line
- Returning signals are analyzed according to amplitude:
  - Above a threshold—grey shade
  - Below the threshold—defined as Doppler data and assigned color
- Color assigned by direction of the flow
  - Towards the transducer—red
  - Away from the transducer—blue
- Limitations
  - Regurgitant jets are three dimensional structures—chamber constraints and direction of flow may cause masking and underestimation
  - Instrument settings (e.g. color scale, filters, gain) can affect the visualization of the jet
  - Jet size is determined by volume but may also be influenced by jet momentum, which depends on flow rate as well as flow velocity
  - Color jet differs from angiographic jet—color Doppler records velocities

1.5 Image Resolution

Resolution is the ability to distinguish between two objects in close proximit

- Spatial resolution—Discerning two objects close in space
- Temporal resolution—Discerning two events close in time

1.5.1 Spatial Resolution (Fig. 1.10)

- In order for two reflectors to be separated on the echocardiographic image, they need to create two separate echoes
- Spatial resolution is the minimum required separation between reflectors that will produce separate echoes
- When describing resolution in numerical terms—the smaller the number the better the resolution
- There are two aspects of spatial (or "detail") resolution:
  - Axial resolution—differentiating objects along the direction of the US beam

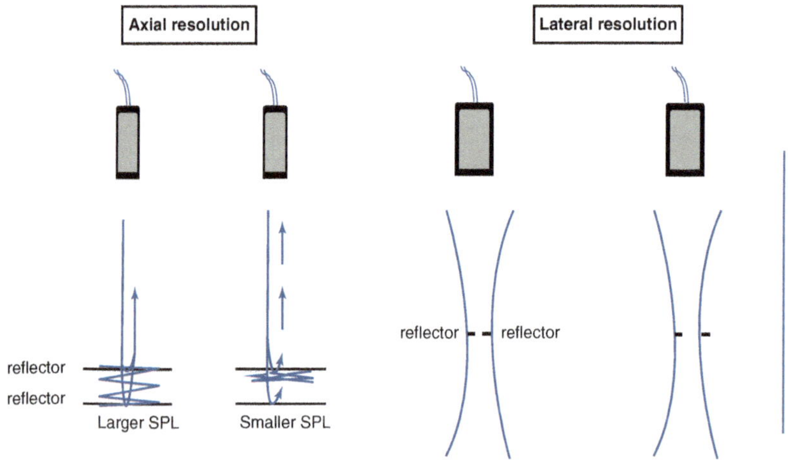

Fig. 1.10 Components of spatial resolution. In order for two reflectors to be separated on the echocardiographic image, they need to create two separate echoes. Two aspects of spatial resolution: axial and lateral resolution. Axial resolution is the ability to separate reflectors that are close to each other along the path of the beam; it depends on spatial pulse length. Lateral resolution is the ability to separate reflectors that are side by side to each other (perpendicular to the direction of the beam); it depends mainly on beam width

- Lateral resolution—differentiating objects perpendicular the direction of the US beam

1.5.1.1 Axial Resolution

- Axial resolution is determined by the spatial pulse length (SPL)
- In order for two reflectors (along the path of the US beam) to produce two separate echoes their distance has to be more than half the SPL

$$\text{Axial resolution}(\text{mm}) = \frac{\text{SPL}(\text{mm})}{2}$$

- In order to improve axial resolution, SPL must be reduced
  SPL = Number of cycles in a pulse x wavelength
  SPL can be reduced by:
  - Minimizing the number of cycles in a pulse
    This is accomplished by damping the ringing of the crystal
    Minimum cycles in a pulse—1-3
  - Reducing the wavelength
    This is accomplished by imaging with higher frequency US wave

  Note: higher frequency improves image resolution however lowers penetration as attenuation increases as frequency increases

1.5.1.2 Lateral Resolution

- Lateral resolution is determined by the beam width
- In order for two reflectors that are side by side relative to the US beam to produce two separate echoes, their distance has to be wider than the beam width
- In order to improve lateral resolution, beam width needs to be reduced
- Beam width is reduced by focusing

1.5.2 Temporal Resolution

- Temporal resolution is determined by the frame rate
- Higher frame rates allow for discerning events that are closely spaced in time
- Frame rate is determined by:
  - Number of scan lines in the imaging sector
  - Required number of focus points
  - Depth of imaging (pulse repetition frequency)
- Increasing number of scan lines, increasing number of focuses or decreasing the PRF will result in reduced frame rate

1.6 US Artifacts

Artifacts are echoes appearing on the sonographic image which do not correspond in location or intensity to actual tissue interfaces in the patient

Types of Artifacts:

- Failure to visualize structures that are present
- Image of a structure that differs in size and/or shape from its actual appearance
- Extraneous US signals that result in the appearance of "structures" that are not actually present (at least not in the displayed location)

Artifacts can occur due to:

- Equipment malfunction
  E.g. broken crystal, electrical interference
- Operator error
  E.g. use of inappropriate color scale, gain misuse or angle correction function
- Violation of assumptions

Basic Assumptions in Echo

1. The depth of the reflector is the only determinant of the go-and-return time
2. Beam dimensions are small, both in lateral direction and section thickness (elevation)
3. The transmitted wave travels along a straight path from the transducer and back to the transducer
4. All detected echoes originate only from the main axis of the beam
5. US wave travels in soft tissue at a constant speed of 1540 m/s

1.6.1 Location Artifacts

1.6.1.1 Axial Direction (Fig. 1.11)

- When a strong reflector is present at the path of the beam, extra “round trips” can be taken by the pulse before it returns to the transducer
- These extra trips increase the measured go-and-return time
- Machine interprets the longer time as a signal returning from deeper structure (assumption 1)
- Additional false image is created behind the true image
- The false image has lower brightness as compared to the true image as energy is lost during the extra trip

  Note:
  - Strong reflector creating this artifact can be on the main path of the beam or encountered by a side lobe of the beam
  - In either case, the false image is placed behind the true image
  - The location of the strong reflector (in front or behind the object imaged) determines whether an extra copy is created vs. a mirror image is created
- Examples include: mirror image artifact, reverberation, comet tail

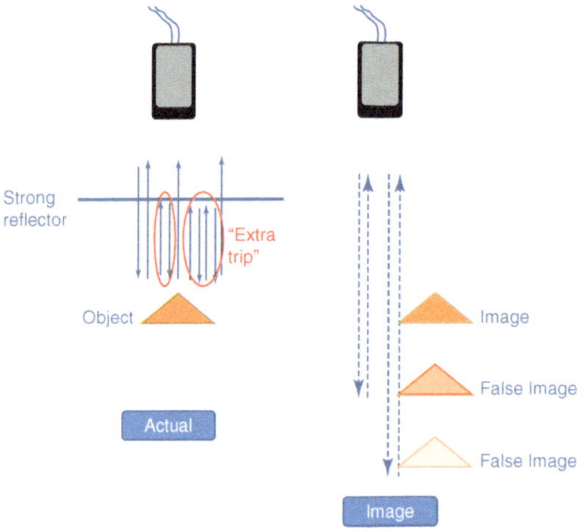

Fig. 1.11 **Location artifacts—Reverberation and mirror image**. When a strong reflector is present along the path of the beam, extra “round trips” can be taken by the pulse before it returns to the transducer. The measured go-and-return time is increased and the machine interprets the longer time as a signal returning from a deeper structure resulting in an additional false image behind the true image

1.6.1.2 Lateral Direction

Side Lobe Artifact (Fig. 1.12)

- A strong reflector can create a returning signal even if it is imaged by a low energy side lobe of the main US beam
- Generally signals created by a side lobe are too weak to create a sufficient returning signal
- However a strong reflector can create a strong enough reflected signal

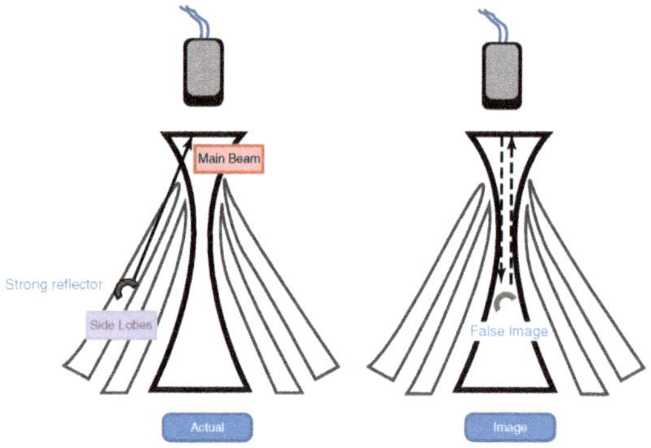

Fig. 1.12 **Location artifacts—Side lobe**. A strong reflector can create a strong enough returning signal even if it is imaged by a low energy side lobe of the main US beam. This signal is interpreted by the machine as if it arrived from the path of the main beam, creating a false image side by side to the true image

- Machine interprets the returned signal as if it arrived from the path of the main beam (assumption 4)
- A false image is created side by side to the true image

Beam Width Artifact
- When two reflectors are side by side (perpendicular to the main beam axis) they may not create separate images
- Reflectors can be separated in the lateral direction or elevational dimension
- If they are separated by less than the beam width, a single image will be created

Refraction Artifact (Fig. 1.13)
- A reflector between the transducer and the object of interest may cause the US beam to refract and continue propagation at an angle
- Interaction between the object of interest and the refracted beam will create a returning signal

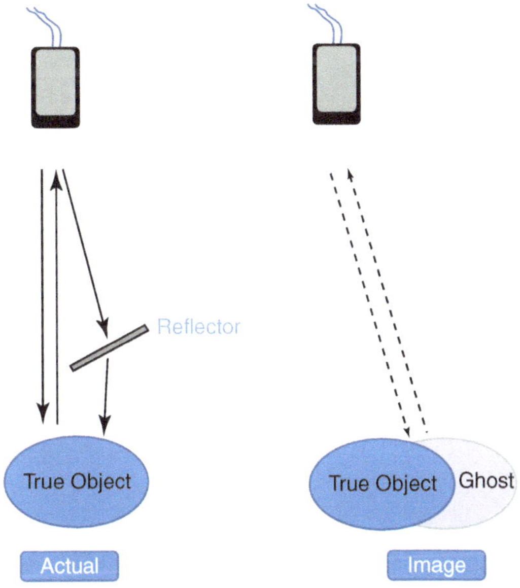

Fig. 1.13 **Location artifacts—Refraction**. A reflector between the transducer and the object of interest may cause the US beam to refract and continue propagation at an angle. However, the machine interprets the returned signal as if it traveled on a straight path from the transducer and back creating a false image side by side to the true image

- Machine interprets the returned signal as if traveled on a straight path from the transducer and back (assumption 3)
- A false image is created side by side to the true image

1.6.2 Attenuation Artifacts

Acoustic Shadowing (Fig. 1.14)
- A structure with marked difference in acoustic impedance anywhere between the transducer and the object of interest may cause acoustic shadowing
- Marked difference in acoustic impedance blocks transmission of all ultrasound beyond it
- Any structure behind the "shadower" will not be imaged at all

Echo Drop Out (Fig. 1.15)
- A structure is interrogated by a beam at a near parallel angle
- Too little or no reflected ultrasound reaches the transducer back
- No image or very faint image is created

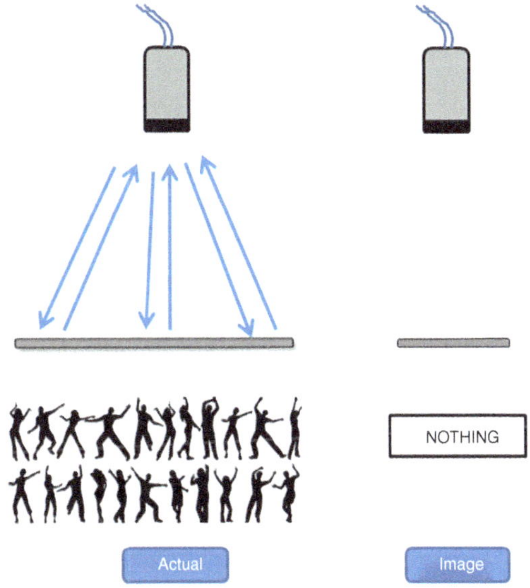

Fig. 1.14 **Attenuation artifacts—Acoustic shadowing**. A structure with marked difference in acoustic impedance anywhere between the transducer and the object of interest may cause acoustic shadowing such that any structure behind the "shadower" will not be imaged at all

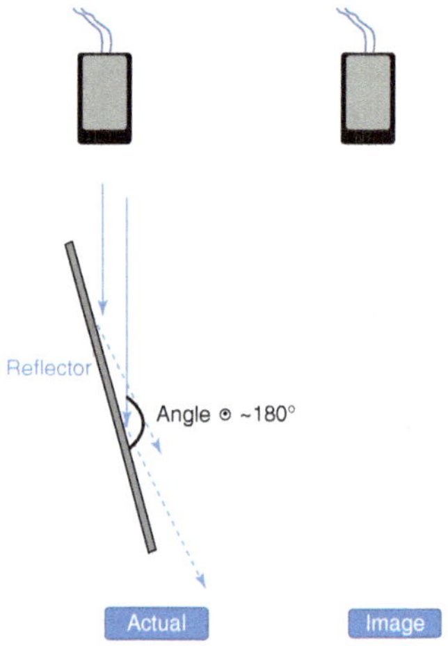

Fig. 1.15 **Attenuation artifacts—Echo drop out**. When a structure is interrogated by a beam at a near parallel angle, too little or no reflected ultrasound reaches the transducer back such that no image or very faint image is created

Further Reading

Edelman SK, editor. Understanding ultrasound physics: fundamentals and exam review. 2nd ed. Woodlands, TX: ESP; 1994.

Kremkau FW. Diagnostic ultrasound: principle and instruments. 6th ed. Philadelphia, PA: W.B Saunders; 2002.

2 TTE and Chamber Quantification

Learning Objectives

- Learn the basic windows and views of transthoracic echocardiogram (TTE)
- Become familiar with the standard TTE protocol
- Know how to perform and interpret basic measurements for proper chamber quantification

General Considerations

- Echo is a tomographic technique—every image is a thin "slice" of the heart
- Echo windows—positions on the chest where echo probe can be placed to obtain images
- There are four standard echo windows (Fig. 2.1)
  - Parasternal—to the left of the sternum, generally at third or fourth intercostal space
  - Apical—under the left breast where the apical impulse is felt
  - Subcostal—immediately below the sternum
  - Suprasternal—immediately superior to the manubrium of the sternum

A fifth echo window, the right parasternal is utilized for specific indications (e.g. interrogating velocities across aortic valve)

Index marker—ultrasound transducers have an index marker on them such that every view can be defined by imaging window and direction of the index marker

Transducer Maneuvers
- Rotate: transducer is fixed in place, index marker is rotated to point towards a different direction
- Tilt: transducer is fixed in place; tip of the transducer is rocked/tilted such that it faces new structures in the same imaging plane
- Slide/move: transduced is moved up or down several intercostal spaces

2.1 Standard Echocardiographic Views

2.1.1 Parasternal Window

Parasternal Long Axis View (PLAX) (Fig. 2.2, Video 2.1)

- Transducer position: third or fourth intercostal space, left of the sternum
- Index marker: pointing towards the patient's right shoulder

---

Electronic Supplementary Material The online version of this chapter (https://doi.org/10.1007/978-3-030-47041-8_2) contains supplementary material, which is available to authorized users.

T. Rambhatla, G. Perk, *The Echocardiography Companion*,
https://doi.org/10.1007/978-3-030-47041-8_2

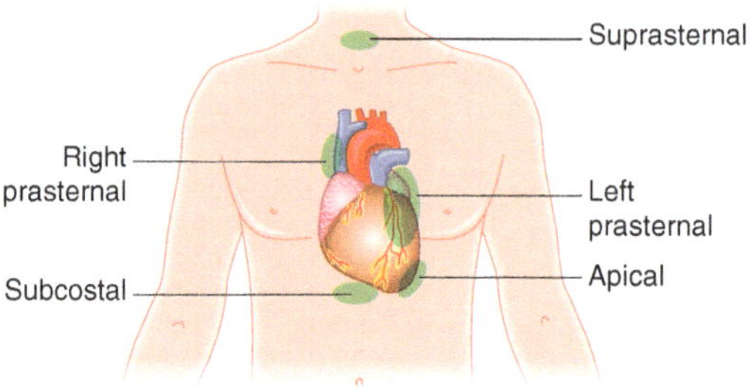

Fig. 2.1 **Echo windows.** Echo window—the place on the chest the transducer is placed. There are four standard echo windows: parasternal, apical, subcostal and suprasternal. In special circumstances and indications, a right parasternal window is utilized as well (e.g. assess maximal velocity across the aortic valve)

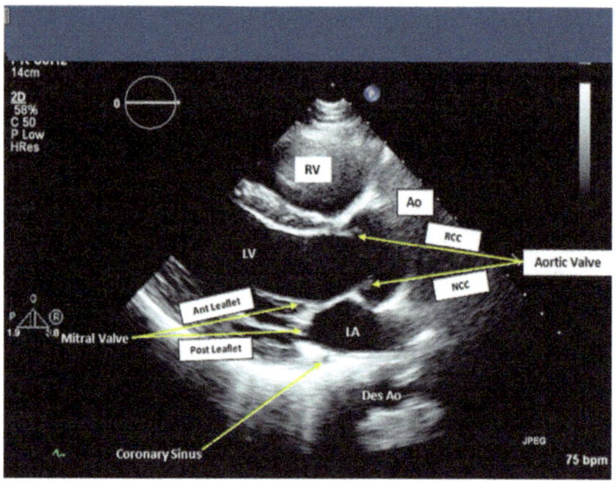

Fig. 2.2 **PLAX view.** 2D echocardiographic image of the parasternal long axis view (PLAX). The PLAX view visualizes the RV, ascending aorta, the anteroseptum, and the inferolateral wall of the LV, the mitral valve, the aortic valve, and the descending aorta. *Ant* anterior, *Ao* aorta, *LV* left ventricle, *NCC* non-coronary cusp, *Post* posterior, *RCC* right coronary cusp, *RV* right ventricle

Imaging points:

- The left ventricle should be perpendicular to the US beam
- The LV apex should not be visualized on PLAX view

Chambers

- Right ventricle (RV)
  - Most anterior structure on PLAX view
  - Generally—right ventricular outflow tract is seen

  Note: if a catheter/wire is seen on this view, likely a Swan Ganz catheter (less likely a pacemaker wire)

Measurement	Timing	Location	Normal values (cm)
RVOT	End diastole	Between RV anterior wall and septal-aortic junction	2.5 ± 0.25

- Ascending aorta
  - The aortic annulus, sinuses of Valsalva, sino-tubular junction and proximal 3–4 cm of tubular ascending aorta can be seen

  Note: to image more of the ascending aorta, transducer can be moved up 1–2 intercostal spaces

Measurement	Timing	Technique	Location	Normal values (cm)
Aortic annulus	Mid systole	Inner edge to inner edge	Between right and non-coronary cusps insertion points	Men 2.6 ± 0.3 Women 2.3 ± 0.2
Ao sinuses	End diastole	Leading edge to leading edge	Maximum diameter of the sinuses	Men 3.4 ± 0.3 Women 3.0 ± 0.3
Sino-tubular junction	End diastole	Leading edge to leading edge	Junction of distal sinuses and proximal tubular aorta	Men 2.9 ± 0.3 Women 2.6 ± 0.3
Ascending aorta	End diastole	Leading edge to leading edge	Largest dimension seen above the sinuses	Men 3.0 ± 0.4 Women 2.7 ± 0.4

- Left ventricle
  - Walls visualized—antero-septum and inferolateral wall (previously posterior wall)
  - End diastolic measurements should be performed at the frame immediately following mitral valve closure or at the peak of the R wave of the QRS complex

Measurement	Timing	Location	Normal range (cm)
Wall thickness	End diastole	At the tips of the mitral leaflets	Men 0.6–1.0 Women 0.6–0.9
LV diastolic dimension	End diastole	At the tips of the mitral leaflets	Men 4.2–5.8 Women 3.8–5.2
LV systolic dimension	End systole, LV smallest	At the tips of the mitral leaflets	Men 2.5–4.0 Women 2.2 ± 3.5
LVOT	Mid systole, valve max open	3–10 mm below the valve plane	Men 2.2 ± 2.1 Women 2.0 ± 1.7

- Left atrium
  - Anteroposterior diameter of the LA can be measured on the PLAX view
  - Measurement done at end systole; leading edge to leading edge; between the posterior aspect of the sinus of Valsalva to the posterior wall (perpendicular to the long axis of the left atrium)
  - Nowadays, left atrial size assessment is based on volumetric measurements from apical views (see below) making 2D linear measurements obsolete.

Valves

- Aortic valve
  - Most commonly, the right (anterior) and the non-coronary (posterior) cusps are visualized
  - With normal tri-leaflet valve, the closure line is at the center of the aortic root
  - Aorto-mitral curtain (fibrous tissue between the aortic root and anterior mitral leaflet) can be visualized

  Note: presence of aorto-mitral curtain identifies the morphologic left ventricle in complex congenital heart disease.
- Mitral valve
  - Both the anterior and posterior leaflets are seen on PLAX view
  - The surface area of both leaflets is similar; the anterior leaflet is longer, the posterior leaflet has a larger annular attachment
  - Both leaflets are connected to both papillary muscles (which should not be visualized on a proper PLAX view)

M-mode

M-mode tracings have been largely replaced by 2D imaging; however, it is notable that the temporal resolution of m-mode recordings is superior and event timing can be accurately assessed on certain M-modes

Typically a standard transthoracic echocardiogram will include several m-mode recordings from the PLAX view

- Aortic valve and left atrium (Fig. 2.3)
  - Obtained at the level of the aortic valve tips

  Note: Anterior and posterior aortic root displacement is caused by atrial filling and emptying; high volume states (e.g. mitral regurgitation) cause increased root displacement; low flow states (e.g. low cardiac output,

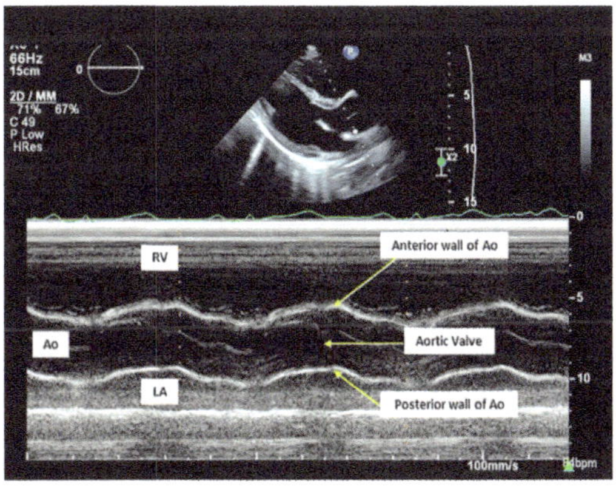

Fig. 2.3 **Aortic Root M-mode.** M-mode echocardiogram at the aortic valve level showing the aortic valve opening and closing during systole and diastole. *Ao* aorta, *LA* left atrium, *RV* right ventricle

mitral stenosis) cause decreased aortic root motion
- Mitral valve (Fig. 2.4)
  - Obtained at the level of the mitral valve tips
  - Motion of the mitral valve leaflets during systole and diastole can be observed
- Left ventricle (Fig. 2.5)
  - Obtained at a mid-ventricular level, distal to the mitral valve tips
  - End diastolic and end systolic dimensions can be measured if the m-line bisects the image at a perpendicular angle (otherwise, 2D based measurements are preferred)

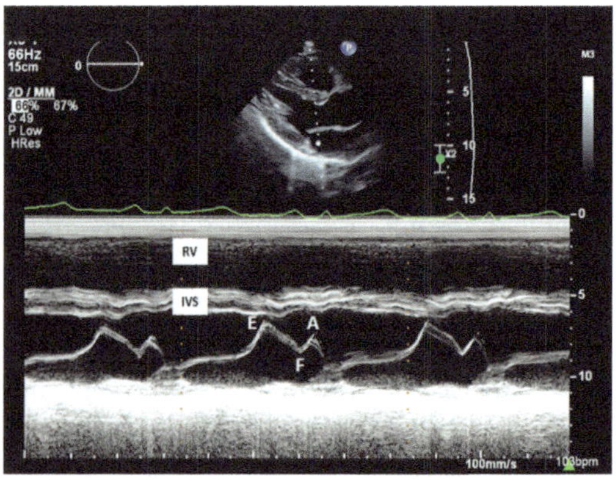

Fig. 2.4 **Mitral Valve M-mode**. M-mode echocardiogram of the mitral valve: E, peak of early opening; F, end of rapid ventricular filling; A, peak late opening with atrial kick. *IVS* interventricular septum, *RV* right ventricle

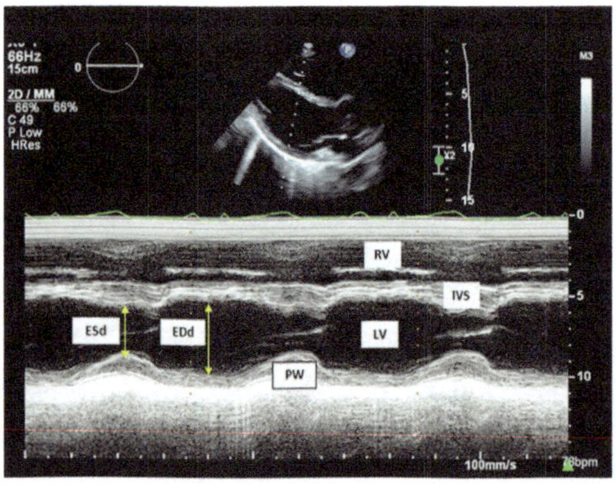

Fig. 2.5 **Basal LV M-mode.** M-mode echocardiogram at the basal LV level. *EDd* end diastolic dimension, *ESd* end systolic dimension, *IVS* interventricular septum, *LV* left ventricle, *PW* posterior wall, *RV* right ventricle

Doppler
- Color Doppler
  - Laminar inflow through the mitral valve and outflow through the aortic valve can be seen
  - Turbulent regurgitant flow in either valve can be identified on PLAX view
- Spectral Doppler
  - Blood flows that are imaged on PLAX view are suboptimally angled for spectral Doppler interrogation
  - Typically no measurements of flow velocities are performed from this view
- Tissue Doppler
  - No standard tissue Doppler measurements are done on PLAX view

Parasternal Right Ventricular Inflow (Tricuspid Tilt)
(Fig. 2.6, Video 2.2)

- Transducer position: From PLAX view, transducer is tilted inferiorly; possibly a slight counterclockwise rotation
- Index marker: pointing towards patient's right shoulder or midpoint between right shoulder and mid-torso

Imaging points:
- The tricuspid valve should be in the center of the image

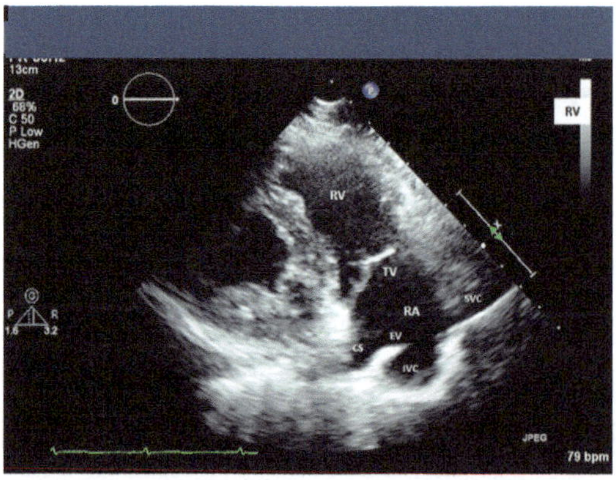

Fig. 2.6 **RV inflow view**. 2D echocardiogram of the RV inflow view showing the right ventricle, tricuspid valve, and right atrial structures. *CS* coronary sinus, *EV* eustachian valve, *IVC* inferior vena cava, *RA* right atrium, *RV* right ventricle, *SVC* superior vena cava, *TV* tricuspid valve

Chambers

- Right ventricle
  - Seen in the upper part of the sector
  - On the upper right part of the sector—anterior wall of RV, upper left part—inferior wall of RV
  - The moderator band may be seen in this view
- Right atrium
  - Coronary sinus is seen entering the right atrium near the AV groove
  - The IVC is seen in the lower part of the sector, as it enters the RA

  Note: The interatrial septum is rarely directly visualized on this view (it is parallel to the imaging plane); may be seen intermittently if there is a septal aneurysm or when a percutaneous closure device is present (e.g. post percutaneous ASD/PFO closure)

Valves

- Tricuspid valve
  - Visualized at the center of the sector
  - Two leaflets are seen: anterior leaflet (leaflet on the right) and either septal or posterior leaflet (depending on transducer orientation)

Doppler

- Color Doppler
  - Laminar inflow through the tricuspid valve can be seen
  - Turbulent tricuspid regurgitation (TR) flow can be recorded when present
- Spectral Doppler
  - Continuous wave Doppler of the TR jet can be obtained for measurement of RV systolic pressure
- Tissue Doppler
  - No standard tissue Doppler measurements are done on RV inflow view

Parasternal Right Ventricular Outflow (Fig. 2.7, Video 2.3)

- Transducer position: From PLAX view, transducer is tilted anteriorly; possibly a slight clockwise rotation
- Index marker: pointing towards patient's right shoulder or midpoint between right shoulder and mid-torso

Chambers

- Right ventricle
  - The RV outflow is visualized on this view
- Proximal pulmonary artery (PA)
  - The proximal main pulmonary artery is seen; occasionally the bifurcation can be seen from this view as well

Valves

- Pulmonic valve
  - Two out of the three leaflets can be seen
  - M mode of the PV may be obtained from this view

Doppler

- Color Doppler
  - Laminar outflow through the pulmonic valve can be seen
  - Turbulent pulmonic insufficiency (PI) flow can be recorded when present
- Spectral Doppler
  - RVOT is often aligned parallel to the US beam on this view, allowing for PW Doppler at the RVOT to be obtained. This may be used for stroke volume calculations (e.g. in cases of left sided regurgitant lesions and calculating regurgitant volume, or when calculating Qp:Qs in cases with intra-cardiac shunts)

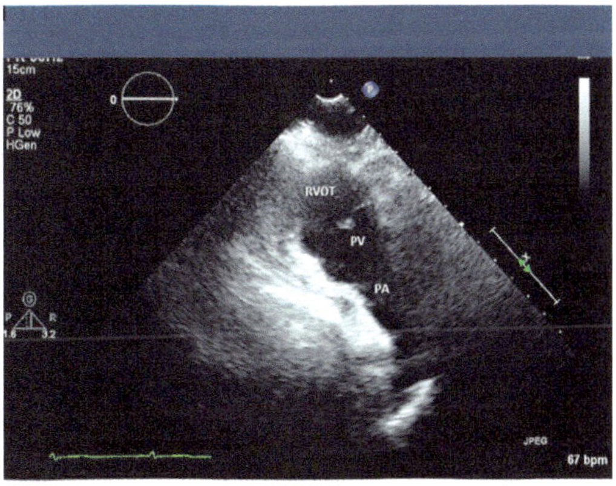

Fig. 2.7 **RV outflow view**. 2D echocardiogram of the RV outflow view showing the right ventricular outflow tract, pulmonic valve, and pulmonary artery. *PA* pulmonary artery, *PV* pulmonic valve, *RVOT* right ventricular outflow tract

- Continuous wave Doppler of the PI jet can be obtained for calculation of PA end diastolic pressure
- Tissue Doppler
  - No standard tissue Doppler measurements are done on RV outflow view

Parasternal Short Axis View (PSAX)

- Transducer position: From PLAX view (third or fourth intercostal space, left of the sternum) transducer rotated 90° clockwise
- Index marker: pointing towards the patient's left shoulder

Imaging points:

- On the PSAX view, the beam is perpendicular to the long axis of the left ventricle
- The transducer is tilted superiorly and inferiorly to obtain the four different levels of the PSAX view: Aortic valve/great vessels, mitral valve leaflets, papillary muscles, LV apex
- Moving the transducer up/down one intercostal space may help optimize the image

PSAX—AV/Great Vessels
(Fig. 2.8, Videos 2.4A and 2.4B)

Chambers

- Right ventricle
  - Most anterior chamber seen on this view
  - On the upper right side of the image, the RVOT is visualized (normal proximal diameter 21–35 mm, distal diameter 17–27 mm)
  - On the upper left side of the image the RV inflow is seen
- Pulmonary artery
  - Proximal pulmonary artery is seen in a long axis orientation
  - Tilting slightly superior/anterior allows visualization of the bifurcation of the main PA and proximal right and left pulmonary arteries
- Right atrium
  - Seen to the left of the aortic valve
  - Occasionally the superior vena cava can be seen entering the RA
  - Interatrial septum is seen posterior to the aortic valve (near the non-coronary cusp)
- Left atrium
  - Posterior to the aortic valve
  - The left atrial appendage may be visualized at the top right side of the visualized LA

Valves

- Aortic valve
  - Seen at the center of the sector
  - All three cusps can be visualized

    Right coronary cusp –most anterior, close to the RV. Careful probe manipu-

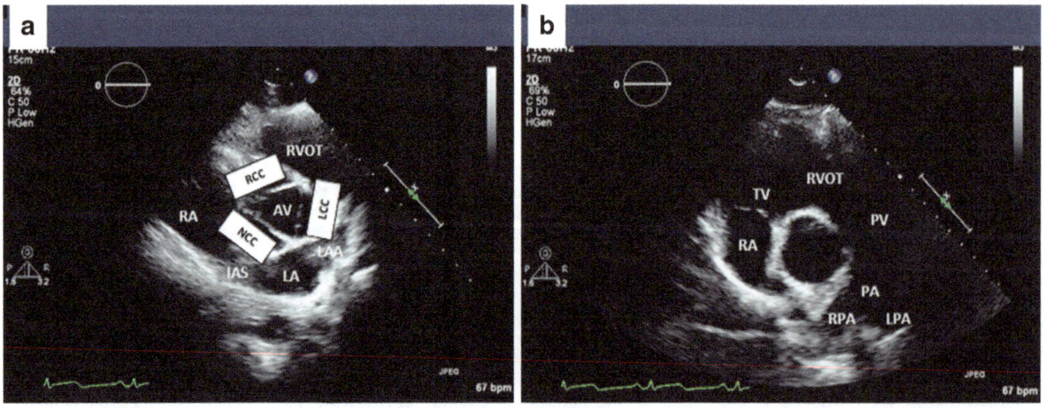

Fig. 2.8 PSAX view AV level. The parasternal short axis (PSAX) view at the aortic level: (**a**) Slight posterior tilt visualizing the left atrial appendage, (**b**) Slight anterior tilt visualizing the main pulmonary artery and its bifurcation. *AV* aortic valve, *IAS* interatrial septum, *LA* left atrium, *LCC* left coronary cusp, *LPA* left pulmonary artery, *NCC* noncoronary cusp, *PA* pulmonary artery, *PV* pulmonic valve, *RA* right atrium, *RCC* right coronary cusp, *RPA* right pulmonary artery, *RVOT* right ventricular outflow tract, *TV* tricuspid valve

lation may allow visualization of the origin of the right coronary artery

Left coronary cusp—on the right side of the AV image, often the origin of the left main coronary artery can be seen, as well as the bifurcation into the left anterior descending and the circumflex artery

Non-coronary cusp—on the left side of the AV image, close to the interatrial septum

Note: to discern the number of cusps of the aortic valve, the image should be assessed during systole. With the aortic valve open, the number of commissures should be evaluated. During diastole, a raphe between two fused cusps of a bicuspid aortic valve may appear as a coaptation area of a third leaflet.

- Tricuspid valve
  - Seen on the left side of the sector
- Pulmonic valve
  - Seen on the right side of the image
  - The pulmonic and aortic valve lie in perpendicular planes—when one is seen in short axis the other is seen in long axis. On PSAX AV level, AV is seen in short axis ("en face") and pulmonic valve in long axis
  - In adults, only 1–2 leaflets of the pulmonic valve can be visualized

Doppler

- Color Doppler
  - Laminar inflow through the tricuspid and laminar outflow through pulmonic valve can be seen
  - Turbulent tricuspid regurgitation and pulmonic insufficiency can be recorded when present
  - Aortic regurgitation can be seen when present; may be possible to locate the origin of the AI jet
- Spectral Doppler
  - PW Doppler at the RVOT may be obtained
  - Continuous wave Doppler of the PI jet can be obtained
  - Continuous wave Doppler of the TR jet can be obtained for measurement of RV systolic pressure
- Tissue Doppler
  - No standard tissue Doppler measurements are done on PSAX view

PSAX—Mitral Leaflets Level

(Fig. 2.9, Video 2.5)

Chambers

- Right ventricle
  - Appears as crescent shaped, at the upper left portion of the sector
- Left ventricle
  - The anterior, lateral, inferior wall and interventricular septum are seen on this view

Valves

- Mitral valve
  - Both leaflets are visualized on the PSAX view
  - Maximal excursion/opening of the mitral valve can be assessed on the PSAX view

  Note: if measuring mitral valve area, care must be taken to image precisely at the tips of the mitral valve (vs. more proximal) in order to make sure the smallest valve area is measured—avoid overestimation of the mitral valve area. Utilizing the biplane view (from a PLAX view) can help verify the accurate location of the short axis plane

  - Medial and lateral commissures of the mitral valve are seen

Doppler

- Color Doppler
  - Mitral regurgitation jet may be seen "en face"
  - May help localize the origin of MR jet

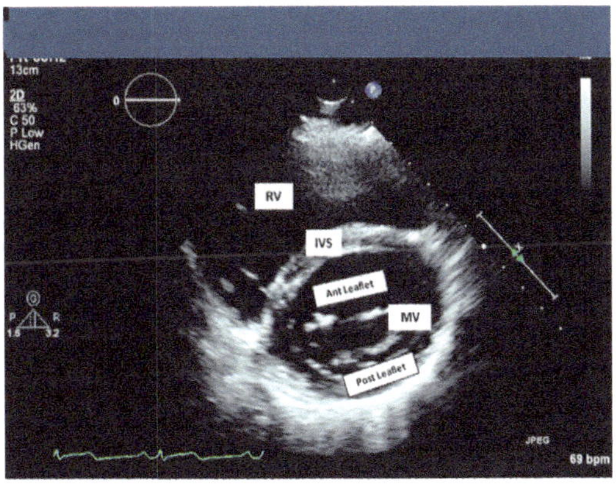

Fig. 2.9 **PSAX view MV level**. The parasternal short axis view at the basal level shows the mitral valve at its orifice. *Ant/Post* anterior/posterior, *IVS* interventricular septum, *MV* mitral valve, *RV* right ventricle

- Spectral Doppler
  - Blood flows that are imaged on PSAX-MV level view are suboptimally angled for spectral Doppler interrogation.
  - Typically no measurements of flow velocities are performed from this view
- Tissue Doppler
  - No standard tissue Doppler measurements are done on RV outflow view

PSAX—Papillary Muscle Level
(Fig. 2.10, Video 2.6)

Chambers

- Right ventricle
  - Seen at the upper medial portion of the sector
- Left ventricle
  - Both papillary muscles should be seen; anterolateral and posteromedial
  - The ventricle should appear circular on this view (mid-ventricular level)
  - Assessment of inward motion and wall thickening of the LV is important for evaluating LV systolic function

  Note: elliptical appearance of the LV at this level usually implies non-perpendicular cross section of the LV. Slight movement of the transducer (angulation and/or superior movement) can help better orient the image. Patients with history of coronary artery disease with scarring/aneurysm of LV segments may in fact have a non-circular appearing LV, despite proper orientation.

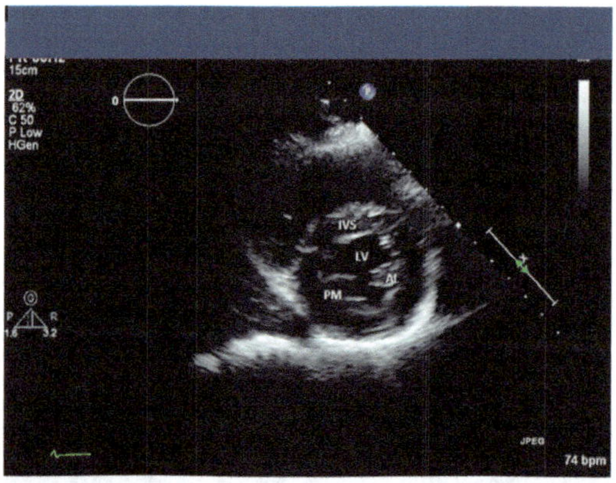

Fig. 2.10 **PSAX view papillary muscles level.** The parasternal short axis view at the midventricular level shows the interventricular septum and the two papillary muscles. *AL* anterolateral papillary muscle, *IVS* interventricular septum, *LV* left ventricle, *PM* posteromedial papillary muscle

Valves

- No valves are seen on this view

Doppler

- No standard color, spectral or tissue Doppler assessments are done on the PSAX view at the papillary muscle level.

PSAX—Apex Level
(Fig. 2.11, Video 2.7)

Further tilting the transducer inferiorly, possibly moving down 1–2 intercostal spaces and angulating the transducer may allow a short axis view at the apical third of the left ventricle.

Chambers

- Left ventricle
  - Only the LV is seen on this view. The apical segments can be visualized and assessed for endocardial thickening and inward motion

Valves, Doppler

- No valve are seen on this view
- No standard color, spectral or tissue Doppler assessments are done on the PSAX view at the apical level

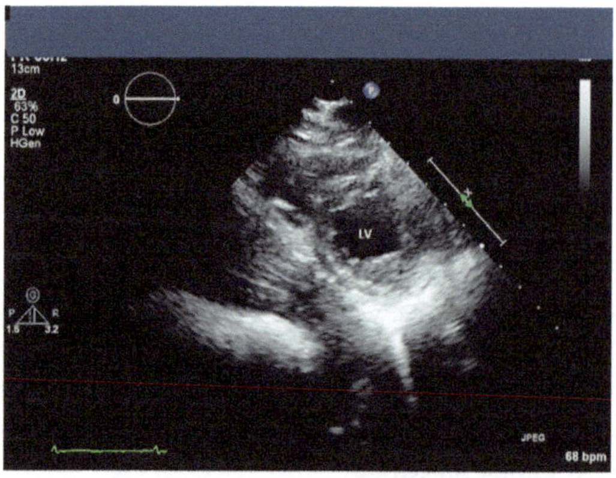

Fig. 2.11 **PSAX view apical level.** Parasternal short axis view at the left ventricle apical level. *LV* left ventricle

2.1.2 Apical Window

Apical Four Chamber View
(Fig. 2.12, Video 2.8)

- Transducer position: starting point can be at the point of maximal apical impulse however can be adjusted as needed to optimize the image
- Index marker: pointing left (patient's lateral aspect of the left chest/back)

Imaging points:

- There may be more than one apical window that can be used for proper imaging
- The left heart appears on the right side of the image, the right heart appear on the left side
- As a general rule of thumb: the LV should occupy approximately $\frac{2}{3}$ of the image, the LA about $\frac{1}{3}$.
- The left ventricle tapers towards an elliptical shape at the apex; a spherical appearance should raise suspicion for foreshortening of the image (unless there is a pathology that causes the LV to become more spherical—e.g. severe aortic insufficiency)
- Repositioning of the transducer throughout the exam may be required to optimize the image
- After initial acquisition of the entire 4-chamber view, sector size and imaging depth should be changed to concentrate on the LV/RV size and function

Chambers

- Left ventricle
  - Walls visualized—lateral wall, inferior septum, and true apex
  - Assessment of global and segmental LV function should be done
  - End diastolic and end systolic volume are measured by the Simpson's rule (method of discs) to obtain the 4-chamber stroke volume and ejection fraction (see normal values below for bi-plane assessment)
- Right ventricle
  - The right ventricle is normally smaller in size and has a triangular shape on this view
    Note: the RV should NOT be apex forming; RV dilatation may manifest as apex-forming RV
  - The right ventricle is normally more trabeculated than the LV
  - For RV measurements, RV focused view is recommended; from the apical four chamber, transducer is rotated slightly counterclockwise such that RV area is maximized. Tilting towards the RV or moving more medially may be required
  - Tricuspid annular plane systolic excursion (TAPSE) is measured from dedicated RV view, for assessment of RV systolic function (normal value ≥17 mm)

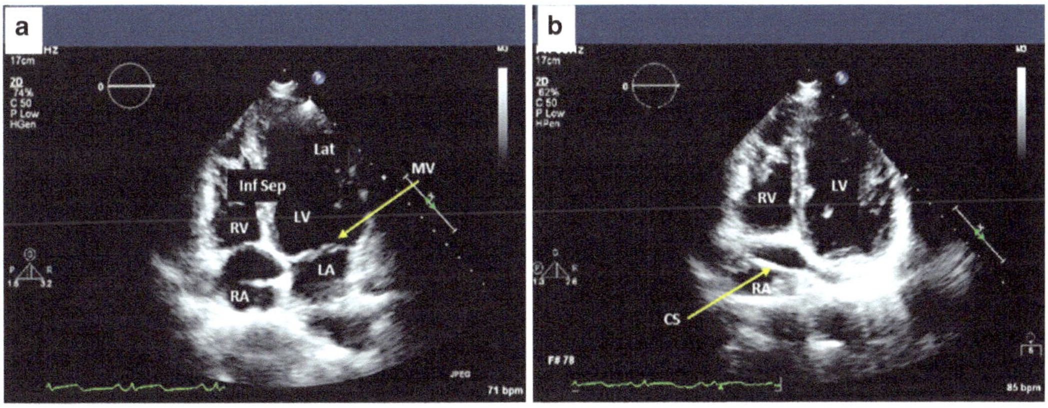

Fig. 2.12 **Apical 4-chamber View.** (**a**) This view shows both atria and ventricles; LV walls visualized are the basal and mid inferior septum, lateral wall, and true apex. (**b**) Slight posterior tilt of the transducer can visualize the coronary sinus at the atrio-ventricular groove. *CS* coronary sinus, *Inf Sep* inferior septum, *LA* left atrium, *Lat* lateral wall, *LV* left ventricle, *MV* mitral valve, *RA* right atrium, *RV* right ventricle

Measurement	Timing	Location	Normal range
RV basal diameter	End diastole	Maximal dimension at the basal third of RV	25–41 mm
RV mid diameter	End diastole	Halfway between maximal diameter and RV apex	19–35 mm
RV longitudinal diameter	End diastole	From midpoint of the tricuspid annulus to the RV apex	59–83 mm
RV end diastolic area (EDA)	End diastole	Tracing of the blood-endocardium border Note: include trabeculations, papillary muscles and moderator band in cavity	Men 10–24 cm^2 Women 8–20 cm^2
RV end systolic area (ESA)	End systole		Men 3–15 cm^2 Women 3–11 cm^2
RV fractional area change (FAC)	—	Calculated from EDA and ESA	FAC < 35% → reduced RV systolic function

- Left atrium
  - Left atrial volume should be measured on apical four chamber view and apical two chamber view to obtain biplane evaluation of LA volume
    Note: left atrial appendage and pulmonary veins should be excluded from LA volume measurements
  - Method of discs is recommended for calculating LA volume; area-length method may also be used
  - Indexing the obtained volume to body surface area is the recommended method for grading LA dilatation
  - See below for normal range and grading of left atrial dilatation
- Right atrium
  - Right atrial volume should be measured (from a dedicated RA view)
    Note: SVC, IVC, right atrial appendage should be excluded from RA volume measurement
  - Summation of discs method is used to calculate RA volume
  - A single plane volume, indexed to BSA, is used to assess RA size (normal values: men 25 ± 7 ml/m^2, women 21 ± 6 ml/m^2)
  - Eustachian valve and Chiari network (normal variants) may be seen on this view
    Note: the interatrial septum is parallel to the US beam on the apical four chamber view; dropout of the septum may occur and should not be confused with atrial septal defect
- Coronary sinus
  - Tilting the transducer posteriorly from the apical 4 chamber view can bring the coronary sinus into view
  - The coronary sinus appears as a tubular structure ending at the right atrium

Valves

- Mitral valve
  - The mitral annulus is seen (major axis)
  - Both mitral leaflets are visualized—anterior leaflet (close to the septum), posterior leaflet (near the lateral wall)
  - Full diastolic opening of the leaflets is seen during diastole; "flat" closure line is seen during systole
- Tricuspid valve
  - The tricuspid valve is slightly apically displaced as compared to the mitral valve
  - Two tricuspid leaflets are visualized—septal leaflet close to the septum, and either anterior or posterior leaflet close to the free wall of the RV
  - Full diastolic opening of the leaflets is seen during diastole

Doppler

- Color Doppler
  - Laminar inflow through mitral and tricuspid valve can be seen
  - When present, TR/MR turbulent jets are seen during systole

  - Occasionally, vena cava inflow can be seen in the RA
- Spectral Doppler
  - Pulse Doppler of the mitral inflow is performed at the tips of the mitral valve (for assessment of diastolic function and filling pressure)
    Note: the sample volume should be placed slightly towards the lateral wall as normal mitral inflow is directed laterally
  - Pulse Doppler of the pulmonary vein may be attempted
    Note: the pulmonary veins are in the very far field of the sector on the apical views; limits the maximal Nyquist limit as well as quality of the signal
  - Pulse Doppler at the level of the mitral annulus should be performed when calculation of inflow volume is necessary (e.g. for volumetric calculations of regurgitant volumes)
  - Continuous wave Doppler of the mitral inflow is performed on this view, for assessment of mean mitral inflow gradient, pressure half time
  - When clinically relevant (e.g. post TV surgery) continuous wave Doppler of the tricuspid inflow is performed on this view, for assessment of mean tricuspid inflow gradient
  - Continuous wave Doppler of TR and MR jet should be performed; assess for density of the signal, peak MR/TR velocity, shape of the signal
- Tissue Doppler
  - Pulsed Doppler at the mitral annulus
    - Performed both at the lateral and medial aspects of the annulus
    - Diastolic e' velocity important for assessment of diastolic function and filling pressures
    - Systolic s' velocity correlates with global LV systolic function
  - Pulsed Doppler at the tricuspid annulus
    - Performed at the lateral aspect of the tricuspid valve
    - Systolic s' velocity correlates with global RV systolic function (s' < 9.5 cm/s suggests RV systolic dysfunction)

Apical Five Chamber View
(Fig. 2.13, Video 2.9)

- Transducer position: Starting from the apical four chamber view, transducer is tilted anteriorly until LVOT/AV/proximal aortic root come into view
- Index marker: pointing left (patient's lateral aspect of the left chest/back)

Imaging points:
- In some adults, further anterior tilt of the transducer may bring into view the pulmonary artery as it comes out of the RV (more easily obtained in children)

Chambers
- Left ventricle
  - Walls visualized—similar to the apical four chamber view; more anterior segments of the interventricular septum and lateral wall are visualized
  - LVOT is visualized
    Note: on this view the LVOT is more parallel to the US beam making it suboptimal for diameter measurement, however suited for Doppler interrogation

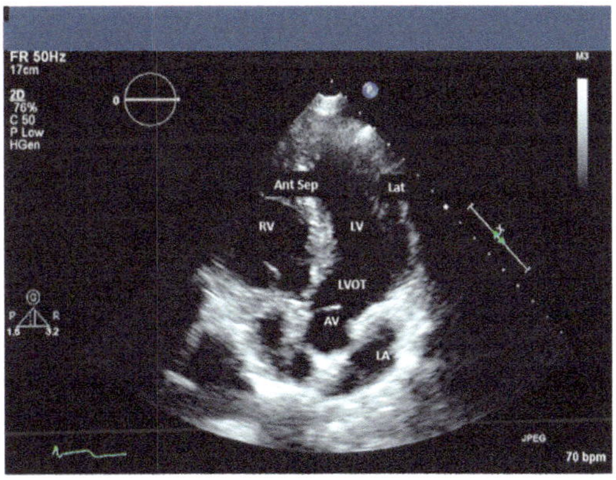

Fig. 2.13 **Apical 5-chamber view.** Apical 5 chamber view visualizing the four chambers plus left ventricular outflow tract and the aortic valve. Walls visualized are the antero-septum, lateral wall, and true apex. The atria are not fully visualized on this view (not suitable for atrial volume measurement) *Ant Sep* antero-septum, *AV* aortic valve, *LA* left atrium, *Lat* lateral wall, *LV* left ventricle *LVOT* left ventricular outflow tract, *RV* right ventricle

- Right ventricle
  - The RV is seen on this view, however measurements should not be obtained from this angulation
- Aortic root
  - The proximal aortic root can be seen with its anatomical relationship with surrounding structures

Valves

- Mitral valve/Tricuspid valve
  - The anterior leaflet of the mitral is seen near the aortic valve/aortic root, posterior leaflet near the lateral wall of the LV
  - Diastolic excursion of the valves may not be fully visualized on this view
- Aortic valve
  - Only two cusps of the aortic valve can be seen on this view (most commonly the left coronary cusp is seen and either the right or the non-coronary cusp)
  - The view is particularly suitable for spectral Doppler evaluation (see below) as the flow is most often parallel to the US beam

Doppler

- Color Doppler
  - Inflow through TV/MV can be seen, however suboptimally on this view
  - TR/MR jet may be seen; interrogation at all views is important so eccentric jets are not overlooked
  - Laminar outflow through LVOT/AV can be seen
  - Turbulent AI jet can be visualized if present
- Spectral Doppler
  - Apical five chamber view is especially important for interrogation of flow through the LVOT and aortic valve
  - Pulsed Doppler in the LVOT is performed (calculation of stroke volume, exclude LVOT obstruction)
  - Continuous wave Doppler through aortic valve is performed; peak and mean gradients across aortic valve are acquired
  - Spectral tracing of AI jet when present is obtained (for jet density, slope, pressure half time and end diastolic gradient calculation)
- Tissue Doppler
  - No standard tissue Doppler measurements are done on apical five chamber view

Apical Two Chamber View
(Fig. 2.14, Video 2.10)

- Transducer position: Starting from the apical four chamber view, transducer is rotated approximately 60° counterclockwise
- Note: when using a 3D TTE probe, rather than physically rotating the probe, the imaging angle can be changed to obtain a different view from the same transducer position
- Index marker: pointing approximately towards patient's left shoulder

Imaging points:

- Transducer may need to be moved up or down one intercostal space to optimize the view
- Papillary muscles should not be seen on this view

Chambers

- Left ventricle
  - Walls visualized—anterior wall, inferior wall, and true apex

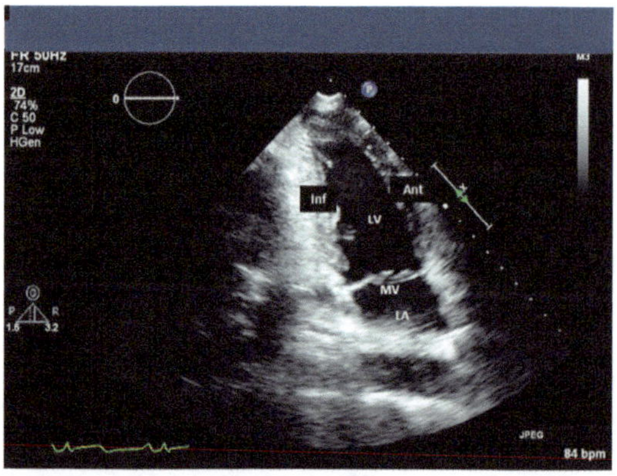

Fig. 2.14 **Apical 2-chamber view**. Walls visualized are the anterior wall, inferior wall, and apex. *Ant* anterior, *Inf* inferior, *LA* left atrium, *LV* left ventricle, *MV* mitral valve

- Assessment of global and segmental LV function should be done
- End diastolic and end systolic volume are measured by the Simpson's rule (method of discs) to obtain the 2-chamber stroke volume and ejection fraction
- Biplane volumes and ejection fraction can then be calculated

Measurement	Normal range—men	Normal range—women
LV EDV (ml)	62–150	46–106
Indexed LV EDV (ml/m²)	34–74	29–61
LV ESV (ml)	21–61	14–42
Indexed LV ESV (ml/m²)	11–31	8–24
LVEF (biplane, %)	52–72	54–74

- Left atrium
  Left atrial volume should be measured on apical four chamber view and apical two chamber view to obtain biplane evaluation of LA volume.
  Note: left atrial appendage and pulmonary veins should be excluded from LA volume measurements

LA volume range	Maximal LA volume (ml/m²)
Normal range	16–34
Mildly dilated	35–41
Moderately dilated	42–48
Severely dilated	> 48

Valves

- Mitral valve
  - The anterior leaflet is seen "en face" in the two chamber view
  - The coaptation area of the anterior and posterior leaflets is visualized "en face" as well

Doppler

- Color Doppler
  - Inflow through MV can be seen
  - MR jet may be seen; interrogation at all views is important so eccentric jets are not overlooked

  Note: due to the orientation of the closure line on this view, mitral regurgitation vena contracta should not be measured on the apical two chamber view
- Spectral Doppler
  - Continuous wave Doppler through mitral inflow and MR jet can be obtained; important when eccentric jets/prosthetic valves are in place and flow directions may be unusual
- Tissue Doppler
  - No standard tissue Doppler measurements are done on apical two chamber view

Apical Three Chamber View
(Fig. 2.15, Video 2.11)

- Transducer position: Starting from the apical two chamber view, transducer is rotated approximately 60° counterclockwise (alternatively, with 3D TTE probe—imaging angle can be changed)
- Index marker: pointing approximately towards patient's right shoulder

Imaging points:

- Image is very similar to the PLAX view, however since imaging is done from the apical window, the LV apex is visualized on this view

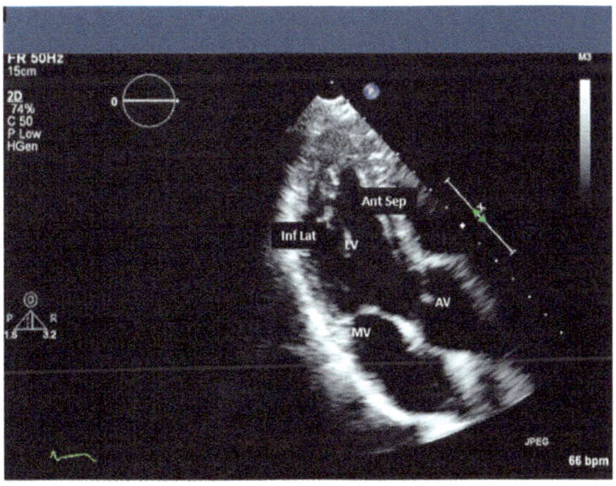

Fig. 2.15 **Apical 3-chamber view**. Apical 3 chamber view is very similar to the PLAX view (tilted 90°). Walls visualized are the anterosetpum, inferolateral wall, and apex. *Ant Sep* anterosetpum, *AV* aortic valve, *Inf Lat* inferolateral, *LV* left ventricle, *MV* mitral valve

Chambers

- Left ventricle
  - Walls visualized—antero-septum, infero-lateral wall, and true apex
  - Assessment of global and segmental LV function should be done
- LVOT/Proximal aortic root
  - Due to parallel angle of imaging, 2D measurements should be performed on the PLAX view rather than the apical three chamber
- Left atrium
  - Seen at the far field of the sector
- Right ventricle
  - Part of the RV is seen on this view
  - Measurements should not be obtained from this view

Valves

- Mitral valve
  - The anterior leaflet is seen near the aorta, the posterior leaflet near the inferolateral wall

Doppler

- Color Doppler
  - Inflow through MV can be seen
  - MR jet may be seen; interrogation at all views is important so eccentric jets are not overlooked
- Spectral Doppler
  - Continuous wave Doppler through mitral inflow and MR jet can be obtained
  - Pulsed Doppler in the LVOT is performed
  - Continuous wave Doppler through aortic valve is performed; peak and mean gradients across aortic valve are acquired
  - Spectral tracing of AI jet when present is obtained (for jet density, slope, pressure half time and end diastolic gradient calculation)
- Tissue Doppler
  - No standard tissue Doppler measurements are done on apical three chamber view

2.1.3 Subcostal Window

Subcostal Four Chamber View (Fig. 2.16, Video 2.12)

- Transducer position: patient's abdomen, immediately below the Xiphoid process. Transducer should point towards the patient's left shoulder
- Index marker: pointing towards patient's left side (approximately 3 o'clock position, similar to apical four chamber orientation)

Imaging points:

- Images are commonly acquired with patient supine with abdominal muscles relaxed (bending the knees can help relax the abdominal muscles)

Chambers

- All four chambers are visualized on the subcostal 4-chamber view
  - Walls visualized—RV free wall, interventricular septum and LV lateral wall
  - RV free wall thickens is measured from this view; performed at end diastole, below the tricuspid annulus (distance approximately

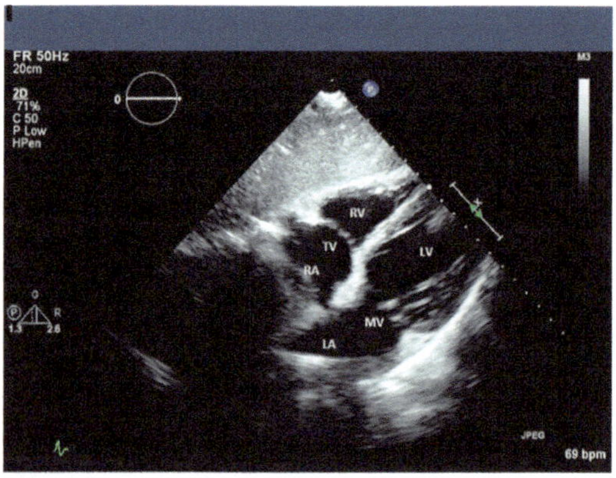

Fig. 2.16 **Subcostal long axis view**. All four chambers are visualized on this view. The right heart is seen anterior to the left heart and near the liver. *LA* left atrium, *LV* left ventricle, *MV* mitral valve, *RA* right atrium, *RV* right ventricle, *TV* tricuspid valve

the length of the TV leaflet), care should be taken to avoid trabeculae, papillary muscle, or epicardial fat (normal range 1–5 mm)
Note: both the interventricular septum and interatrial septum are perpendicular to the US beam in this view, making is suitable for assessment for septal defects

Valves

- Mitral valve and tricuspid valve are visualized
- Slight anterior tilt can bring the aortic valve into view

Doppler

- Color Doppler
  - MR/TR jet may be seen; interrogation at all views is important so eccentric jets are not overlooked
- Spectral Doppler
  - Blood flows that are imaged on subcostal view are typically suboptimally angled for spectral Doppler interrogation.
  - Generally no measurements of flow velocities are performed from this view
    Note: occasionally, outflow through aortic valve is well angled for interrogation; when obtaining maximum velocity is essential (e.g. aortic stenosis patients), continuous wave Doppler interrogation should be performed from this view as well
- Tissue Doppler
  - No standard tissue Doppler measurements are done on subcostal view

Subcostal Short Axis View/IVC View
(Fig. 2.17, Videos 2.13A and 2.13B)

- Transducer position: From the long axis view, transducer rotated approximately 90° counterclockwise and then tilted inferiorly
- Index marker: pointing towards patient's chest center (or slightly left of the center)

Imaging points:

- Short axis views of the heart from this window are similar to those from parasternal window
- In cases where parasternal images are suboptimal, some chamber linear measurements may be obtained from this view

Chambers/Valves

- See description above for parasternal short axis views (PSAX)
- IVC and hepatic veins

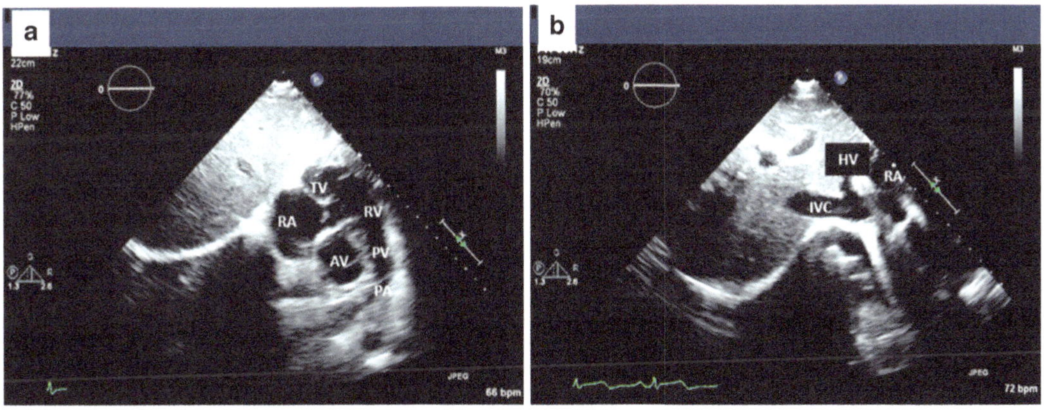

Fig. 2.17 **Subcostal Short Axis view and IVC.** Subcostal short axis view can be acquired at several levels. (**a**) Short axis at the aortic valve level. (**b**) Angulation of the transducer from the short axis orientation shows the inferior vena cava and the hepatic veins. *AV* aortic valve, *HV* hepatic vein, *IVC* inferior vena cava, *PA* pulmonary artery, *PV* pulmonary valve, *RA* right atrium, *RV* right ventricle, *TV* tricuspid valve

- Tilting the transducer inferiorly from the short axis view (such that it points towards patient's liver) brings the IVC and hepatic veins into view
  - IVC size is measured 1–2 cm distal to the IVC-RA junction
  - Inspiratory decrease in IVC size should be looked for; if needed, patient should be asked to "sniff" and IVC size should be recorded
  - Hepatic veins (mainly the central hepatic vein) can be seen draining into the IVC
- Abdominal aorta
  - The abdominal aorta can be seen running parallel to the IVC

Doppler

- Color Doppler
  - Continuous laminar flow should be seen in the IVC
  - Forward laminar flow from hepatic veins into IVC can be seen often
  - Systolic flow should be seen in the abdominal aorta
- Spectral Doppler
  - Pulsed Doppler of the hepatic veins should be performed (to assess for flow reversal in cases with significant tricuspid regurgitation)
- Tissue Doppler
  - No standard tissue Doppler measurements are done on subcostal view

2.1.4 Suprasternal Window

Suprasternal View
(Fig. 2.18, Video 2.14)

- Transducer position: Suprasternal notch or right supraclavicular area
- Index marker: Straight up towards patient's chin (12 o'clock position). Slight clockwise rotation, towards the 1 o'clock position, may be required.

Imaging points:

- Images should be acquired with patient in supine position; neck extension (including relative hyperextension with a pillow placed under patient's shoulders) can help better position the probe

Chambers

- Aorta
  - Ascending aorta, aortic arch and proximal descending aorta are visualized
  - Arch vessels may be visualized
- Pulmonary artery
  - The right pulmonary artery is visualized in cross section under the aortic arch

Valves

- No valves are visualized from the suprasternal view

Doppler

- Color Doppler
  - Systolic laminar flow should be seen in ascending aorta, arch and descending aorta
- Spectral Doppler
  - Continuous wave Doppler at the ascending/descending thoracic aorta should be recorded; flow should be systolic only, approximately 1 m/s
  - Routine pulsed Doppler should be done at the descending aorta, below the origin of the subclavian artery; flow should be non-turbulent and systolic only; early diastolic reversal may be a normal variant (longer diastolic reversal can be seen with significant AI)
  - High velocity anywhere (>2 m/s) should prompt a search for the origin of the

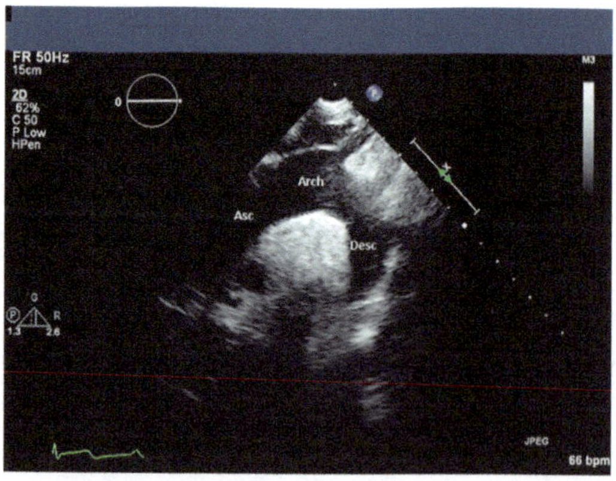

Fig. 2.18 **Suprasternal view.** This view shows the ascending aorta (Asc), aortic arch and the proximal descending aorta (Descn). Arch vessels may be occasionally seen

obstruction by using pulsed Doppler at various locations until the point of flow acceleration is identified
- Tissue Doppler
  - No standard tissue Doppler measurements are done on subcostal view

2.2 Additional Imaging Techniques

2.2.1 Agitated Saline (Bubble) Injection

- Although not routinely performed on every TTE, agitated saline injection can be done to assess for intra-cardiac shunt, intra-pulmonary shunt or evaluation for presence of persistent left superior vena cava
- Optimal view for acquisition is determined by the indication for the bubble study as well as the patient's optimal echo window
- Acquisition should start before opacification of the right heart and continue for a long enough period (typically ~10–15 beats) to evaluate for late appearance of bubbles in the left chambers
- When performing bubble injection with Valsalva maneuver, patient should be instructed to perform Valsalva without taking a deep breath before in order to avoid losing the image while the patient inhales
- It can be helpful to "train" the patient in performing Valsalva prior to the injection and verifying image quality remains adequate
- Location of the injection (right/left upper/lower extremity) should be documented
- Known significant right to left shunt is a contraindication for bubble injection

2.2.2 Ultrasound Enhancing Agents—UEA ("Contrast STUDY")

- Current approved indication for use of echo contrast—improve LV endocardial delineation
- Echo contrast should be used when image quality is suboptimal; defined as inability to delineate two or more contiguous LV segments in any of the three apical views
- In addition, off label common uses of UEA include evaluation of intra-cardiac masses and thrombi

  Note: for detailed description of usage of UEA please refer to the specific guideline

2.2.3 Strain Imaging

- Currently, the most useful clinical data is the global longitudinal strain, as obtained by 2D speckle tracking technique
- If patients are followed serially with strain imaging, it is important to perform repeat strain analysis on the same US system to reduce variability that is due to different equipment and software

  Note: for detailed description of strain imaging please refer to the specific guideline

Further Reading

Kou S, Caballero L, Dulgheru R, et al. Echocardiographic reference ranges for normal cardiac chamber size: results from the NORRE study. Eur Heart J Cardiovasc Imaging. 2014;15(6):680–90. https://doi.org/10.1093/ehjci/jet284.

Lang RM, Badano LP, Mor-Avi V, et al. Recommendations for cardiac chamber quantification by echocardiography in adults: an update from the American Society of Echocardiography and the European Association of Cardiovascular Imaging. J Am Soc Echocardiogr. 2015;28(1):1–39.e14. https://doi.org/10.1016/j.echo.2014.10.003.

Lopez-Candales A, Hernandez-Suarez DF. Strain imaging echocardiography: what imaging cardiologists should know. Curr Cardiol Rev. 2017;13(2):118–29. https://doi.org/10.2174/1573403X12666161028122649.

Mitchell C, Rahko PS, Blauwet LA, et al. Guidelines for performing a comprehensive transthoracic echocardiographic examination in adults: recommendations from the American Society of Echocardiography. J Am Soc Echocardiogr. 2019;32(1):1–64. https://doi.org/10.1016/j.echo.2018.06.004.

Porter TR, Mulvagh SL, Abdelmoneim SS, et al. Clinical Applications of Ultrasonic Enhancing Agents in Echocardiography: 2018 American Society of Echocardiography Guidelines Update. J Am Soc Echocardiogr. 2018;31(3):241–74. https://doi.org/10.1016/j.echo.2017.11.013.

Transesophageal Echocardiography 3

Learning Objectives

- Learn the basic windows and views of transesophageal echocardiogram
- Become familiar with a TEE protocol
- Understand the benefits, as well as shortcomings of TEE exam
- Know how to prepare a patient for a TEE exam

General Considerations

- Like TTE, TEE provides tomographic views of the heart
- Image quality on TEE is superior compared to TTE for several reasons:
  - Close proximity between the probe and the heart
  - Higher frequency transducer; as imaging is relatively shallow, less attenuation allows for higher frequency to be used
- TEE does not replace TTE imaging as some data are better acquired by TTE
  - Chamber quantification is standardized as per TTE imaging
  - Anterior structures may be better visualized with TTE
  - Some intra-cardiac flows are better interrogated by TTE due to more optimal angle of incidence
- TEE is more invasive than TTE; knowledge of indications, risks, and contraindications is of utmost importance to avoid complications

3.1 Indications

It is impossible to list all conceivable indications for TEE; it's more prudent to understand the principles that should guide decision to obtain a TEE

- Evaluation of posterior structures like left atrium, left atrial appendage or thoracic aorta
- Detailed evaluation of structural heart disease, when TTE images are inadequate or insufficient (e.g. evaluation for endocarditis—known TTE sensitivity low, ~50%—if clinical suspicion justifies, TEE is indicated)
- Evaluation of prosthetic heart valves
- Patient's characteristics preclude proper assessment by TTE (e.g. chest wall trauma, body habitus, ventilated patients)
- Guidance of transcatheter structural interventions
- Monitoring during open heart surgeries or during non-cardiac surgery when there is a known cardiac condition which may affect outcomes

Electronic Supplementary Material The online version of this chapter (https://doi.org/10.1007/978-3-030-47041-8_3) contains supplementary material, which is available to authorized users.

T. Rambhatla, G. Perk, *The Echocardiography Companion*,
https://doi.org/10.1007/978-3-030-47041-8_3

- Important to understand when TEE may not be helpful; e.g. evaluation of anterior structures or the apical segments of the LV (which are in the far field of TEE sector)

Most commonly, TEE is utilized as adjunct to TTE (except of course when it is procedure/surgery related). There may be situations where TEE is the first test of choice. Examples include (but not limited to):

- Suspected acute aortic pathology—e.g. dissection/transection
- Diagnosis of endocarditis when there is at least moderate pre-test clinical suspicion
- Re-evaluation of prior TEE finding where interval change may alter clinical management
- Pre cardioversion in patients with atrial fibrillation/flutter

3.2 Risks/Possible Complications of TEE

- In general, the rate of complications from TEE is very low; overall mortality risk is estimated at less than 1 in 10,000 and significant morbidity risk is estimated at less than 1%.

Risks of esophageal intubation	Risks of moderate sedation
Dental trauma (0.1%)	Respiratory depression
Lip injury (13%)	Hypotension
Minor pharyngeal bleeding (0.01–0.2%)	Heart failure (0.05%)
Dysphagia (1.8%)	Arrhythmias (0.06–0.3%)
Severe odynophagia	
Major bleeding (<0.01%)	
Esophageal perforation (<0.01%)	**Major morbidity—0.2%**
Hoarseness (12%)	**Mortality— < 0.01–0.02%**
Laryngospasm/ bronchospasm (0.2%)	
Aspiration	
Endotracheal tube dislodgment	
Tracheal intubation (0.02%)	

- When obtaining the pre-procedure H&P it is imperative to specifically ask about any possible condition that might increase the risk of the TEE (e.g. h/o GI bleed, GI surgery, significant neck arthritis)
- If any high risk condition is identified, appropriate consultation should be obtained prior to the TEE
- Pre-procedure exam should focus on vital signs, oxygen saturation, cardiac findings, breathing status, and assessment for appropriateness for moderate sedation (e.g. oropharyngeal exam, Malampati score, assessment of anesthesia risk, dental exam etc.)
- Specific institution protocols regarding required training and proper use of moderate sedation should be followed

3.3 Contraindications to TEE

Absolute contraindications	Relative contraindications
Active GI bleed	Cervical joint disease (limited neck mobility)
Severe esophageal pathology: • Stricture • Perforation • Laceration • Diverticulum • Tumor • Recent surgery	GI pathology: • H/o neck/mediastinal radiation • Recent GI bleed • Remote history of esophageal surgery • Dysphagia • Esophageal varices, Barrett's esophagus • Active esophagitis
Perforated viscus	Coagulopathy/severe thrombocytopenia
Uncooperative/ non-consenting patient	Sleep apnea
Non NPO status	

Note: when assessing an unstable patient for TEE, risks and benefits should be considered. Although the risk of TEE might be increased, if the benefit outweighs the risk (e.g. making a diagnosis that will alter/expedite proper management) then TEE should be considered

3.4 Post Procedure

Upon completion of a TEE:

- Patient should be examined for any possible complications

- Patient should be monitored for a while post procedure to verify vitals/respiratory status are stable.
- Probe should be examined for any blood or unusual debris
- Images should be stored properly and transferred to the appropriate server
- Clear discharge instructions should be given; precise time when food intake can be resumed, possible warning signs for any complications, contact information for the lab
- Findings should be reported in a timely manner, in particular if emergent attention is required (Table 3.1)

Table 3.1 TEE checklist

Pre procedure—H & P	**Intra procedure—Sedation**
• Identify patient (two methods)	• Time out immediately pre sedation
• Indication for the study, relevant medical history	• Double check pre-procedure vitals/O_2 sat
• Last food and drink	• Specify meds to be used & estimated doses
• Swallowing problems	• Monitor vitals/O_2 sat after every dose
• H/o GI bleed	**Post procedure**
• Prior endoscopy/GI work up/GI surgery	• End study on the machine
• H/o liver disease, EtOH abuse	• Check for bleeding/pain/difficulty swallowing
• Restriction of neck mobility (e.g. severe arthritis)	• Report important results to referring MD in timely manner
• Allergies (sedatives/sleeping meds)	• Procedure note/full report in patient's chart (including sedation doses, any complications, issues with passing probe)
• Dentures, loose teeth	• Sign all required procedure documents
• Most recent echo results	
• Check coagulation studies, platelet count	
• Informed consent	
Pre procedure—Probe	
• Connect and select TEE probe	
• Verify all controls are working (flexion/rotation/angle)	
Pre procedure—Other equipment	
• Connect ECG, verify proper tracing	
• Suction, oxygen	
• Patient positioning	

3.5 Instrument Settings (Fig. 3.1)

Several controls are available on every TEE probe.Various manipulations are available in order to optimize image acquisition and quality

- Superior/inferior movement
  - The probe can be pulled up (withdrawing; towards the patient's head) or pushed down (advancing; towards the feet)
- Rotation
  - The probe can be rotated (using both hands) towards the patient's left side or right side
- Flexion/retro-flexion
  - Utilizing the large-wheel control, the probe tip can be flexed anteriorly (anteflexion) or posteriorly (retro flexion)

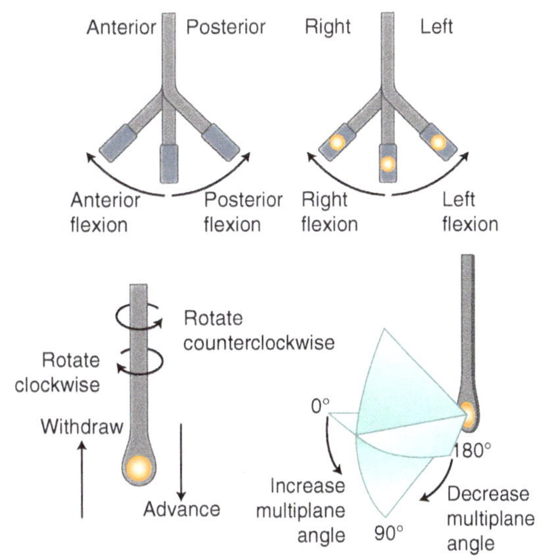

Fig. 3.1 **Transesophageal echo probe—Controls and maneuvers.** Transesophageal echo probe showing various maneuvers utilized to obtain images: withdraw/advance—superior/inferior movement; rotation—using both hands, turning the probe towards the patient's left side or right side; flexion/retro-flexion—utilizing the large-wheel control, the probe tip can be flexed anteriorly (anteflexion) or posteriorly (retro flexion); side to side flexion (tip flexion)—utilizing the smaller wheel, the probe tip can be flexed either to the left or to the right; angle rotation—the imaging sector can be electronically rotated from 0° to 180°

- Side to side flexion (tip flexion)
  - Utilizing the smaller wheel, the probe tip can be flexed either to the left or to the right
- Angle rotation
  - The imaging sector can be electronically rotated from 0° to 180°. Note—no physical change in the probe/tip or the probe occurs when the angle is changed

3.6 Image Display

- Images are displayed with the probe position at the top of the image; near field structures are close to the transducer at the upper part of the screen, far field structures are at the bottom of the screen
- At 0° with sector directed anteriorly (to the heart)—displayed image shows the patient's right side at the left part of the screen and the left side on the right side of the screen
- At 90° with sector directed anteriorly—displayed image shows inferior structures on the left side of the screen and superior structures at the right side of the screen
  Note: to move a structure to the center of the region of interest (ROI), different probe manipulations should be carried out at different angles; at 0°—in order to bring a structure that is visualized at the side of the screen to the center, the probe needs to be rotated; to center a structure at 90°—the probe needs to be advanced or withdrawn. At in-between angles, a combination of these maneuvers should be carried out.
- Biplane views (available on 3D TEE probes) allow simultaneous visualization at two imaging planes, typically two orthogonal planes
  - The primary view is displayed on the left side, the secondary view is displayed on the right (typically 90° rotation relative to the primary view, although the rotation can be changed to any degree between 0° and 180°)
  - The rotated view is oriented like a "forward" rotation from the primary view (e.g. +90° to the primary view if orthogonal planes are used). If the primary view is at above 90° angle, the secondary view may appear reversed compared to standard views

3.7 Standard Echocardiographic Views

3.7.1 General Imaging Considerations

- Anatomic variability exists such that relationship between the esophagus and the cardiac structures can vary; basic views on standard TEE exam will be describe, however fine tuning and probe adjustments should be done to optimize image quality and structure visualization.
- Probe manipulations should be carried out according to the displayed image, rather than by targeting a specific depth, rotation or angle; these should be used only as rough estimates for the proper location of a certain view.
- Although it is good practice to follow a standard protocol while performing a TEE exam to assure that all structures are visualized and interrogated adequately, the protocol may need to be adjusted depending on the specific indication and the patient's clinical status.
- TEE protocol can be "view based" or "structure based"
  - View based—at any given position/view, all structures are interrogated (by 2D/3D, color and spectral Doppler)
  - Structure based—each structure (e.g. chamber/valve) is interrogated at all views before proceeding to the next structure
- Typically, four imaging "windows" are used on TEE:
  - Deep trans-gastric (deep TA)
  - Trans-gastric (TG)
  - Mid-esophageal (ME)
  - Upper esophageal (UE)

At any window the transducer can be manipulated to obtain the various standard views. Important to remember that off angle/nonstandard views may be important in certain situations (e.g. assessing for post TAVR PVL)

The main views from the various transducer position are described and shown; for more detailed description, as well as structure-based discussion, please refer to specific TEE guidelines

3.7.2 Deep Trans-Gastric Window (Fig. 3.2, Video 3.1)

TG Five Chamber View

- Position: deep in the stomach
- Transducer tip: anteflexion and occasional left tip flexion
- Imaging angle: 0–20°
- On this view, the LVOT and AV are parallel to the US beam; ideal window for spectral Doppler interrogation of LVOT/AV
- Mitral valve also visualized and can be assessed anatomically and by color Doppler

3.7.3 Trans-Gastric Window

TG Basal Short Axis View

- Position: in the stomach
- Transducer tip: anteflexion
- Imaging angle: 0–20°
- Short axis of the LV at the level of the mitral valve is seen
- "En face" view of the MV is obtained; anterior leaflet on the left, posterior leaflet on the right; medial commissure in the near field, lateral commissure in the far field

TG Midpapillary Short Axis View (Fig. 3.3, Video 3.2)

- Position: in the stomach, slightly distal to the basal view, at the level of the papillary muscles
- Transducer tip: relaxed or slight anteflexion
- Imaging angle: 0–20°
- LV seen; global and segmental function can be assessed

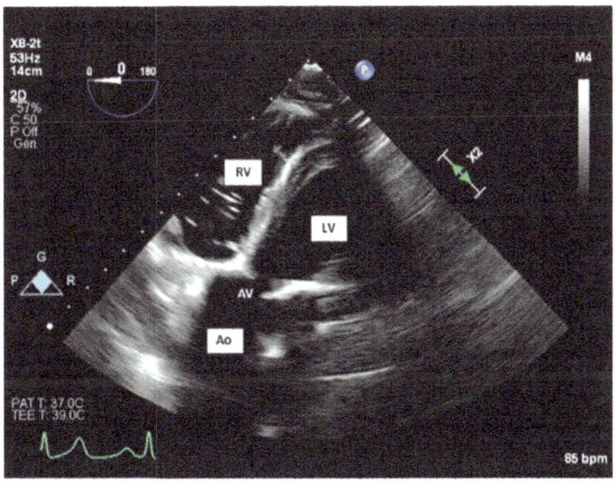

Fig. 3.2 **Deep transgastric view**. The deep transgastric view is obtained by advancing the probe deep in the stomach (near the LV apex) and anteflexing until the aortic valve is visualized. *Ao* aorta, *AV* aortic valve, *LV* left ventricle, *RV* right ventricle

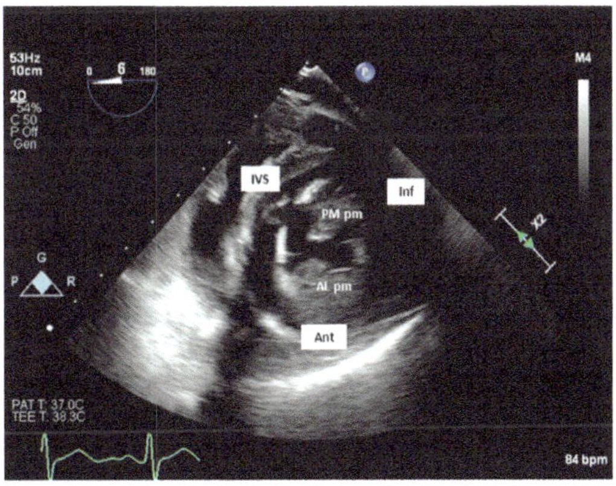

Fig. 3.3 **Transgastric LV view**. Advancing the probe past the upper stomach at 0 degrees will display the left ventricle in short axis at the mid papillary level. The posteromedial papillary muscle is seen between 11–12 0'clock and the anterolateral papillary muscle is seen around 5 0'clock. *Ant* anterior, *AL pm* anterolateral papillary muscle, *Inf* inferior, *IL* inferolateral, *IVS* interventricular septum, *PM pm* posteromedial papillary muscle

TG Apical Short Axis View

- Position: in the stomach, slightly distal to the mid ventricular level
- Transducer tip: anteflexion
- Imaging angle: 0–20°
- LV and RV apex are visualized
- Biplane imaging allows for further wall motion/LV function assessment

TG RV Basal View

- Position: in the stomach, level of basal short axis or slightly distal, probe rotated towards patient's right
- Transducer tip: anteflexion
- Imaging angle: 0–20°
- LV/RV can be seen on this view
- TV/PV visualized

TG RV View
(Fig. 3.4, Video 3.3)

- Position: in the stomach, level of basal short axis or slightly distal, probe rotated towards patient's right
- Transducer tip: anteflexion, maximal right flexion
- Imaging angle: 0–20°
- TV and PV visualized
- RVOT/PV may be parallel to the US beam (probe advancement may be necessary) allowing spectral Doppler interrogation (e.g. for shunt calculation)

TG Two Chamber View

- Position: in the stomach, mid ventricular level
- Transducer tip: neutral
- Imaging angle: 90–110°
- LV seen in long axis; Walls visualized: anterior wall (far wall), inferior wall (near wall)
- Papillary muscles, cords and MV leaflet are seen
- Left atrial appendage may be visualized, however not adequately for full evaluation

TG Long Axis View
(Fig. 3.5, Video 3.4)

- Position: in the stomach, mid ventricular level, possible slight rotation to the right
- Transducer tip: neutral
- Imaging angle: 120–140°
- LV seen; wall visualized: inferolateral and anteroseptum
- LVOT/AV /proximal aortic root can be seen

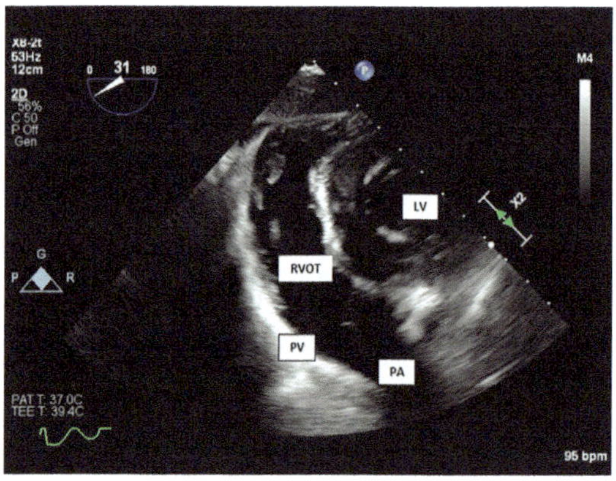

Fig. 3.4 **Transgastric RV view.** Transgastric RV view at 0–20° is obtained by probe rotation towards patient's right and slight anteflexion of the transducer tip. *LV* left ventricle, *PA* proximal pulmonary artery, *PV* pulmonic valve, *RVOT* right ventricular outflow tract

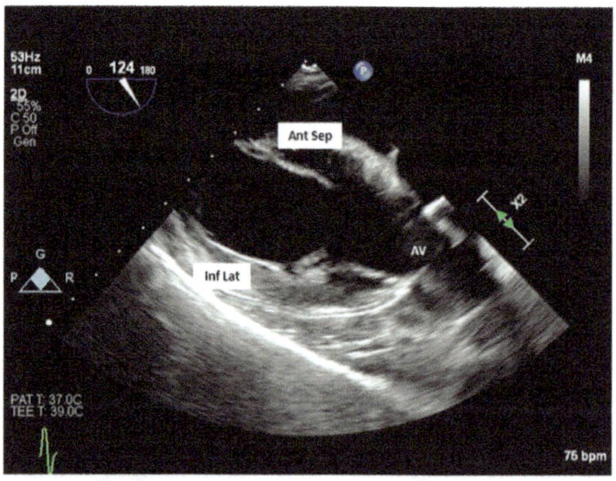

Fig. 3.5 **Transgastric LV long axis view.** Rotation to 110–120° (and rightward turn of the probe) will produce the long axis view with the aortic valve on the right side. Walls visualized: inferolateral and anteroseptum. In this view, the left ventricular outflow tract and aortic valve are more parallel with the ultrasound beam, allowing possible spectral Doppler measurements. *Ant Sep* anteroseptum, *AV* aortic valve, *Inf Lat* inferolateral

- Doppler angle may be parallel; if so, spectral evaluation of LVOT/AV may be carried out

TG RV Inflow View
(Fig. 3.6, Video 3.5)

- Position: in the stomach, mid ventricular level, transducer rotated towards patient's right
- Transducer tip: neutral
- Imaging angle: 90–110°
- RV/RA, tricuspid and pulmonic valves are visualized

3.7.4 Mid Esophageal Window

ME Four Chamber View
(Fig. 3.7, Video 3.6)

- Position: mid-esophageal (may be slightly deeper than the 5 chamber view—see below)
- Transducer tip: neutral or retroflexion
- Imaging angle: 0–20°
- AV/LVOT should not be visualized on this view
- All four chambers are visualized
- Interatrial septum and interventricular septum are seen
- TV/MV can be seen and interrogated with 2D/3D imaging and color Doppler
  Note: advancing the probe slightly allows visualization of the coronary sinus as it enters the right atrium

ME Five Chamber View
(Fig. 3.8, Video 3.7)

- Position: mid-esophageal
- Transducer tip: slight anteflexion
- Imaging angle: 0–20°
- Four cardiac chambers + LVOT/AV are seen on this view
  Note: the LV (and RV) may be foreshortened on this view, limiting accurate assessment of global and segmental function
- Further anteflexion of the probe tip brings the left atrial appendage and the left pulmonary veins into view

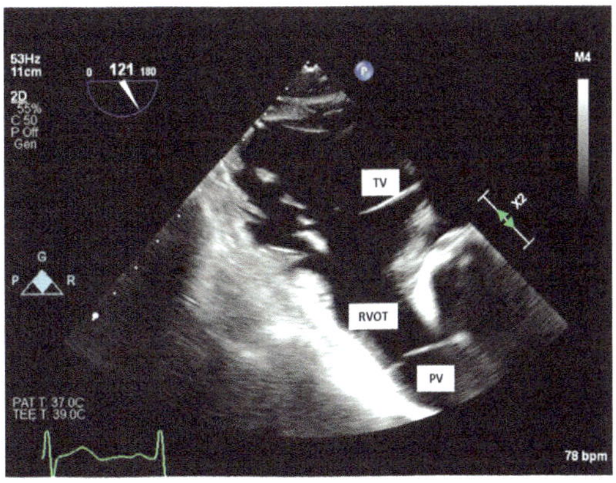

Fig. 3.6 **Transgastric RV inflow-outflow view**. The transgastric right ventricular inflow/outflow view is obtained by rightward turn of the probe from the long axis view at 120 degrees. The inferior (diaphragmatic) portion of the right ventricle is visualized at the top of the image and the right ventricular outflow tract and pulmonic valve are visualized at the bottom. *PV* pulmonic valve, *RVOT* right ventricular outflow tract, *TV* tricuspid valve

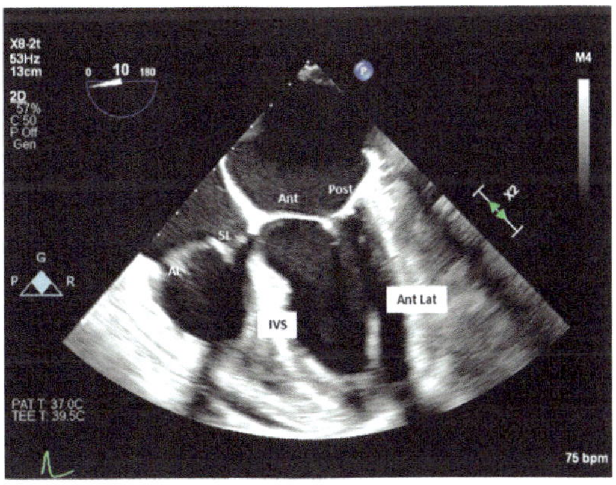

Fig. 3.7 **Mid-esophageal four chamber view**. The mid-esophageal four chamber view is obtained at 0–20°. Retroflexion of the probe and occasionally slight rotation of the angle past 0° may be required to have the ventricles elongated and aortic valve removed from the view. *Ant* anterior leaflet of mitral valve, *Ant Lat* anterolateral, *IVS* interventricular septum, *Post* posterior leaflet of mitral valve

ME Mitral Commissural View
(Fig. 3.9, Video 3.8)

- Position: mid-esophageal, similar to four-chamber level
- Transducer tip: neutral
- Imaging angle: 50–70°
- Important view for mitral valve anatomy

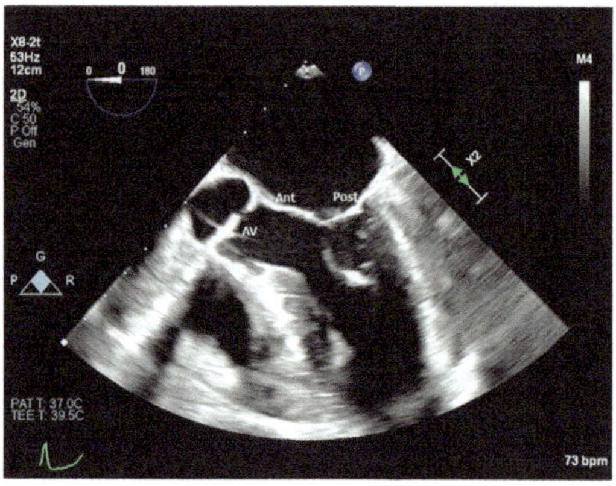

Fig. 3.8 **Mid-esophageal five chamber view**. Mid-esophageal five chamber view is obtained at 0–20° with anteflexion of the probe tip and possible slight withdrawal of the probe. The more anterior structures, the aortic valve and left ventricular outflow tract are visualized. *Ant* anterior leaflet of mitral valve, *AV* aortic valve, *Post* posterior leaflet of mitral valve

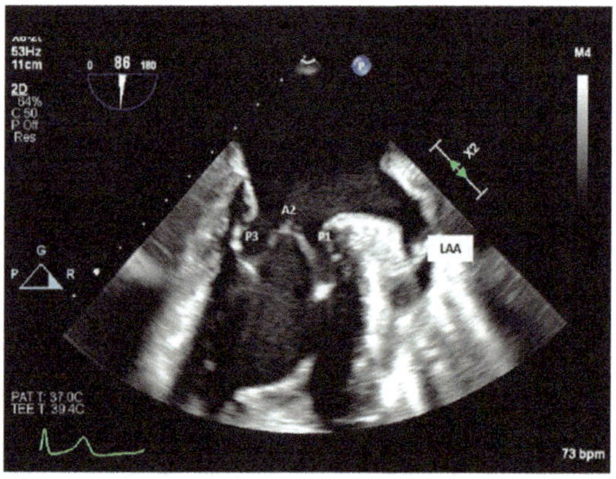

Fig. 3.9 **Mid-esophageal commissural view**. The mid-esophageal commissural view is obtained by rotating the angle to ~60–70° with a slightly leftward turn of the probe. This view allows visualization of the mitral scallops P1-A2-P3. *LAA* left atrial appendage

- Lateral and medial commissures are seen
- Clear identification of mitral leaflets scallops is available on this view; from right to left the scallops imaged are P1-A2-P3
- Chords and papillary muscles can be seen as well

ME Two Chamber View
(Fig. 3.10, Video 3.9)

- Position: mid-esophageal, similar to four-chamber level
- Transducer tip: neutral

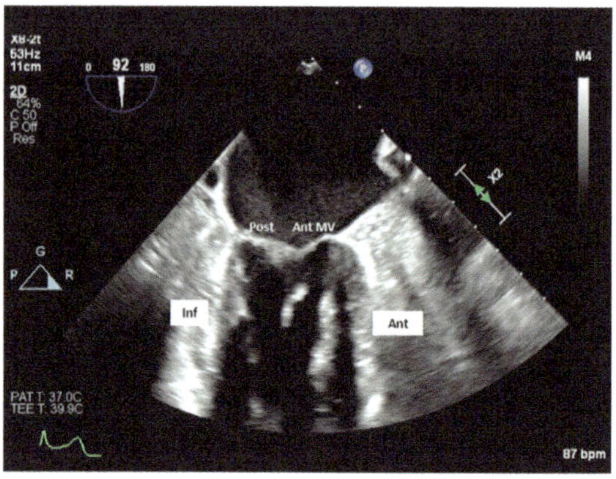

Fig. 3.10 **Mid-esophageal Two Chamber View**. The mid-esophageal two chamber view is obtained with rotation to ~90°. The right atrium and ventricle are not visualized. LV walls visualized: anterior and inferior wall. *Ant* anterior, *Ant MV* anterior mitral valve leaflet, *Inf* inferior, *Post* posterior mitral valve leaflet

- Imaging angle: 80–100°
- LV seen; walls visualized: anterior wall (right side of the image), inferior wall (left side)
- LA, LAA, MV can be seen
- Coronary sinus can be visualized in cross section, at the AV groove, above the basal inferior wall

ME Long Axis LVOT View
(Fig. 3.11, Video 3.10)

- Position: mid-esophageal, similar to four-chamber level
- Transducer tip: neutral
- Imaging angle: 120–140°
- This view is "upside down" parasternal long axis view from TTE
- LV seen; walls visualized: anteroseptum (on the right) inferolateral (on the left)
- MV seen, typically the central part of the valve (A2/P2); to confirm, biplane view can be obtained showing the orthogonal view ("reversed" commissural view)
- Slight withdrawal of the probe (and possibly small rotation of the probe) can optimize the view for the LVOT/AV in long axis
- Further probe withdrawal can bring into view the ascending aorta; occasionally lowering the imaging angle (to approximately 110°) can optimize the ascending aorta view

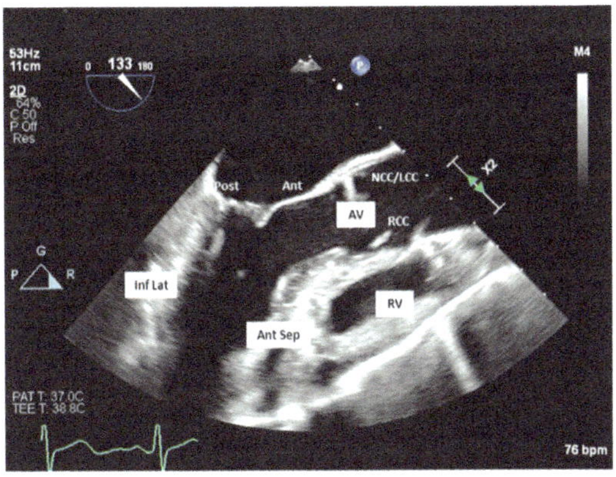

Fig. 3.11 **Mid-esophageal LVOT view**. The mid-esophageal long axis view is seen at 120–140° with a slight rightward (clockwise) turn of the probe. The left ventricular outflow tract, aortic valve, and aorta are brought into view. *Ant Sep* anteroseptum, *Ant* anterior mitral valve leaflet, *AV* aortic valve, *Inf Lat* inferolateral, *RCC* right coronary cusp, *NCC* non-coronary cusp, *LCC* left coronary cusp, *RV* right ventricle

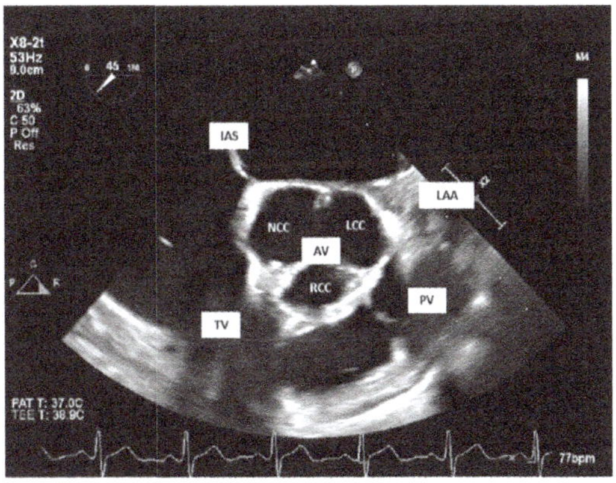

Fig. 3.12 **Mid-esophageal short axis AV-level view**. The mid-esophageal short axis view of the aortic valve is visualized at ~50°. The coronary cusp adjacent to the interatrial septum is the non-coronary cusp. *AV* aortic valve, *IAS* interatrial septum, *LAA* left atrial appendage, *LCC* left coronary cusp, *NCC* non-coronary cusp, *PV* pulmonic valve, *RCC* right coronary cusp, *TV* tricuspid valve

ME AV Short Axis View
(Fig. 3.12, Video 3.11)

- Position: mid-esophageal, similar to four-chamber level
- Transducer tip: slight anteflexion
- Imaging angle: ~50°
- Essentially "upside down" parasternal short axis view at the AV level
- The AV is seen "en face" in the center
- The left coronary cusp is seen at the near field and on the right of the valve, the non-coronary cusp at the near field and to the left, the right coronary cusp at the far field of the valve
- Left atrium in the near field, superior part of interatrial septum in the upper left part of the sector, right atrium to the left of the AV, RV/ROVT below the aortic valve
- Advancing the probe slightly from the AV short axis view can optimize the view for RVOT/PV

ME Bicaval View
(Fig. 3.13, Video 3.12)

- Position: mid-esophageal, transducer rotated towards the patient's right
- Transducer tip: neutral
- Imaging angle: 90–110°
- Structures visualized—left atrium (near field), right atrium, right atrial appendage interatrial septum, IVC, SVC
- Further rotation of the probe to the right, and possibly slight withdrawal brings into view the right pulmonary veins (at the right side of the image, near the SVC)

3.7.5 Upper Esophageal Window

Ascending Aorta Sort Axis View
(Fig. 3.14, Video 3.13)

- Position: upper-esophageal
- Transducer tip: strong anteflexion
- Imaging angle: 0–30°

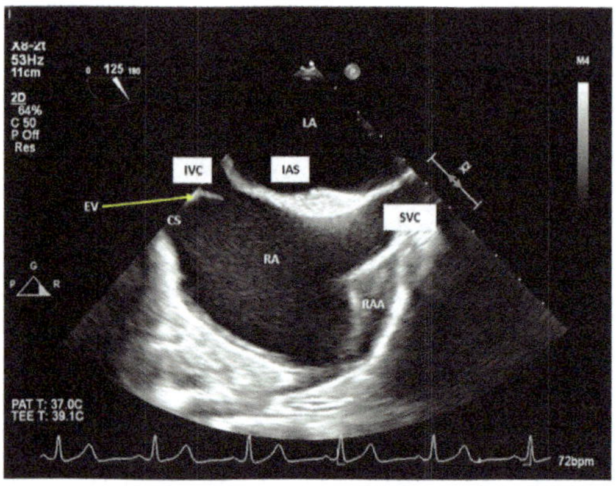

Fig. 3.13 Mid-esophageal bicaval view. Mid-esophageal bicaval view is obtained at ~120° angle with rightward turn (clockwise) of the probe. The IVC is visualized on the left and the SVC on the right. *CS* coronary sinus, *EV* eustachian valve, *IAS* interatrial septum, *IVC* inferior vena cava, *LA* left atrium, *RA* right atrium, *RAA* right atrial appendage, *SVC* superior vena cava

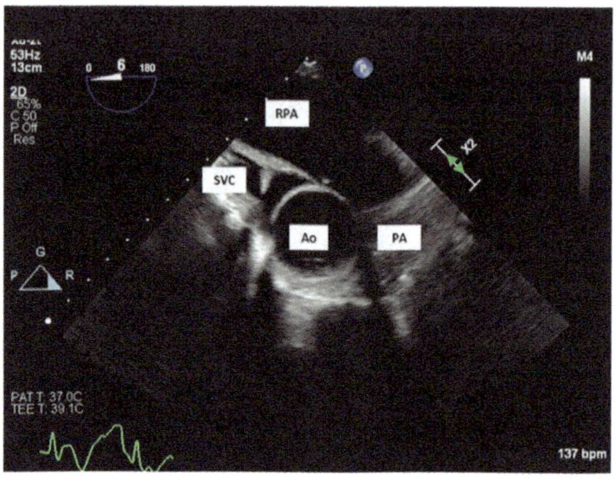

Fig. 3.14 Upper esophageal great vessel view. The upper esophageal great vessel view is obtained at 0° with a strong ante-flexion of the probe. Aortic arch, superior vena cava, the main pulmonary artery, and the right pulmonary artery are visualized. *Ao* aorta, *PA* pulmonary artery, *RPA* right pulmonary artery, *SVC* superior vena cava

- The main pulmonary artery, bifurcation, proximal ~2 cm of the left PA and proximal ~4 cm of the right PA can be seen
- The ascending aorta is seen in cross section below the pulmonary artery
- The SVC is seen in cross section, to the left of the aorta

3.7.6 Thoracic Aorta Imaging

- The thoracic aorta is imaged from several different TEE "windows", however typically it is done in continuous fashion, at the end of the study (Fig. 3.15, Video 3.14)
- Imaging starts by turning the probe (from a TG or low esophageal view) to the patient's left (counterclockwise) at imaging angle of 0–10°
- The descending aorta is adjacent to the esophagus, posterior and slightly to the left of it
- At 0° imaging, the descending aorta is imaged at a short axis (appears as a circular structure)
- Once the aorta appears on the display, the probe should be advanced until the aorta and the esophagus separate (marking the transition from the thoracic to the abdominal aorta, as the diaphragm is crossed)
- Image optimization should include lowering the depth, adjusting the focus and the gain controls
- Long axis views of the descending aorta can be obtained by changing the imaging angle to 90° or by simultaneous biplane imaging

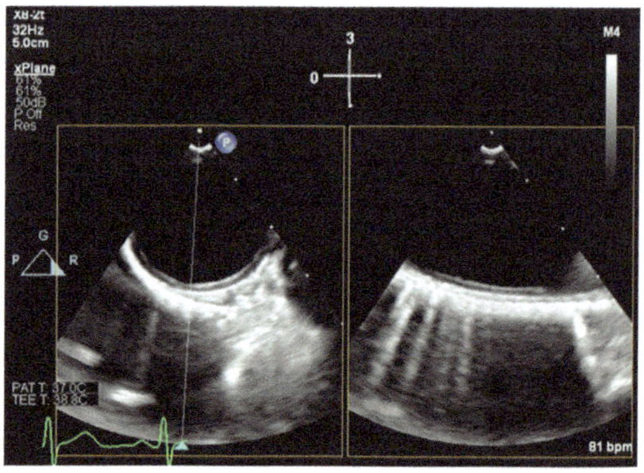

Fig. 3.15 Thoracic aorta. Thoracic aorta is visualized with leftward turn of the probe (counterclockwise) from the mid-esophageal view at 0°until the aorta is seen in short axis as a circular image in the center of the field. Rotation of the angle to 90–100° or the use of bi-plane imaging allows visualization of the aorta in long axis

- The probe is slowly withdrawn in the esophagus and the aorta is inspected
- Upon reaching the arch, the image elongates → the probe is then rotated towards the patient's right (clockwise) to inspect the mid aortic arch
- Typically the left main bronchus crosses between the esophagus and the aorta such that there is a "blind spot" at the proximal arch/ distal ascending aorta which is not visible by TEE

Further Reading

Hahn R, Abraham T, Adams MS, et al. Guidelines for performing a comprehensive transesophageal echocardiographic examination: reccomendations from the American society of echocardiography and the society of cardiovascular anesthesiologists. J Am Soc Echocardiogr. 2013;26:921–64.

Purza R, Ghosh S, Walker C, et al. Transesophageal echocardiography complications in adult cardiac surgery: a retrospective cohort study. Ann Thorac Surg. 2017;103(3):795–802. https://doi.org/10.1016/j.athoracsur.2016.06.073.

4 Left Ventricular Systolic Function

Learning Objectives

- Understand the different parameters by which left ventricular systolic function can be described
- Learn various methods by which to measure or estimate the systolic function parameters
- Review the key concepts of stress echocardiography

General Considerations

- The heart functions as a pump that produces cardiac output.
  - Cardiac output (CO)—volume of blood pumped out of the heart every minute
  - Stroke volume (SV)—volume of blood pumped out of the heart every beat
  - CO = SV × Heart Rate
- Several factors affect the ability of the heart to produce a cardiac output:
  - Intrinsic myocardial contractility
  - Preload (ventricular volume/pressure immediately prior to systole initiation)
  - Afterload (the pressure against which the heart has to work in order to eject blood during systole)
- Ejection fraction (EF)—Fraction of the end diastolic volume that gets ejected during systole
  - $EF = \frac{EDV - ESV}{EDV} \times 100$

    EDV—end diastolic volume, ESV—end systolic volume
  - Can also be written as:
  - $EF = \frac{SV}{EDV} \times 100$

Note: although EF is an important measure of cardiac function with prognostic significance, it is in fact a "non-physiologic" measure which does NOT equal cardiac output.

Hearts with different ejection fractions can produce similar cardiac outputs and hearts with the same ejection fraction can produce different cardiac outputs.

4.1 Measuring Stroke Volume and Cardiac Output

4.1.1 VTI Based Method (Fig. 4.1)

- If area can be measured or calculated at a place that pulse wave (PW) Doppler can be obtained → flow at that area can be calculated by:
  - Flow volume (ml) = CSA(cm^2) × VTI(cm)

    CSA—Cross Sectional Area, VTI—Velocity Time Integral

T. Rambhatla, G. Perk, *The Echocardiography Companion*,
https://doi.org/10.1007/978-3-030-47041-8_4

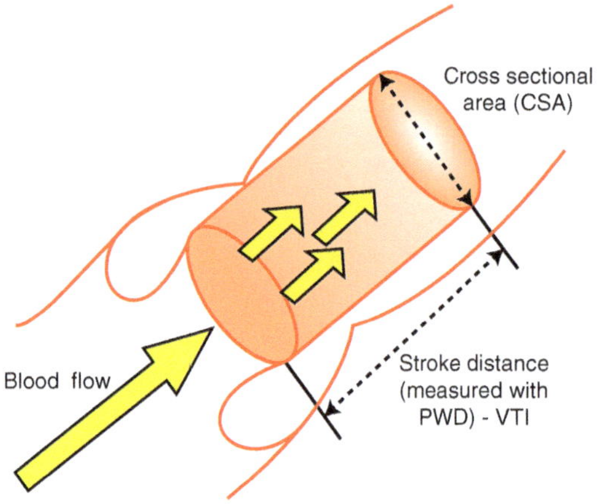

Fig. 4.1 VTI based method for stroke volume calculation. The flow across a fixed orifice is equal to the product of the orifice cross sectional area (CSA) and the velocity time integral (VTI). The VTI represents the "stroke distance" and can be measured with the built-in calculation packages in the echocardiography unit. At any point that CSA area and VTI can be measured (e.g. LVOT), stroke volume can be calculated. If preformed across the LVOT, stroke volume = LVOT CSA × LVOT VTI. *CSA* cross sectional area, *VTI* velocity time integral

- For SV calculation, this can be done at LVOT, RVOT, mitral/tricuspid annulus level
  Note: if there is a regurgitant lesion, important to understand which flow volume is calculated (e.g. total stroke volume including regurgitant volume vs. forward stroke volume)
  Example:
  - Significant aortic regurgitation → LVOT stroke volume includes aortic regurgitant volume and does NOT represent forward SV.
  - To measure true systemic stroke volume → use RVOT SV (assuming no intracardiac shunt).

4.1.2 2D LV Volume Based Method (Fig. 4.2)

- Endocardial border is traced
- Volume is calculated based on the Simpson's rule (method of discs):
  - The left ventricle is divided into a "stack" of cylinders
  - For each cylinder, the radius (r) and height (h) are measured automatically
  - The radius of each cylinder is measured from two orthogonal view
  - Volume of each cylinder is calculated as: $V = \pi r_1 r_2$
    r_1, r_2 – cylinder radii as measured on the two orthogonal views
  - LV volume is calculated as the sum of all the cylinders' volumes
- LV volume is calculated from two orthogonal views (four-chamber and two-chamber), both at end diastole and end systole
  - SV = EDV – SV
    Note—this method calculates TOTAL stroke volume. In the presence of significant MR or AI—calculated SV includes regurgitant volume

4.1.3 3D LV Volume Based Method (Fig. 4.3)

- Utilizes full volume acquisition of the left ventricle
- No geometric assumptions needed
- The endocardial border is traced at end diastole and end systole

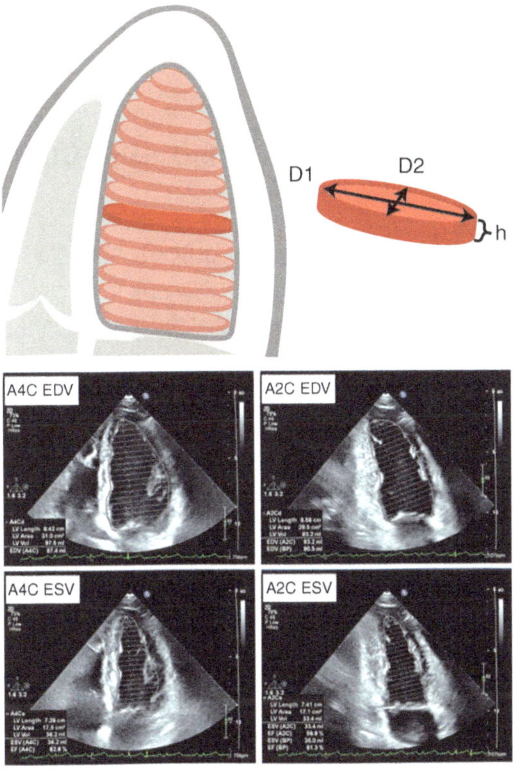

Fig. 4.2 **LV volume based method for stroke volume calculation. (Simpson's rule/Method of Discs).** Apical four chamber and two chamber views are used to measure the left ventricular end-diastolic and end-systolic volumes; the endocardial border needs to be clearly visualized. The traced area is divided into a stack of cylinders of equal height. The volume of all the cylinders is summed to calculate LV volume and end diastole (EDV) and end systole (ESV). Subtracting ESV from EDV gives the stroke volume. Results from the two orthogonal planes are used to provide the LV stroke volume

- Volume is directly measured by the software Note: no geometric assumptions are made for calculating volume. Like the 2D based, this method also calculates total stroke volume.

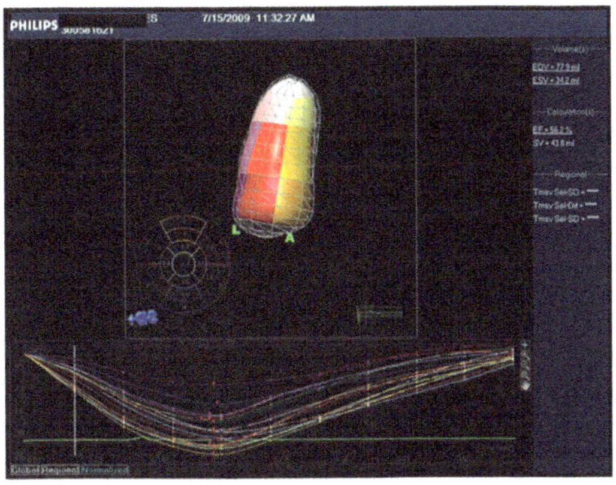

Fig. 4.3 **3D volume based method for stroke volume calculation.** Utilizing a 3D probe, a large data set can be acquired, which includes the entire LV volume. Automatic tracing of the endocardial borders and volume calculations at end diastole (EDV) and end systole (ESV) are performed. No geometric assumptions are required, as the software calculates the volumes based on the traced endocardium. Segmental analysis can also be performed (each segment is displayed with different color); individual segments' volume changes can be analyzed

4.2 Measuring Ejection Fraction

4.2.1 Volume Based Method

- 2D or 3D based LV volume measurements can be used to calculate LV EF.
- $EF = \frac{EDV - ESV}{EDV} \times 100$
- If 2D volumes are used, 2 orthogonal views should be used to calculate the EF
- Normal ejection fraction: male 52–72%, female 54–74%

4.2.2 Visual Estimation

- Based on qualitative assessment of wall thickening and endocardial inward motion
- Experienced echocardiographers can visually estimate LV EF with reasonable accuracy

4.2.3 EF Related Measurements

Fractional Shortening (FS)

- Based on linear measurements of the LV at the mid-ventricular level
- LV internal dimension at end diastole (LVIDd) and end systole (LVIDs) are measured
- $FS = \frac{LVIDd - LVIDs}{LVIDd} \times 100$
- FS normal range: 25–45%
  Note—in patients with segmental abnormalities in LV function, FS may misrepresent global LV function. Volumetric methods are hence preferred over linear methods.

EPSS (E point septal separation)

- Measurement performed on left ventricular M mode tracing at level of the mitral valve leaflets
- The distance between the tip of the mitral E point and the ventricular septum (endocardial-blood border) is measured
- Increased EPSS (>7 mm) occurs due to a combination of LV dilatation and reduced stroke volume (which causes decreased excursion of the mitral valve leaflets) and has good sensitivity and spcecificity to identify reduced LVEF

4.3 Measuring LV Contractility

- Ideally, contractile function would be measured independent of other parameters that effect LV systolic function (e.g. preload and afterload)
- Currently available measures are all influenced by loading conditions.

4.3.1 Tissue Doppler Imaging (TDI) (Fig. 4.4)

- The velocity of myocardial contraction is measured by pulsed wave Doppler
- Sample volume is placed at the mitral annulus (lateral and medial aspect)
- Myocardial velocity is measured based on the Doppler principle
  Note: Tissue velocity signal is a lower frequency higher amplitude signal as compared to blood flow velocity signal
- Measured velocity—velocity by which the myocardium moves towards and away from the transducer during systole and diastole respectively

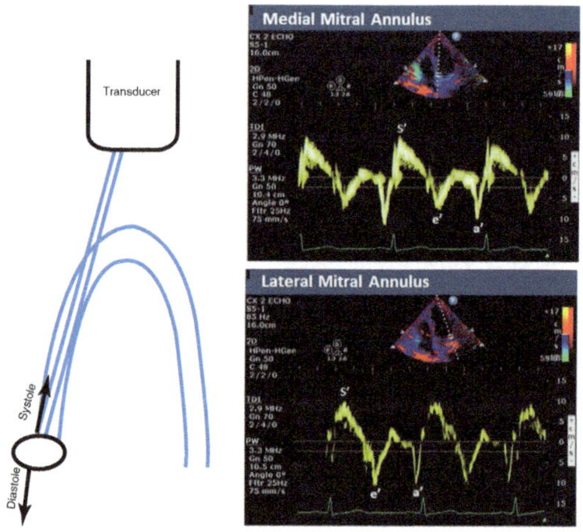

Fig. 4.4 Tissue Doppler imaging method for assessing systolic function. Tissue Doppler imaging (TDI) is based on the Doppler principle—utilizing Doppler shift to calculate the target's velocity. TDI of the medial and lateral mitral annulus allows acquisition of the systolic (s') and diastolic (e', a') components. S′ represents the longitudinal velocity of myocardial contraction, during which the myocardium moves towards the transducer. S′ correlates with global left ventricular systolic function; S′ velocity > than 5.5 cm/s suggests normal systolic function. Note: as the technique is Doppler based, optimal data is obtained when myocardial velocity is interrogated at a parallel angel to the US beam

- TDI signal has three components—systolic component (s`), early diastolic (e`) and late diastolic/ atrial contraction (a`)
- Systolic tissue velocity (s`) correlates with global systolic LV function; s` > 5.5 cm/s suggests normal systolic function

4.3.2 Strain Imaging

- Definition: measurement of the deformation; calculated as the change in a segment's length relative to its original length
- Strain = $\frac{L_1 - L_0}{L_0}$

  L_0—original length, L_1—length after deformation
- Strain is a dimensionless number; generally presented as percent change: $\frac{L_1 - L_0}{L_0} \times 100$
- By convention—lengthening is marked as positive strain and shortening as negative strain
- Strain can be measured for the various components of myocardial deformation; longitudinal systolic shortening, radial thickening and circumferential shortening.
- Absolute values of strain differ for the various deformation components
- Two ways to measure tissue strain:
  - Tissue Doppler based strain

    Measured parameter: tissue velocity (based on Doppler principle)

    A velocity gradient is present between the base of the heart and the apex of the heart

    Strain rate (change in strain over time, SR) is calculated based on the velocity gradient

    $$SR = \frac{V_2 - V_1}{D}$$

    Integrating SR over time gives the strain value

    Only strain in the direction of the ultrasound beam can be calculated since the measured parameter is based on the Doppler principle, which requires parallel angle of incidence
  - Speckle tracking based strain

    Measured parameter: tissue "speckle" motion over several consecutive frames

    Speckle motion represents tissue motion → derived parameters include tissue velocity, strain and strain rate.

    Strain in all directions can be measured as this method is independent of angle of incidence

    Most robust data exists for measuring Global Longitudinal Strain (GLS)

    Commonly, longitudinal strain is measured from three apical views and presented as a bullseye view (Fig. 4.5)

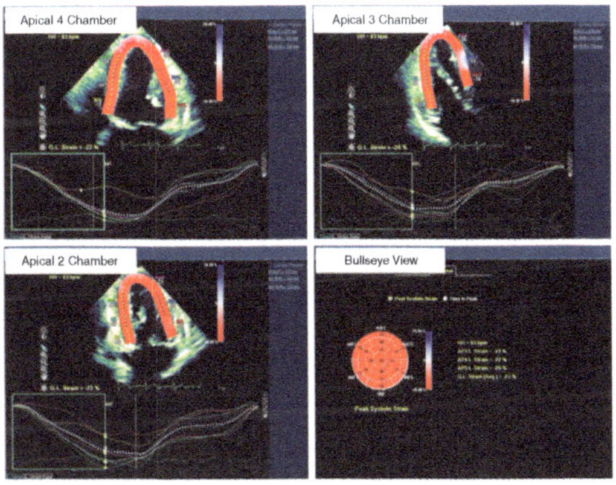

Fig. 4.5 **Speckle tracking strain analysis.** Strain analysis is the measurement of a deformation; calculated as the change in a segment's length relative to its original length. Strain can be measured for the various components of myocardial deformation; longitudinal systolic shortening, radial thickening and circumferential shortening. Commonly, longitudinal strain is measured from three apical views and presented as a bullseye view; each segment's longitudinal strain is presented on the bullseye map, and an average global longitudinal strain is calculated for the LV

Note: Standardization of strain values among different vendors is still evolving; serial strain measurements should be performed on the same echocardiographic system to avoid inter-vendor differences

4.3.3 dP/dT

- Measurement of the rate of ventricular pressure rise at early systole (Fig. 4.6)
- Utilizes mitral regurgitation spectral envelope
- On MR envelope: points where MR velocity reaches 1 m/s and where velocity reaches 3 m/s are marked.
- Pressure gradient between LV and LA at these points is 4 mmHg and 36 mmHg respectively
- The change in ventricular pressure between these two points: 36–4 = 32 mmHg

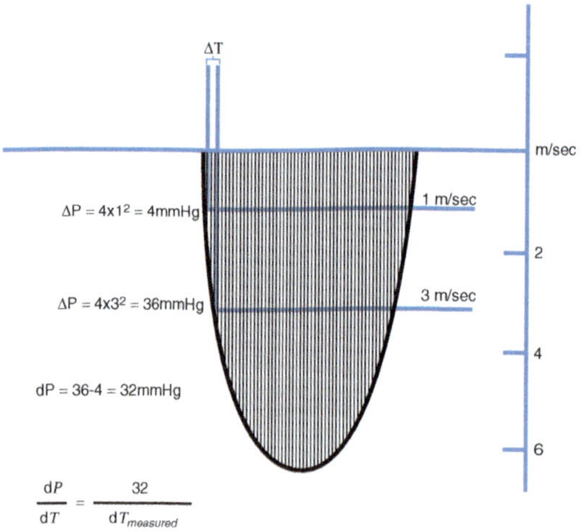

Fig. 4.6 Ventricular pressure rise, dP/dT. The rate of the rise of ventricular pressure is an index of contractility and can be measured with continuous wave Doppler assessment of a mitral regurgitation jet. The time it takes for the MR jet velocity to increase from 1 m/s to 3 m/s is measured. This correlates with a LV-LA pressure gradient rise from 4 mmHg to 36 mmHg, meaning LV dP of 32 mmHg. Dividing the dP (32 mmHg) by the measured time (dT) gives an estimate of systolic function. dP/dT greater than 1000 mmHg/s correlates with normal systolic function. Note: the same technique can be applied to the right ventricle using tricuspid regurgitation jet

- The time it takes to reach from V = 1 m/s to V = 3 m/s is measured on the spectral envelope
- dP/dT is calculated as the LV pressure change (32 mmHg) divided by the time it took (in seconds)
- Normal dP/dT > 1000 mmHg/s

4.3.4 Myocardial Performance Index (MPI) (Fig. 4.7)

- Ratio between isovolumetric contraction and relaxation periods to systolic ejection period
- Can be obtained by measuring time intervals on standard Doppler (from apical 5-chamber

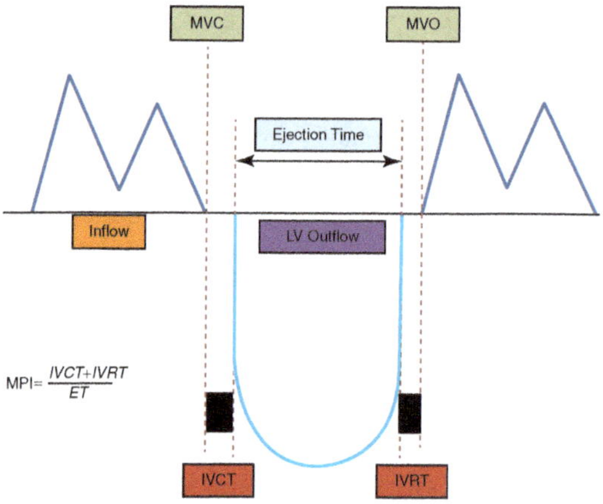

Fig. 4.7 Left ventricle myocardial performance index (MPI). Simultaneous capture of mitral inflow and LV outflow Doppler tracings allows the calculation of the LV MPI (apical five chamber view is utilized). The MPI is the sum of isovolumetric contraction time and isovolumetric relaxation time divided by ejection time. The sum of isovolumetric contraction and relaxation times can be calculated by subtracting ejection time from the time between mitral valve closure to opening. Systolic dysfunction causes an increase in both isovolumetric contraction time and isovolumetric relaxation time, which then results in an overall shortening of ejection time and an increase in the MPI. MPI values that correlate with normal systolic function are ~0.4; higher values (typically 0.6–1) suggest systolic dysfunction. *ET* ejection time, *IVCT* isovolumic contraction time, *IVRT* isovolumic relaxation time, *MPI* myocardial performance index, *MVC* mitral valve closure, *MVO* mitral valve opening

view capturing both mitral inflow and aortic outflow) or from tissue Doppler tracing

- Systolic dysfunction causes increase in isovolumetric contraction time; diastolic dysfunction typically increases isovolumetric relaxation time
- Normal MPI ≈ 0.4
- LV dysfunction can prolong IVCT and IVRT resulting in increased MPI (typically between 0.6–1)

4.4 Assessing LV Segmental Function

- For detailed evaluation and for ease of communication, the LV is divided into segments
- Most commonly used—17 segments model
- Coronary distribution follows a predictable pattern such that in most cases of segmental wall motion abnormalities the ischemic vessel can be identified with acceptable accuracy
- On the long axis, the LV is divided into three parts—basal mid and apical
- The basal and mid parts are divided into 6 segments each, the apical third is divided into 4 segments plus apical cap (Fig. 4.8)
- Each segment is assessed for wall thickening as well as endocardial inward motion

  Note: tethering of myocardial segments can appear as segmental motion and hence important to concentrate on thickening/shortening while analyzing segmental function

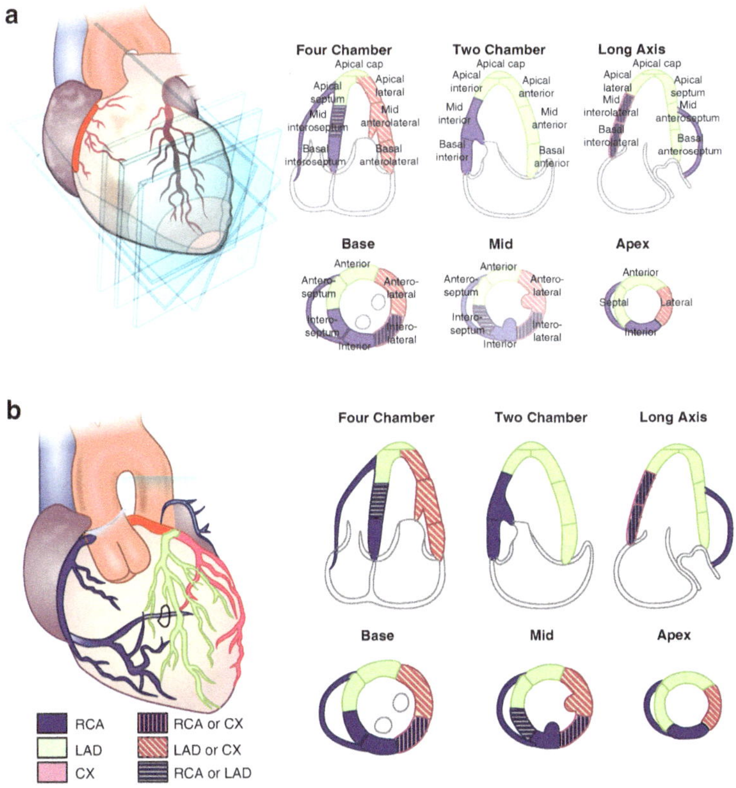

Fig. 4.8 Seventeen segment model with corresponding blood supply. The left ventricle is divided into 17 segments; on the long axis, each wall is divided into three sections: basal and mid and apical. The basal and mid sections of the LV are divided into 6 segments, and the apical third is divided into 4 segments. A separate apical "cap" is the 17th segment. Coronary blood supply typically follows a predictable distribution such that segmental wall motion analysis often allows for identification of the culprit vessel

- For each segment, function can be defined as: normal, hyperkinetic, hypokinetic, akinetic, or dyskinetic
- Semi-quantitative scoring can be utilized:
  - Each segment is graded: normal (or hyperkinetic)—1, hypokinetic—2, akinetic—3, dyskinetic—4. The sum of all segments' score is then divided by the number of scored segments.
  - Normal ventricle—wall motion score index—1
  - The higher the score → the more abnormal the LV
- Strain imaging can also be used to assess segmental LV function; parameters that are looked at include strain, strain rate, tissue velocity.
  Note: tissue velocity measures velocity relative to the transducer and hence may be affected by tethering. Strain/strain rate are preferable.

4.5 Stress Testing

- The underlying concept of stress echocardiography is that various cardiac conditions manifest cardiac abnormalities and/or symptoms when workload is increased, but not necessarily at rest
- For example, flow limiting coronary artery stenosis without a prior infarction will not cause resting wall motion abnormalities.
- Increase in cardiac workload can be achieved in several ways:
  - Exercise (treadmill, upright bicycle, supine bicycle)
  - Pharmacologic agents (dobutamine, vasodilators)
  - Atrial pacing

Exercise stress testing allows for physiologic data to be obtained:

- Hemodynamic and clinical data can be obtained
- Symptoms during/following stress
- Test duration on standard exercise protocol
- Heart rate and blood pressure response
- Workload achieved (maximal heart rate × maximal systolic blood pressure)
- Estimated maximal METs achieved

Note:

- Treadmill stress test imaging is done immediately post exercise, whereas with bicycle stress testing continuous imaging is done
- If treadmill protocol is used, immediate post-stress images should be acquired within 1 minute of effort termination
- Different workloads can be achieved by treadmill vs. bicycle exercise
- Cardiac output increase is mainly dependent on heart rate with bicycle exercise, larger increases in stroke volume are noted with treadmill exercise.

Pharmacological stress testing allows for:

- Continuous imaging throughout the various stress stages
- Can be utilized when effort tolerance is decreased due to cardiac or non-cardiac causes

Note:

- Choosing stress modality (effort vs. pharmacological) mainly depends of patient's characteristics
- Choice between the various modalities of stress or various modalities of pharmacologic tests is generally by specific lab protocols
- Regardless of the stress modality, stress images are compared side by side with images obtained at rest
- For wall motion assessment, cine loops of systole only are utilized; this allows for side by sides comparison despite different heart rates at rest and stress
- Depending on the stress test indication, additional data can be obtained and compared between rest and stress (e.g. pulmonary artery pressure, mitral inflow gradient, aortic valve velocities, diastolic function parameters)

Evaluation for Ischemia

- The most common indication for stress echocardiography is evaluation for inducible ischemia
- Although some variability exists in coronary artery anatomy and distribution, in most cases segmental wall motion abnormalities correlate well with coronary distribution:
  - Left anterior descending (LAD)—anteroseptum, anterior wall, commonly apical cap, apical lateral wall (via Diagonal branches)
  - Right coronary artery (RCA)—is most commonly the origin of the PDA (80%—right dominant circulation)
  - Posterior descending artery (PDA)—inferior septum and inferior wall
  - RCA can also supply the inferolateral wall and right ventricle
  - Circumflex artery/marginal branches—lateral wall, inferolateral wall

Possible responses to stress:

Resting wall motion	Stress wall motion	Interpretation
Normal	Normal/hyperkinetic	Normal
Normal	Hypokinesis/akinesis/dyskinesis	Ischemia
Akinesis	Normal or hypokinesis	Viable
Akinesis	Akinesis/dyskinesis	Scar

Overall LV function should be assessed—normal response includes:

- Decreased end systolic volume
- Increased ejection fraction

Note:

- Endocardial resolution is of paramount importance for proper interpretation of stress echocardiograms. Contrast agents should be used if endocardial border recognition is suboptimal.
- The sensitivity and specificity of stress echocardiography for the diagnosis of significant CAD is similar to other non-invasive modalities (approximately 85%).

False negative causes:

- Inadequate stress (less than 85% of target heart rate achieved or overall low workload)
- Long delay in obtaining immediate post-stress images (for treadmill stress protocol)
- Single vessel coronary disease (in particular left circumflex disease)
- Concentric remodeling or hypertrophy of the left ventricle
- Baseline hypercontractile LV

False positive causes:

- Hypertensive response
- Hypertrophic cardiomyopathy ± LVOT obstruction (apical wall motion abnormalities can be seen despite lack of obstructive CAD)
- Reduced myocardial perfusion reserve as seen in microvascular disease, LV hypertrophy, diabetes, myocarditis, idiopathic cardiomyopathy
- Coronary spasm
- Abnormal septal motion due to ventricular pacing, post-operative state or conduction abnormalities

Other Indications for Stress Echocardiography

- Evaluation for possible cardiac cause of dyspnea
  - In addition to wall motion analysis to rule out ischemia, other parameters to be assessed:
    - Diastolic function parameters
    - Pulmonary artery pressure response to stress
- Valvular heart disease
  - Discrepancy between patient's symptoms and resting echo findings
    - Symptoms despite non-severe disease on resting echo (e.g. "mild" mitral ste-

nosis on resting echo with symptoms of dyspnea on exertion)

No symptoms despite severe disease on resting echo (e.g. patient denies symptoms despite severe aortic stenosis on resting echocardiogram)

- Risk stratification in various cardiac diseases (e.g. known CAD, hypertrophic cardiomyopathy)
- Viability assessment

Further Reading

Lopez-Candales A, Hernandez-Suarez DF. Strain Imaging echocardiography: what imaging cardiologists should know. Curr Cardiol Rev. 2017;13(2):118–29. https://doi.org/10.2174/1573403X12666161028122649.

Mitchell C, Rahko PS, Blauwet LA, et al. Guidelines for performing a comprehensive transthoracic echocardiographic examination in adults: recommendations from the American Society of Echocardiography. J Am Soc Echocardiogr. 2019;32(1):1–64. https://doi.org/10.1016/j.echo.2018.06.004.

Pellikka PA, Arruda-Olson A, Chaudhry FA, et al. Guidelines for performance, interpretation, and application of stress echocardiography in ischemic heart disease: from the American Society of Echocardiography. J Am Soc Echocardiogr. 2020;33(1):1–41.e8. https://doi.org/10.1016/j.echo.2019.07.001.

Porter TR, Mulvagh SL, Abdelmoneim SS, et al. Clinical applications of ultrasonic enhancing agents in echocardiography: 2018 American Society of Echocardiography Guidelines Update. J Am Soc Echocardiogr. 2018;31(3):241–74. https://doi.org/10.1016/j.echo.2017.11.013.

5 Left Ventricular Diastolic Function

Learning Objectives

- Understand the phases of diastole
- Review the stages of diastolic dysfunction
- Review the echocardiographic parameters available for assessing diastolic function and filling pressures
- Provide a simple algorithm for echocardiographic evaluation of diastolic function

General Considerations

Phases of diastole (Fig. 5.1)

- Isovolumetric relaxation
- Rapid filling
- Diastasis
- Atrial contraction

Components of LV diastolic function:

- LV relaxation
- Restoring forces
- LV compliance

Filling pressures include

- Mean left atrial pressure (LAP)
- LV pre-A pressure
- Mean LV diastolic pressure
- Left ventricular end diastolic pressure (LVEDP)

Since the clinically relevant filling pressure is mean LAP, the echocardiographic assessment concentrates on identifying what is the mean LAP.

5.1 Echocardiographic Evaluation of Diastolic Function

Step 1

- Clinical, hemodynamic, and echocardiographic data must be considered;
  - Age, blood pressure, heart rate, arrhythmias, LV volume, wall thickness, global LV function, LA volume, presence and severity of mitral valve disease

Step 2

- When evaluating diastolic function, the clinical questions are different for patients with preserved EF vs. those with reduced EF.
- Preserved EF clinical questions:
  - Is there diastolic dysfunction? If so, what grade?
  - What are the filling pressures?
- Reduced EF results from myocardial dysfunction hence diastolic function is always abnormal when there is systolic dysfunction.

T. Rambhatla, G. Perk, *The Echocardiography Companion*,
https://doi.org/10.1007/978-3-030-47041-8_5

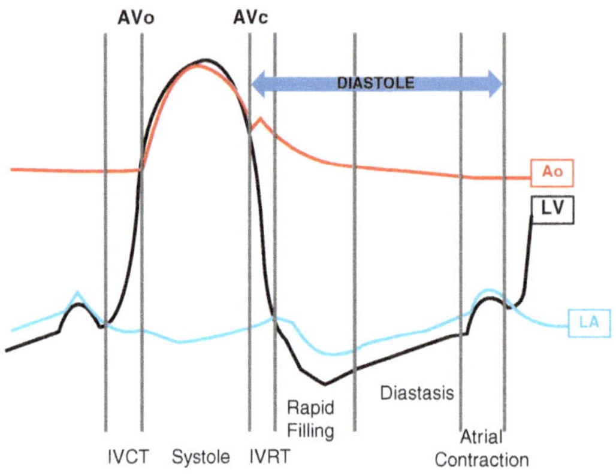

Fig 5.1 **Phases of diastole**. Wiggers diagram of intracardiac pressures during the cardiac cycle showing simultaneous pressure tracings of the left ventricle, left atrium, and the aorta. *Ao* aorta, *AVc* aortic valve closure, *AVo* aortic valve opening, *IVCT* isovolumic contraction time, *IVRT* isovolumic relaxation time, *LA* left atrium, *LV* left ventricle

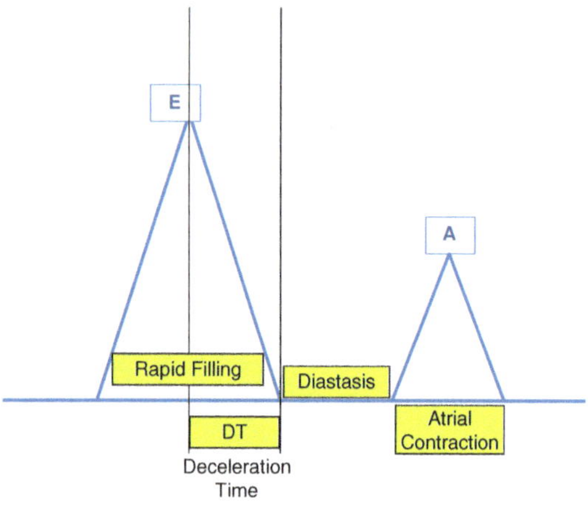

Fig 5.2 **Normal mitral inflow pattern**. Diastolic filling pattern is assessed by the early rapid filling wave (E), the late filling wave due to atrial contraction (A), the ratio of the velocities of the E and A wave, and the deceleration time of the E wave. *DT* deceleration time

- Reduced EF clinical question:
  - How severe is the diastolic dysfunction (what grade)?
  - What are the filling pressures?
- Note: The steps that follow can be used if none of these conditions are present
  - Atrial fibrillation
  - Significant mitral valve disease (more than moderate annular calcification)
  - Any degree of mitral stenosis
  - More than moderate mitral regurgitation
  - Mitral valve repair
  - Prosthetic mitral valve
  - Presence of LVAD
  - Post heart transplant
  - Presence of left bundle branch block
  - Ventricular paced rhythm

Step 3
Mitral inflow pattern

- Normal mitral inflow pattern (Fig. 5.2)
  - E wave during rapid filing
  - Period of minimal flow between left atrium and left ventricle (diastasis)
  - A wave during atrial contraction
  - In normal hearts E > A (most of the LV filling occurs during the rapid filling phase)
- Check E/A ratio
  - E/A ≤ 0.8, or E/A ≥ 2 → definitely abnormal

  Note: in young (<40 years old) healthy individuals, E/A > 2 may be normal → use other parameters to discern whether diastolic dysfunction is present.
- If E/A ≤ 0.8 AND peak E velocity ≤ 50 cm/s → grade I diastolic dysfunction with normal or low LAP
- If E/A ≥ 2 → grade III diastolic dysfunction with elevated mean LAP

  Deceleration time (DT) is usually short (<160mSec) in these situations however may not be below 160mSec if the peak E very high (> 120 cm/s) → more time needed for deceleration

  DT (and other diastolic parameters) should be used in patients with recent conversion from atrial fibrillation to sinus rhythm; in these cases, A velocity may be low due to atrial stunning, making the E/A ratio high even if LAP is not elevated.

Step 4

- If E/A ratio is between 0.8 and 2 and E velocity > 50 cm/s, further assessment required.
- If EF normal → decide if diastolic function is normal or abnormal

Parameters to measure (Fig. 5.3):	Cutoff for abnormal value
Septal and lateral TDI e` velocity	Septal <7 cm/s, lateral <10 cm/s
E/e` ratio (average septal and lateral)	> 14
Maximal LA volume	> 34 cc/m^2
Peak TR jet velocity	>2.8 m/s

- If more than 2 parameters reach abnormal cutoff → diastolic dysfunction is present
- If more than 2 parameters are in the normal range → diastolic function is normal
- If 2 parameters are normal and 2 abnormal → cannot determine diastolic function

Step 5

- If normal EF and diastolic dysfunction present (based on step 4) or if EF abnormal—decide grade of diastolic dysfunction and estimate LAP
- In most patients, three parameters can be used to assess severity of diastolic dysfunction and filling pressures

Parameters to measure:	Cutoff for abnormal value
E/e` ratio (average septal and lateral)	> 14
Maximal LA volume	> 34 cc/m^2 (A-L method or MOD)
Peak TR jet velocity	>2.8 m/s

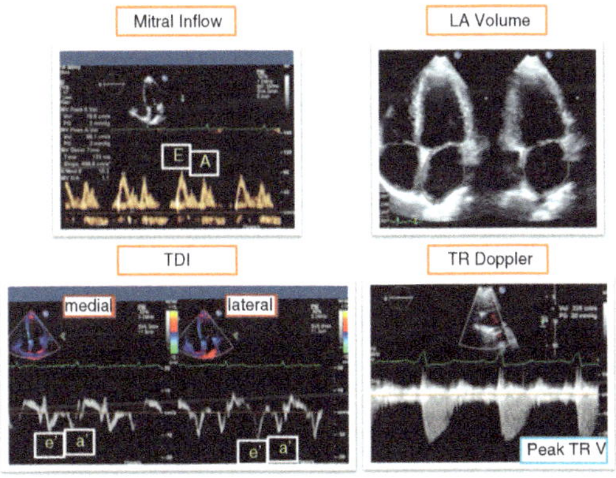

Fig 5.3 **Parameters for diastolic dysfunction assessment.** In addition to mitral inflow pattern, left atrial size, tissue Doppler imaging, and tricuspid regurgitation velocity are all used to grade diastolic dysfunction. *LA* left atrium, *TDI* tissue Doppler imaging, *TR* tricuspid regurgitation, *V* velocity

- If 2 or more parameters reach abnormal cutoff → grade II diastolic dysfunction with elevated mean LAP
- If 2 or more parameters are in the normal range → grade I diastolic dysfunction with normal mean LAP
- If only 2 parameters are available for interpretation and one meets abnormal threshold and one does not → use secondary parameters (see below)

Step 6

Secondary parameters for diastolic dysfunction assessment in cases of discrepancy or lack of primary parameters

- Mitral L wave (Fig. 5.4)
  - Ongoing filling of the LV during mid diastole due to elevated left atrial pressure and delayed LV relaxation (velocity generally >20 cm/s)
  - Sensitivity is overall low, however when present with known cardiac disease it is specific for elevated filling pressures.
- Isovolumetric relaxation time (IVRT) (Fig. 5.5)
  - Normal subjects—IVRT ≤70mSec
  - Impaired relaxation and normal LAP → IVRT prolongs
  - Increased LAP → IVRT shortens (IVRT duration—inversely related to LV filling pressures)
  - Needs to be combined with other diastolic parameters
  - Can be affected by heart rate and blood pressure

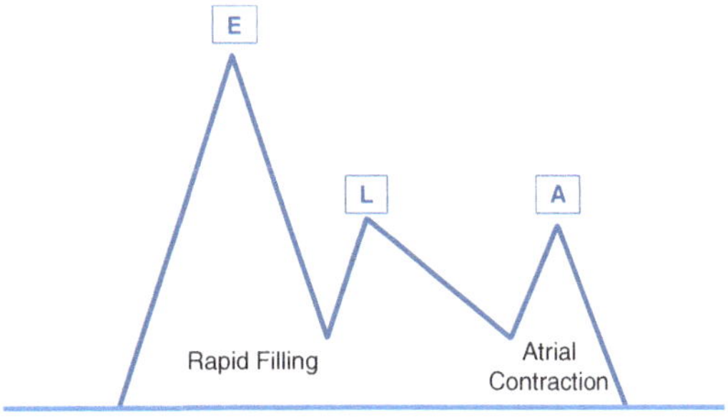

Fig 5.4 **Mitral L wave.** The presence of an L wave in the mitral inflow spectral Doppler is due to ongoing LV filling during diastasis and suggests elevated left atrial pressure

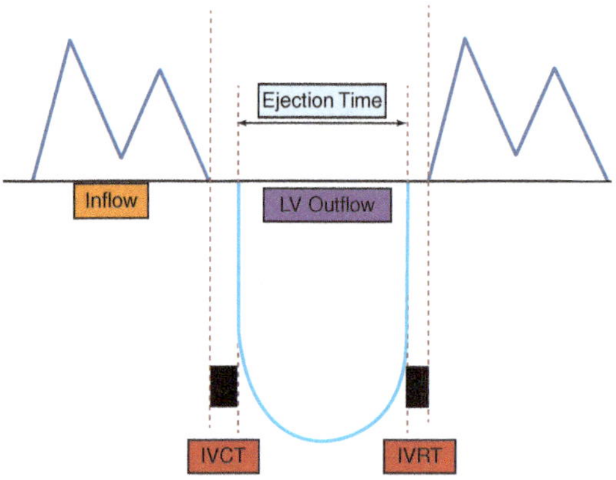

Fig 5.5 **Isovolumetric relaxation time (IVRT)**. Normal IVRT ≤70 ms. Impaired relaxation with normal left atrial pressure prolongs IVRT. With increasing left atrial pressure, IVRT shortens such that IVRT is inversely correlated with LV filling pressures. *IVCT* isovolumic contraction time, *IVRT* Isovolumic relaxation time

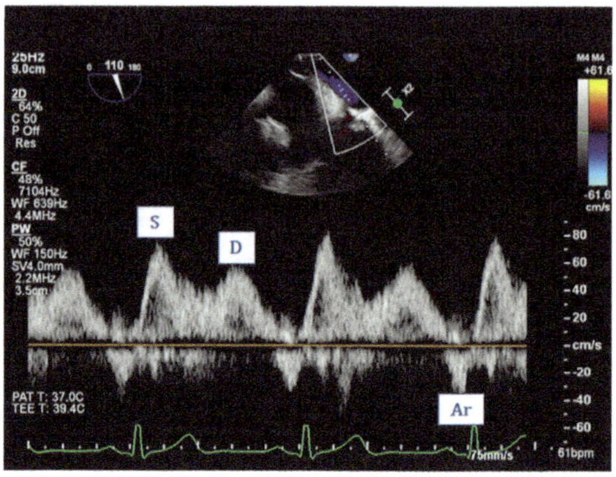

Fig 5.6 **Pulmonary vein spectral Doppler**. Normal pulmonary vein flow consists of three waves: S wave—triggered by atrial relaxation (during ventricular systole) and apical displacement of the mitral annulus; D wave—triggered by atrial emptying during ventricular diastole; Ar wave—small backwards flow into the pulmonary veins due to atrial contraction

- $T_{E\text{-}e`}$ Interval
  - Obtained by:
    - Measuring time interval between QRS and E wave onset
    - Measuring time interval between QRS and e` onset
    - Subtracting second interval from first to calculate the delay between onset of E and onset of e`
    - Impaired LV relaxation → low and delayed e` velocity
    - Elevated LAP → early onset E
    - From above—the worse the diastolic dysfunction the longer $T_{E\text{-}e`}$ Interval

  Note: must use matching R-R intervals
- IVRT/ $T_{E\text{-}e`}$ Interval ratio
  - The ratio correlates well with LAP
  - Ratio < 2 highly specific for elevated LAP

    Note: can be used in patients with mitral valve disease
- Pulmonary vein flow (Fig. 5.6)
  - S wave:
    - Caused by atrial relaxation and motion of mitral annulus towards LV apex
    - Affected by changes in LAP, LA contractility, LV/RV contractility
  - D wave:
    - Caused by atrial emptying during ventricular diastole
    - Affected by early diastolic filling and ventricular compliance
  - Ar wave:
    - Caused by atrial contraction and "back flow" into pulmonary veins
  - PV flow patterns changes with diastolic dysfunction
    - Ar-A duration (time difference between Ar duration and mitral A duration) > 30 ms indicates elevated LVEDP
    - Note: can be used in patients with mitral valve disease and patients with HOCM
  - Additional parameters to use, in patients with reduced LVEF
    - Reduced S velocity
    - S:D ratio < 1 correlated with increased left atrial pressure
    - Note: S:D ratio may be <1 in young healthy individuals
    - Systolic filling fraction

      $$\left(\frac{\text{S wave VTI}}{\text{total forward VTI}}\right)$$

      <40% indicates increased left atrial pressure
    - Note: PV flow pattern may be challenging to obtain on TTE

5.2 Diastolic Stress Test

- Diastolic dysfunction may manifest at stress, despite normal hemodynamics at rest
- Stress response in healthy individuals with normal diastolic function:
  - Mitral E velocity increases (increased LV "suction")
  - Annular e` velocity increases
    Note: stress e` velocity correlates well with exercise capacity
  - E/e` ratio remains unchanged

- Stress response in patients with diastolic dysfunction:
  - Annular e` does not increase (myocardial relaxation does not augment normally)
  - E/e` ratio increases

Indications:

- Patients with symptoms of heart failure or dyspnea on exertion with resting echocardiogram showing grade I diastolic dysfunction with normal LAP

Test should not be performed:

- Patients with normal EF and no evidence of diastolic dysfunction (with preserved annular TDI velocities)—unlikely to develop diastolic dysfunction with stress
- Patients with resting evidence of elevated LAP—cause for dyspnea presumably already exists

Test protocol:

- Exercise preferred over dobutamine to mimic everyday physiologic stress
- Treadmill protocol or supine bicycle can be used
- Baseline E, e` and TR peak velocity are obtained at all possible stages
  Note: at high heart rates, mitral inflow waves, as well as diastolic TDI waves may fuse and interfere with interpretation. Repeat acquisition of data during recovery, after heart rate slowed a little, may be helpful.
- If stress test performed both for evaluation of suspected or known CAD as well diastolic function assessment → wall motion data should be acquired first
- If echo contrast agent is used, only TR peak velocity can be utilized (TDI signals are not useful)

Test results:

Abnormal diastolic function test	Normal diastolic function test
All the following:	All the following:
Stress average E/e` > 14, or septal E/e` > 15	Average or septal E/e` <10
Peak TR velocity > 2.8 m/sec	Peak TR velocity < 2.8 m/sec
Septal e` < 7 cm/sec or lateral e` < 10 cm/sec	

- If only TR velocity is abnormal at peak stress → indeterminate test (normal individuals may have increased pulmonary blood flow with exercise)
- If not all parameters are abnormal → indeterminate test

Further Reading

González-Vilchez F, Ayuela J, Ares M, Mata NS, González AG, Durán RM. Comparison of Doppler echocardiography, color M-mode Doppler, and Doppler tissue imaging for the estimation of pulmonary capillary wedge pressure. J Am Soc Echocardiogr. 2002;15(10 Pt 2):1245–50. https://doi.org/10.1067/mje.2002.125752.

Nagueh SF, Smiseth OA, Appleton CP, et al. Recommendations for the evaluation of left ventricular diastolic function by echocardiography: an update from the American Society of Echocardiography and the European Association of Cardiovascular Imaging. Eur Heart J Cardiovasc Imaging. 2016;17(12):1321–60. https://doi.org/10.1093/ehjci/jew082.

Oh JK, Hatle L, Tajik AJ, Little WC. Diastolic heart failure can be diagnosed by comprehensive two-dimensional and Doppler echocardiography. J Am Coll Cardiol. 2006;47(3):500–6. https://doi.org/10.1016/j.jacc.2005.09.032.

Sorrentino R, Esposito R, Santoro C, et al. Practical impact of new diastolic recommendations on noninvasive estimation of left ventricular diastolic function and filling pressures [published online ahead of print, 2019 Oct 13]. J Am Soc Echocardiogr. 2019;S0894-7317(19):30924–1. https://doi.org/10.1016/j.echo.2019.08.013.

6 Right Ventricular Function and Pulmonary Hypertension

Learning Objectives

- Learn the different parameters by which the right ventricular size and function are evaluated with echocardiography
- Review key concepts of pulmonary hypertension and its effects on the right ventricle, as they pertain to echocardiography

General Considerations

- RV failure is an independent risk factor for mortality in patients with LV failure and carries very important prognostic implications.
- Difficulty in imaging the RV is due to several factors: anterior location, unique crescent shape, and reference values that have not been extensively evaluated.
- The RV is anatomically and functionally different than the LV; typical methods used to assess the LV cannot be used for RV assessment.

6.1 RV Anatomy and Measurements

- The RV is a thin walled crescent shaped structure that wraps around the LV
- The shape of the RV is also largely dependent on the interventricular septum
- In general, the RV is composed of three areas:
  - Inlet—TV and its apparatus
  - Apex—heavily trabeculated and has a prominent moderator band
  - Outlet or infundibulum—region of smooth myocardium and the pulmonic valve

    Note: most RV reference values are not indexed to sex or BSA; as a result, accurate classification into classes (mild, moderate, severe) may not be possible

Imaging Windows

Comprehensive evaluation of the RV should utilize all the following views:

- Parasternal window (Fig. 6.1):
  - Long axis view, short axis view and RV inflow view
- Apical four chamber view
- Modified/RV focused apical four chamber view (Fig. 6.2)
- Subcostal view

Qualitative Parameters

Parameters that suggest RV enlargement:

- RV that appears as large or larger than the LV (apical four chamber view)

Electronic Supplementary Material The online version of this chapter (https://doi.org/10.1007/978-3-030-47041-8_6) contains supplementary material, which is available to authorized users.

T. Rambhatla, G. Perk, *The Echocardiography Companion*, https://doi.org/10.1007/978-3-030-47041-8_6

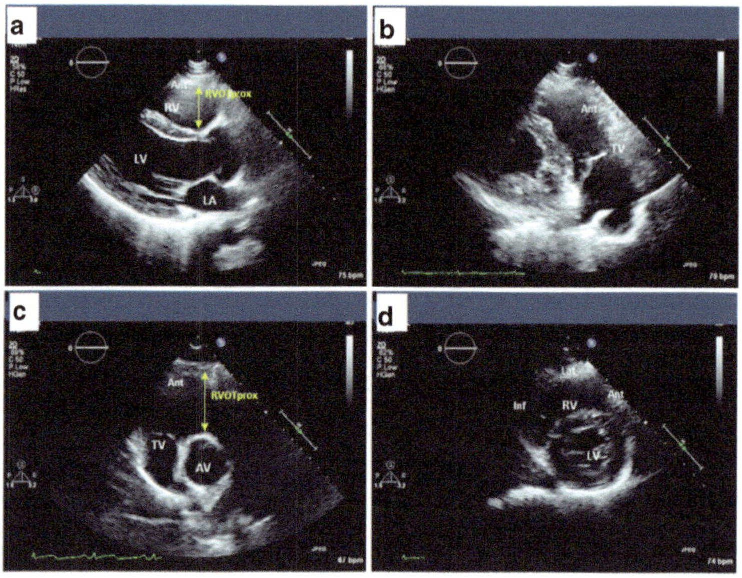

Fig. 6.1 **Parasternal views of the right ventricle.** (**a**) The standard parasternal long axis view visualizes the RV anterior wall; proximal right ventricular outflow tract is measured on this view as well (**b**) Right ventricular inflow view showing the RV anterior and inferior wall (**c**) Parasternal short axis view at the aortic valve level shows the basal anterior RV wall and the right ventricular outflow tract; proximal right ventricular outflow tract can be measured (**d**) parasternal short axis view at the mitral valve level shows the basal level of the inferior, lateral, and anterior wall segments of the right ventricle. The RV maintains its crescent shape with the interventricular septum maintaining a rounded shape. *Ant* anterior, *AV* aortic valve, *Inf* inferior, *LA* left atrium, *LV* left ventricle, *RV* right ventricle, *RVOT* right ventricular outflow tract, *TV* tricuspid valve

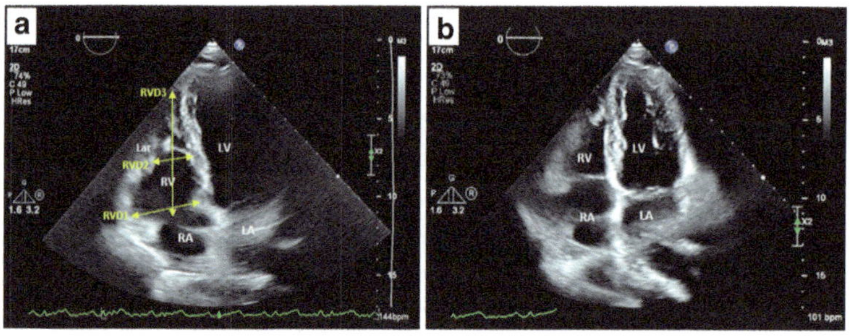

Fig. 6.2 **Apical RV-focused view.** (**a**) RV focused apical four chamber view is the recommended view for assessment and measurement of the dimensions of the right ventricle (RVD1, basal level; RVD2, mid cavity; RVD3, longitudinal). The lateral (free wall) of the right ventricle is visualized. (**b**) Standard apical four chamber view is shown for comparison. *LA* left atrium, *Lat* lateral, *LV* left ventricle, *RA* right atrium, *RV* right ventricle

- RV that is "apex forming"—RV extends to the apex (normally only the LV should form the apex)

Quantitative Parameters

Linear measurements
PLAX
• RVOT prox > 30 mm
PSAX
• RVOT prox > 35 mm
• RVOT distal > 27 mm
RV focused apical 4CH
• RVD_1 base > 41 mm
• RVD_2 mid > 35 mm
• RVD_3 long > 83 mm
Area measurements
RV focused apical 4CH
• RV EDA women > 20 cm^2, men > 24 cm^2
• RV ESA women > 11 cm^2, men > 15 cm^2
Wall thickness
Subcostal, M mode
• >5 mm

6.1.1 RV Blood Supply

RCA and LAD supply the right ventricle (Fig. 6.3)

- RCA
  - Acute marginal branch supplies the anterior and lateral walls of the RV.
  - Conus artery (first branch of the RCA) supplies the RVOT/infundibulum (in 30% of cases the conus artery has a separate coronary ostium from the RCA).
  - PDA supplies the inferior wall of the RV and part of the inferior septum.
- LAD
  - LAD supplies the anterior septum, RV apex, and moderator band (via septal perforators).

  Note: RV infarction due to RCA occlusion can lead to a "pseudo McConnell sign"; if LAD blood supply is normal, the preserved septal and moderator band contractility appears as RV apical sparing

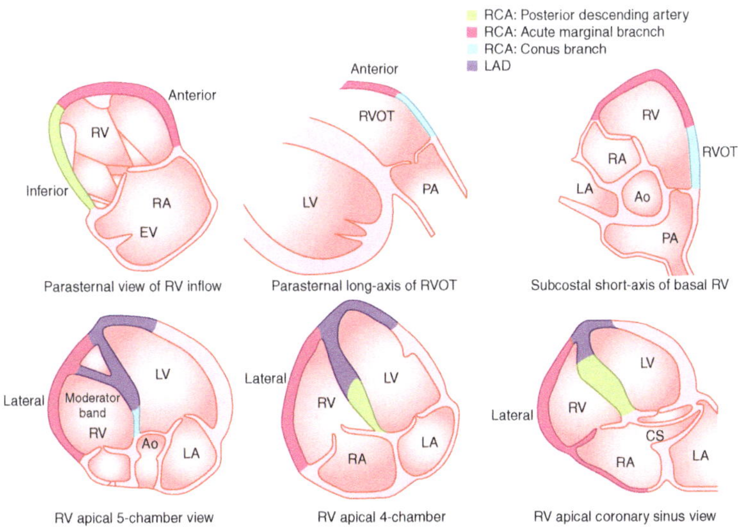

Fig. 6.3 **Right ventricle blood supply**. Right ventricular wall segments with their corresponding coronary blood supply. *Ao* Aorta, *CS* coronary sinus, *LA* left atrium, *LAD* left anterior descending artery, *LV* left ventricle, *PA* pulmonary artery, *RA* right atrium, *RCA* right coronary artery, *RV* right ventricle, *RVOT* right ventricular outflow tract

6.2 RV Systolic Function Assessment

- RV and LV are dependent on each other for preload and have the same stroke volume, despite having vastly different workloads
- The RV requires only ~$\frac{1}{6}^{\text{th}}$ of the workload of the LV while pumping the same amount of blood
- This is accomplished by a more energy-efficient method of contraction, pumping against lower afterload (lower pressure pulmonary system) and generating lower pressures
- As opposed to the LV, where the main work force comes from circumferential constriction and reduction in diameter, the RV ejects blood mostly via longitudinal contraction and RV shortening
- A lower proportion of RV stroke work goes to pressure generation, while much higher proportion goes to generating blood momentum

6.2.1 Qualitative Parameters

Parameters that may suggest RV systolic dysfunction:

- RV size does not decrease in systole
- LV appears under filled/small cavity LV
- Hyperdynamic LV and decreased LV stroke volume

6.2.2 Quantitative Parameters (Table 6.1)

Table 6.1 Reference values for normal RV systolic function

Method	Echocardiographic imaging and limitations
TAPSE ≥ 17 mm	M-mode imaging; measurement of systolic movement of the lateral TV annulus as a surrogate for longitudinal systolic function Accuracy may be limited due to translational motion and tethering
TDI S′ ≥ 9.5 cm/s	Measures myocardial systolic velocity of the lateral TV annulus with TDI as a surrogate for longitudinal systolic function Accuracy is angle dependent (as any Doppler based technique)
FAC ≥ 35%	Based on two-dimensional tracing of RV area (include trabeculae and moderator band in the area traced) $\text{RV FAC} = \frac{EDA - ESA}{ESA} \times 100$ Limited by difficult views and RV geometry; excludes RVOT contributions
RIMP Two techniques: PW ≤ 0.43 TDI ≤ 0.54	$\text{RIMP} = \frac{IVCT + IVRT}{ET} = \frac{TVCOT - ET}{ET}$ Shorter IVCT (pressure generated quicker) and short IVRT (RV relaxes quicker) → short RIMP → better RV systolic function Load dependent; RIMP can be falsely normal in situations that shorten IVRT (e.g. high RAP states)
EF (not routinely used)	Three dimensional volumetric assessment $\text{RV EF} = \frac{EDV - ESV}{EDV} \times 100$ Requires good image quality and post-processing; load dependent
Strain Absolute value: GLS > 20%	Speckle tracking method preferred; acquired from RV focused apical four chamber view Angle independent; vendor specific; load dependent
RV dP/dT ≥ 400	Measurement of the rate of rise of early RV systolic pressure: on the TR envelope, the time of pressure rise from 4 mmHg to 16 mmHg is measured (jet velocity increase from 1 m/s to 2 m/s) Load dependent; can be falsely prolonged in high RAP states

TAPSE tricuspid annulus plane systolic excursion, *TDI* tissue doppler imaging, *FAC* fractional area change, *EDA* end diastolic area, *ESA* end systolic area, *RIMP-RV* index of myocardial performance, *IVCT* isovolumetric contraction time, *IVRT* isovolumetric relaxation time, *ET* ejection time, *TVCOT* tricuspid closure to opening time, *EDV* end diastolic volume, *ESV* end systolic volume, *GLS* global longitudinal strain

6.3 RV Diastolic Function

Evaluation of RV diastolic function is recommended for:

- Suspected RV disease, as a marker of subtle/subclinical dysfunction
- Known RV dysfunction for prognostication

Parameters used to evaluate RV diastolic function:

- Tricuspid inflow E and A velocities (average over several beats due to respiratory variations)
- Tricuspid annulus tissue Doppler velocities—e', a'
- E/A ratio
- E/e'
- Deceleration time
- Right atrial size
- Right atrial pressure estimate from IVC size and respiratory variations
- Hepatic vein flow pattern

Definitions of diastolic dysfunction grades:

- Impaired relaxation
  - Tricuspid E/A < 0.8
- Pseudonormal:
  - Tricuspid E/A 0.8–2.1 and E/e' > 6
  - Predominant diastolic flow in hepatic veins
- Restrictive
  - E/A > 2.1 and DT < 120 ms
  - Late diastolic antegrade flow in pulmonary artery

6.4 Ventricular Interdependence (Fig. 6.4, Video 6.1)

- When pressures in the RV increase (in diastole or systole or both), the LV assumes a 'D' shaped configuration, with flattening of the septum
- The position and configuration of the interventricular septum depends on the pressure gradient between the LV and RV during the cardiac cycle.
  Note: analysis of septal motion for ventricular interdependence requires absence of paradoxical septal motion from other causes (e.g. LBBB, RV pacing, etc.)
- Quantification—eccentricity index:
  - Ratio between LV anteroposterior diameter and LV septal-lateral dimension (on PSAX view)
  - Normal LV/RV relative pressures → LV appears round → index = 1

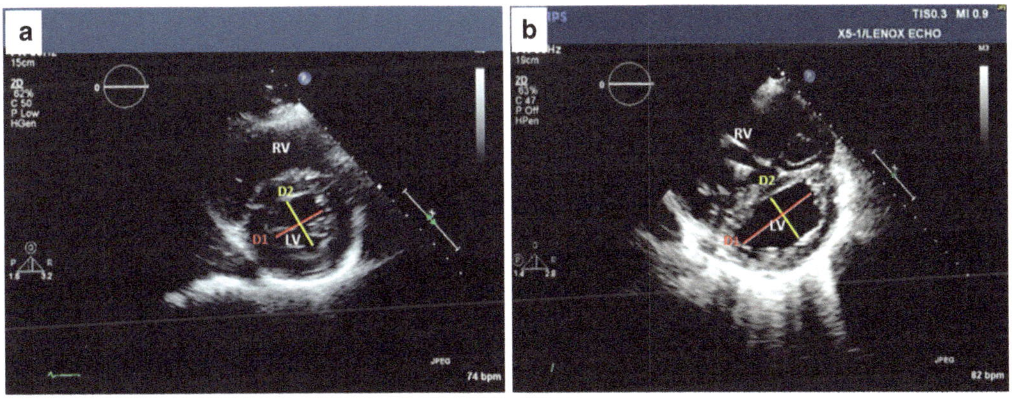

Fig. 6.4 **RV/LV interdependence—Eccentricity index.** (**a**) Normal right and left ventricular morphology: the left ventricle has a round configuration; the ratio of the antero-posterior dimension (D1) to the septal-lateral dimension (D2) is close to 1. (**b**) Right ventricular overload, the LV takes a crescent shape, the interventricular septum flattens, and antero-posterior dimension of the left ventricle is greater than the septal-lateral dimension; eccentricity index >1. *LV* left ventricle, *RV* right ventricle

  - Eccentricity index >1 (antero-posterior diameter larger than septal–lateral diameter) → RV overload
  - Eccentricity index should be evaluated over the cardiac cycle
- RV volume overload:
  - Examples: chronic severe TR, large ASD, severe PI
  - Septal shift noted mainly at end diastole
  - Eccentricity index = 1 at end systole, increased at end diastole
- RV pressure overload:
  - Examples: pulmonary hypertension, pulmonic stenosis
  - Septal shift seen both at end systole and end diastole (most pronounced at end systole)
  - Eccentricity index >1 at end diastole and end systole

6.5 Acute Pressure Overload

- Seen with acute PE (massive/sub-massive)
- The acute increase in RV afterload is not tolerated well; thin walled RV has not had sufficient time to hypertrophy and remodel → cannot compensate for the increased pressure → RV dilatation and failure
- RV cannot generate high pressure → low RVSP/TR jet velocity
- 60:60 sign
  - RVOT acceleration time (AT) < 60 ms
  - Relatively low PA systolic pressure (<60 mmHg)
- McConnel's Sign
  - Severe hypokinesis of basal to mid RV free wall with RV apical sparing (hyperdynamic apical contraction)

6.6 Pulmonary Hypertension (PH)

- Under normal circumstances, the pulmonary circulation is a low resistance circuit (~$\frac{1}{8}$th pressure of the systemic circulation)
- PH develops when pulmonary pressures reach $\frac{1}{4}$th the systemic circulation pressure

6.6.1 Definition

- PH is defined as an increase in mean pulmonary arterial pressure (PAP_{mean}) ≥ 25 mmHg at rest, as assessed by right heart catheterization.
- Pulmonary artery systolic pressure (PASP) ≥ 35 mmHg is suggestive of PH; however, increased pulmonary flow (e.g. with left to right shunt) can cause increased PASP without an increase in pulmonary vascular resistance (PVR)
- A more complete classification of PH includes PAP_{mean}, PASP, and PVR (Tables 6.2 and 6.3)

Table 6.2 Severity of pulmonary hypertension

Severity of pulmonary hypertension			
Severity	PAP_{mean} (mmHg)	PASP (mmHg)	PVR (Wood's Units)
Mild	≥25	≥35	>3
Moderate	≥40	≥50	>3
Severe	≥55	≥75	>3

PAP pulmonary artery pressure, *PASP* pulmonary artery systolic blood pressure

Table 6.3 WHO clinical classification of pulmonary hypertension (PH)

WHO classification of pulmonary hypertension (PH) and etiologies		
Type 1	Pulmonary arterial hypertension (4%)	Idiopathic, genetic, congenital heart disease, drugs/toxins, portal hypertension, Connective Tissue Disease, HIV
Type 2	PH due to left heart disease (80%)	Systolic/diastolic dysfunction, valvular heart disease
Type 3	PH due to intrinsic lung disease (10%)	OSA, COPD, ILD
Type 4	Chronic Thromboembolic PH (1%)	PE, and other causes of PA obstruction other than PS
Type 5	PH with multifactorial mechanisms (6%)	Pulmonary vasculitis, hematologic disorders, chronic renal failure, Glycogen storage disease, thyroid disorders

6.6.2 Echocardiographic Assessment

Anatomic Assessment

1. M-mode of pulmonic valve (PV) (Fig. 6.5)
   - Absent/diminished 'a' (atrial) wave of PV
     - Under normal circumstances, atrial kick causes posterior deflection of PV leaflet, followed by normal systolic opening and closing
     - With pulmonary HTN—downstream pressure elevated → slight increase in RV diastolic pressure during atrial kick is not enough to cause posterior motion of the PV leaflet
   - Note: in Pulmonic stenosis
     - PA pressure is not elevated, but RVEDP and RVSP are elevated
     - Atrial kick increases RVEDP further and easily overcomes the normal PA diastolic pressure → exaggerated posterior motion of PV leaflet
     - Also seen in constrictive pericarditis, or any situation with increased RVEDP and normal PA diastolic pressure
   - 'Flying W'
     - Early systolic partial closure of PV followed by re-opening of the valve once RV re-generates enough pressure to open PV again
2. 2D assessment
   - Enlarged right sided chambers
   - RV to LV ratio—RV larger than the LV suggestive of volume and/or pressure overload
   - RV wall thickness—RVH suggests presence of RV pressure overload state
   - D-shaped septum/septal flattening/paradoxical septal motion

Doppler Assessment

1. TR spectral Doppler
   - Systolic PAP estimate = 4 × (TR Vmax)^2 + RAP
   - Estimate of PAP_{mean} = 0.61 × SPAP +2
2. PI spectral Doppler
   - Diastolic PAP = 4 × (PI_{EDV})^2 + RAP

     Note: once PA systolic pressure is estimated (from TR jet) and PA diastolic pressure is estimated (from PI_{EDV}), PAP_{mean} can be calculated as: $\frac{PAsys + 2xPAdias}{3}$
   - Alternative methods for PAP_{mean}:
     - PAP_{mean} = 4 × (PI_{earlyV})^2 + RAP
     - PAP_{mean} = TR mean gradient + RAP
3. RVOT spectral Doppler
   - RVOT PW morphology
     - Systolic notch/bifid wave—early systolic decrease in RVOT outflow due to high downstream pressure (corresponds to the M-mode 'flying w')
     - Low velocity/small VTI
   - Acceleration Time (AT)

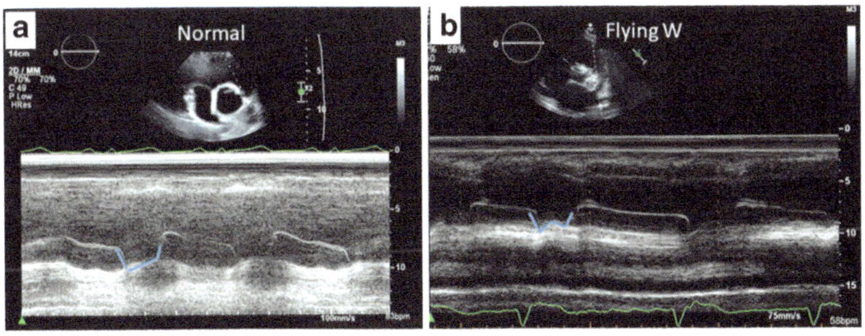

Fig. 6.5 **Pulmonic valve M-mode.** (**a**) Normal pulmonic valve m-mode shows leaflet opening throughout systole, until closure at the end of ejection period. (**b**) With pulmonary hypertension, there is partial early systolic closure of the pulmonic valve, followed by re-opening in later systole once the right ventricle has generated enough pressure to overcome the pulmonary artery systolic pressure, creating the "flying W" configuration

- Measured from the onset of the QRS on ECG to the peak of the pulmonary flow (in sinus rhythm, HR 60–100/min)
- The faster the AT, the higher the PAP
  $PAP_{mean} = 79 - (0.45 \times AT)$
  If $AT < 120_{ms} \rightarrow PAP_{mean} = 90 - (0.62 \times AT)$
  AT <90–100 ~ closely correlates with $PAP_{mean} > 60$

Note: if pulmonary flow is increased (i.e. ASD with significant left to right shunt), AT may underestimate PAP

4. Estimation of pulmonary vascular resistance (PVR)
   - Normal PVR is 1.5 Woods Units (<240 dynes-sec/m)
   - Δ Pressure = Flow × Resistance → $\text{Resistance} = \frac{\Delta \text{Pressure}}{Flow}$
   - If mean PAP can be calculated, mean LAP estimated, and pulmonary-system cardiac output can be measured → above equation can be used to calculate PVR (see Chap. 7—hemodynamics)
   - Alternate method for estimating PVR: $\frac{TR\,Vmax}{RVOT\,VTI} \times 10 + 0.16$

   Note: Calculating PVR helps distinguish between PAHTN from high flow (e.g. high output states like anemia, sepsis, left to right shunt) and high resistance states (e.g. type 1 pulmonary HTN)
5. Mitral inflow pattern
   - If PH is due to type II/left heart disease—MV inflow pattern may be suggestive of increased LAP

Further Reading

Lang RM, Badano LP, Mor-Avi V, et al. Recommendations for cardiac chamber quantification by echocardiography in adults: an update from the American Society of Echocardiography and the European Association of Cardiovascular Imaging. J Am Soc Echocardiogr. 2015;28(1):1–39.e14. https://doi.org/10.1016/j.echo.2014.10.003.

Mitchell C, Rahko PS, Blauwet LA, et al. Guidelines for Performing a Comprehensive Transthoracic Echocardiographic Examination in Adults: Recommendations from the American Society of Echocardiography. J Am Soc Echocardiogr. 2019;32(1):1–64. https://doi.org/10.1016/j.echo.2018.06.004.

Rudski LG, Lai WW, Afilalo J, et al. Guidelines for the echocardiographic assessment of the right heart in adults: a report from the American Society of Echocardiography endorsed by the European Association of Echocardiography, a registered branch of the European Society of Cardiology, and the Canadian Society of Echocardiography. J Am Soc Echocardiogr. 2010;23(7):685–788. https://doi.org/10.1016/j.echo.2010.05.010.

7 Hemodynamics in the Echo Lab

Learning Objectives

- Understand how intracardiac pressures are estimated using echocardiography
- Use a clinical example to demonstrate how to use and investigate unusual hemodynamic echocardiographic data

General Considerations

Basic principles for doing hemodynamics in the echo lab:

- Blood flow velocities are measured based on the Doppler principle
- Velocities and pressure gradients are related through the Bernoulli principle
- Use all available data (e.g. Doppler data, blood pressure in both arms, heart rate) in order to understand hemodynamics.
  1. Doppler echocardiography is used to measure intra-cardiac velocities, both blood flow velocities and tissue velocities
     - Velocities are calculated using the Doppler principle (Fig. 7.1):
       The observed frequency of a wave depends on the relative speed of the source and the observer
       - Sound wave of known frequency is sent from a source (transducer)
       - The returned wave's frequency is detected by the transducer (as the observer)
       - The change between the emitted frequency and the returned frequency is the Doppler shift
       - Velocity of the target is calculated by the Doppler equation
  2. The Bernoulli principle connects the velocity of a flow with a pressure change
     - In echocardiography we use the modified Bernoulli equation:
     - $\Delta P = 4\ V^2$
     - Essentially—once we know the velocity by which blood travels from one chamber to another, we know the pressure gradient between these two chambers.
  3. Wiggers diagrams (Fig. 7.2) show the relationship between the pressures in the various cardiac chambers.
     - Of note, the general appearance of the right heart and left heart pressure curves is similar; however absolute values of pressures are different.

In order to know absolute pressures, as opposed to gradients, we must have some pressures we can independently measure or estimate.

T. Rambhatla, G. Perk, *The Echocardiography Companion*,
https://doi.org/10.1007/978-3-030-47041-8_7

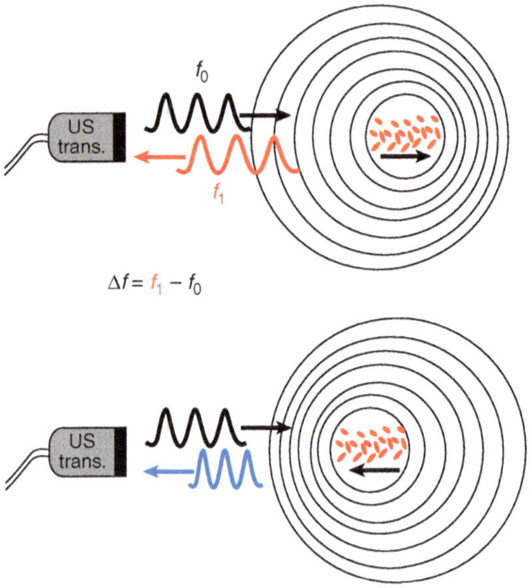

Fig. 7.1 **The Doppler principle**. The Doppler principle states that the observed frequency of a wave depends on the relative speed of the source and the observer. In clinical echo, sound wave of known frequency is sent from a source (transducer), interacts with a moving target and returned to the transducer. The returned wave's frequency is detected by the transducer and is different from the emitted frequency. This difference (the "Doppler Shift") depends on the velocity of the target and the angle between the interrogating beam and the velocity vector. Since the Doppler shift can be measured by the transducer, the velocity of the target can be calculated as $V = \frac{\Delta f \times C}{2 f_0 \times Cos\theta}$.

C propagation velocity of sound within biological tissue, *Δf* Doppler shift, f_0 emitted frequency, *V* velocity of target

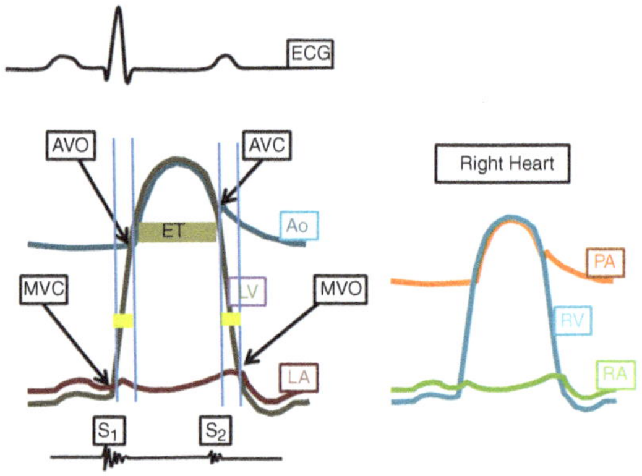

Fig. 7.2 **Wiggers diagrams**. Pressure curves showing the relationship between the pressures in the cardiac chambers. Left panel—left heart pressures, right panel—right heart pressures. Note: the patterns of the pressure curves in the left and right heart are similar, however the absolute values differ. *AVC* aortic valve closure, *AVO* aortic valve opening, *Ao* aorta, *ET* ejection time, *LA* left atrium, *LV* left ventricle, *MVC* mitral valve closure', *MVO* mitral valve opening, *PA* pulmonary artery, *RA* right atrium, *RV* right ventricle

7.1 The Echocardiographic Swan Ganz Catheter

7.1.1 Intra-Cardiac Pressures

Step 1 (Fig. 7.3):

- The aortic pressure is measured directly by measuring blood pressure
- Under normal conditions, LV systolic pressure = aortic systolic pressure
- Right atrial pressure is estimated by measuring IVC size and inspiratory change
- Under normal conditions, RV diastolic pressure = RA pressure

Step 2 (Fig. 7.4):

- TR velocity is used to calculate systolic pressure gradient between RV and RA
- RV systolic pressure = RA pressure + TR systolic gradient
- Under normal conditions, PA systolic pressure = RV systolic pressure

Step 3 (Fig. 7.5):

- PI velocity is used to calculate diastolic pressure gradient between PA and RV
- Since RV diastolic pressure = RA pressure → PA diastolic pressure = PI pressure gradient + RA pressure
- Once PA systolic and diastolic pressures are known, mean PA pressure is calculated by:

$$\text{Mean PAP} = \frac{1}{3}\text{ sys PAP} + \frac{2}{3}\text{ dias PAP}$$

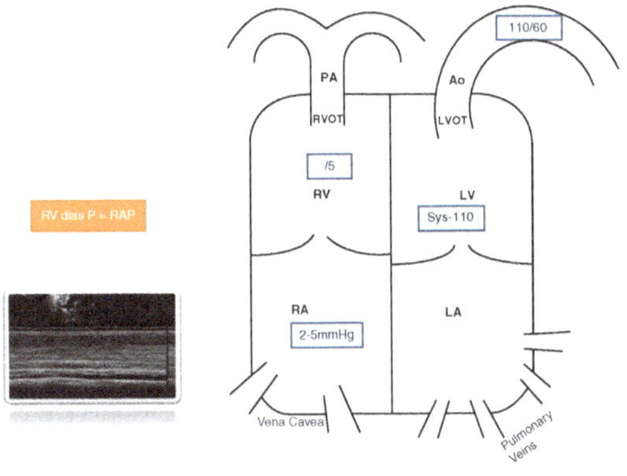

Fig. 7.3 Echocardiographic right heart catheterization—Step 1. Under normal conditions, left ventricular systolic pressure equals the aortic systolic pressure. Right atrial pressure is estimated by evaluation of the inferior vena cava (IVC) from the subcostal view; IVC size and inspiratory change are parameters used to estimate right atrial pressure. Under normal conditions, right ventricular diastolic pressure equals right atrial pressure. *Ao* aorta, *LA* left atrium, *LV* left ventricle, *LVOT* left ventricular outflow tract, *PA* pulmonary artery, *RA* right atrium, *RAP* right atrial pressure', *RV* right ventricle, *RVOT* right ventricular outflow tract

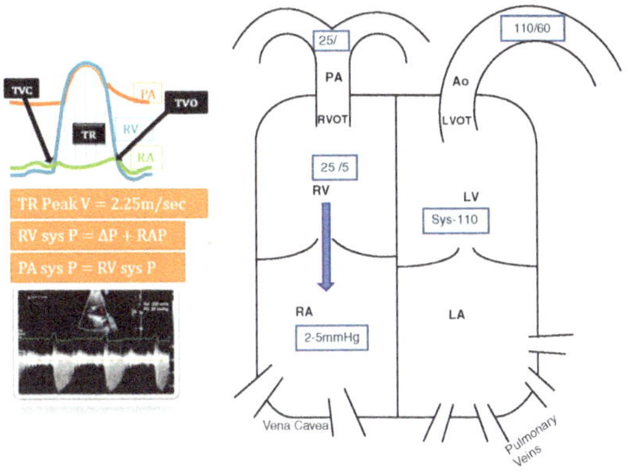

Fig. 7.4 Echocardiographic right heart catheterization—Step 2. Utilizing the tricuspid regurgitation (TR) spectral Doppler, the peak tricuspid regurgitation velocity is measured. Right ventricular systolic pressure equals right atrial pressure + peak TR gradient. Under normal conditions, pulmonary artery systolic pressure equals the right ventricular systolic pressure. *Ao* aorta, *LA* left atrium, *LV* left ventricle, *LVOT* left ventricular outflow tract, *PA* pulmonary artery, *RA* right atrium, *RAP* right atrial pressure', *RV* right ventricle, *RVOT* right ventricular outflow tract, *TVC* tricuspid valve closure, *TVO* tricuspid valve opening, *TR* tricuspid regurgitation

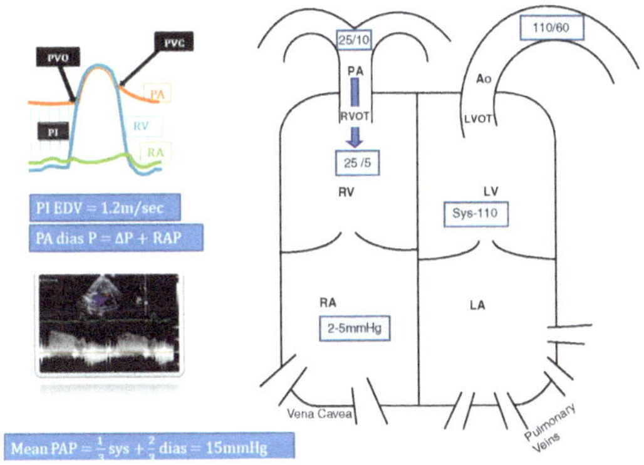

Fig. 7.5 Echocardiographic Right Heart Catheterization—Step 3. Utilizing the pulmonic insufficiency (PI) spectral Doppler envelope, the end diastolic PI velocity is measured. Pulmonary artery end diastolic pressure equals right ventricular diastolic pressure + peak end PI gradient. Once pulmonary artery diastolic pressure is estimated mean pulmonary artery pressure is calculate by: Mean PAP = $\frac{1}{3}$ sys + $\frac{2}{3}$ dias = 15 mmHg. *Ao* aorta, *LA* left atrium, *LV* left ventricle, *LVOT* left ventricular outflow tract, *PA* pulmonary artery, *PA dias o* pulmonary artery diastolic pressure, *PI* pulmonic insufficiency, *PI EDV* pulmonic insufficiency end diastolic velocity, *PVO* pulmonic valve opening, *PVC* pulmonic valve closure, *RA* right atrium, *RAP* right atrial pressure', *RV* right ventricle, *RVOT* right ventricular outflow tract

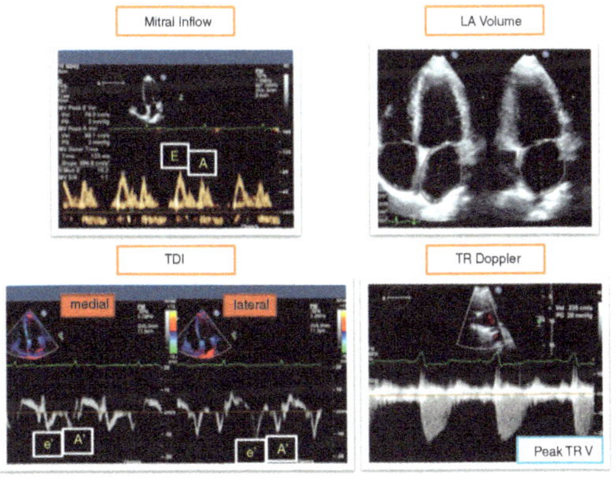

Fig. 7.6 Echocardiographic Right Heart Catheterization—Step 4. Parameters used to estimate left atrial pressure and left ventricular diastolic pressure. *LA* left atrium, *TDI* tissue Doppler imaging, *TR* tricuspid regurgitation, *V* velocity

Step 4 (Fig. 7.6):

- LA pressure and LV diastolic pressure cannot be measured directly on echo
- An estimation of normal vs. elevated pressure can be obtained in many cases
- Parameters to look at:

- Mitral inflow spectral Doppler (PW Doppler at the level of mitral valve tips)
- Tissue Doppler velocity at medial and lateral annulus
- Calculate E/e' ratio
- TR peak velocity
- Left atrial size
- See Chap. 5 for details regarding evaluation of diastolic function and filling pressures

7.1.2 Cardiac Output

1. VTI based method (Fig. 7.7)
   - If area can be measured or calculated at a place that PW Doppler can be obtained → stroke volume (SV) can be calculated by:
     - $SV(ml) = CSA(cm^2) \times VTI(cm)$
       CSA—Cross Sectional Area, VTI—Velocity Time Integral
     - Cardiac output (CO) then is calculated as SV × heart rate

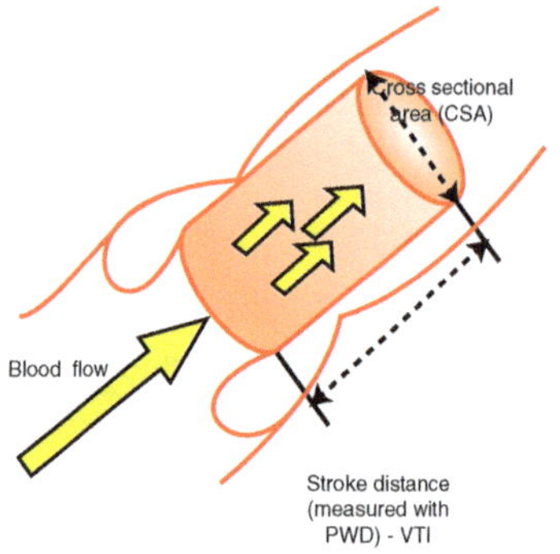

Fig. 7.7 **VTI based method for stroke volume calculation**. The flow across a fixed orifice is equal to the product of the orifice cross sectional area (CSA) and the velocity time integral (VTI). The VTI represents the "stroke distance" and can be measured by PW Doppler and the built-in calculation packages in the echocardiography unit. At any point that CSA area and VTI can be measured (e.g. LVOT), stroke volume can be calculated. If preformed across the LVOT, stroke volume = LVOT CSA × LVOT VTI. *CSA* cross sectional area, *VTI* velocity time integral

     - Cardiac index (CI) = $\frac{CO}{BSA}$
       BSA—Body Surface Area
   - Important considerations:
     - If diameter is measured, the area is calculated based on geometric assumptions (e.g. circular CSA)
     - PW Doppler must be aligned properly such that flow is parallel to beam
     - Regurgitant lesions limit where SV can be measured (e.g. in the presence of significant AI, effective SV cannot be calculated by using LVOT area and VTI as it includes the regurgitant volume).
     - In the presence of shunts - attention should be paid to which SV/CO is being calculated; RV/LV stroke volume measurements can be utilized to calculate Qp:Qs.
2. 2D based method (Fig. 7.8)
   - Utilizing apical 4-chamber and apical 2-chamber view
     - Endocardial border is traced at end diastole and end systole
     - End diastolic volume (EDV) and end systolic volume (ESV) are calculated based on the method of discs (see Chap. 4 on assessing LV systolic function)
     - Stroke volume is calculated as: SV = EDV-ESV
   - Important consideration:
     In the presence of significant AI or MR, the calculated SV will <u>include</u> the regurgitant volume, thus overestimate the effective stroke volume.

7.1.3 Vascular Resistance

Calculation of vascular resistance (R) is based on similar principle to Ohm's law:

$$\text{Flow} = \frac{\Delta P}{R} \rightarrow R = \frac{\Delta P}{\text{Flow}}$$

- ΔP—Pressure drop across the vascular bed of interest
- Flow—flow across the vascular bed of interest

Systemic vascular resistance:
- ΔP = MAP (mean arterial pressure)—RAP (right atrial pressure)
- Flow = systemic cardiac output
- $\text{SVR} = \dfrac{\text{MAP} - \text{RAP}}{\text{C.O.}}$

Pulmonary vascular resistance:
- ΔP = MPAP (mean pulmonary artery pressure)—LAP (left atrial pressure)
- Flow = right heart cardiac output
- $\text{PVR} = \dfrac{\text{MPAP} - \text{LAP}}{\text{Right Heart C.O.}}$

Important consideration:
- Under normal conditions:
- Systemic C.O. = Right Heart C.O
- However in the presence of a shunt, left and right cardiac output differ and the correct cardiac output must be used to calculate the resistance across the vascular bed of interest.

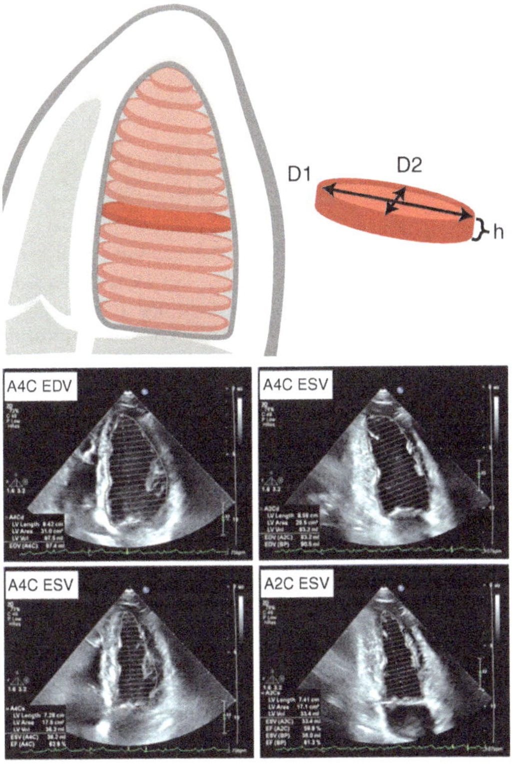

Fig. 7.8 LV Volume based method for stroke volume calculation. (Simpson's rule/Method of Discs). Apical four chamber and two chamber views are used to measure the left ventricular end-diastolic and end-systolic volumes; the endocardial border needs to be clearly visualized. The traced area is divided into 20 cylinders of equal height. The volume of all the cylinders is summed to calculate LV volume and end diastole (EDV) and end systole (ESV). Subtracting ESV from EDV gives the stroke volume. Tracings from the two orthogonal planes are utilized to provide the LV stroke volume

7.2 Sample Case in Echocardiographic Hemodynamics

63 year-old woman, referred for echocardiogram for assessing LV function

- Echo showed normal left ventricular function (EF-65%) and moderate mitral regurgitation
- Spectral Doppler of the mitral regurgitation is shown in Fig. 7.9
- Note—peak MR velocity = 7.6 m/s
- "Usual" MR peak velocity is in the range of 5 m/s (Fig. 7.10).

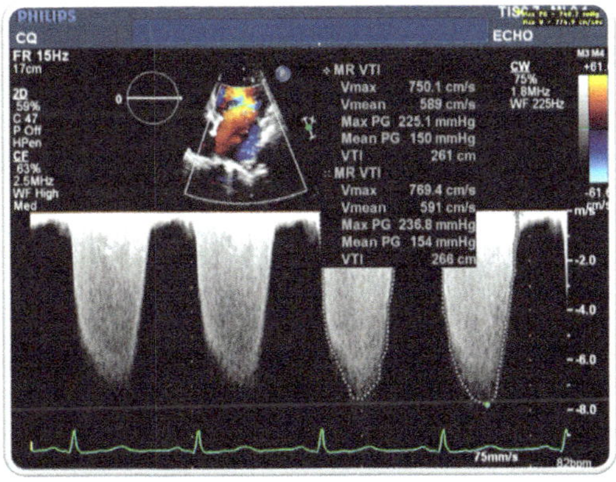

Fig. 7.9 Mitral regurgitation spectral Doppler. Continuous wave spectral Doppler of the mitral regurgitation (MR) jet from the patient presented. Note the peak velocity of the MR is measured to be 7.6 m/s, corresponding to a left ventricle-left atrium pressure gradient of 231 mmHg

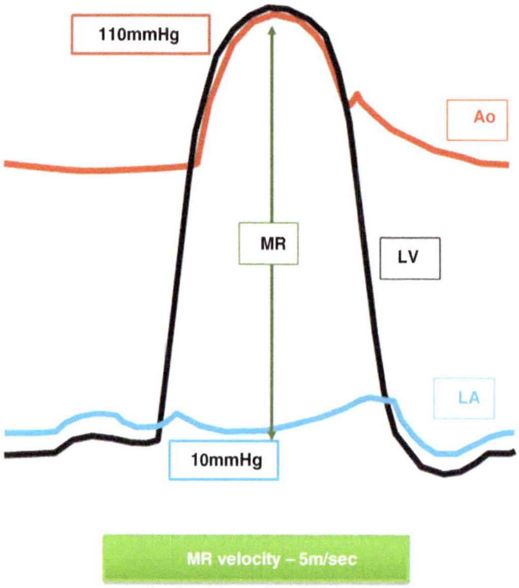

Fig. 7.10 **Typical mitral regurgitation velocity**. The typical mitral regurgitation (MR) peak velocity is in the range of 5 m/s. The driving pressure gradient for MR is the systolic gradient between left ventricle (i.e. systolic blood pressure, normally ~110mmHG) and the left atrium (normally ~10 mmHg); the "usual" systolic pressure difference between the left ventricle and left atrium is thus ~100 mmHg, corresponding to a velocity of 5 m/s. *Ao* aorta, *LA* left atrium, *LV* left ventricle, *MR* mitral regurgitation

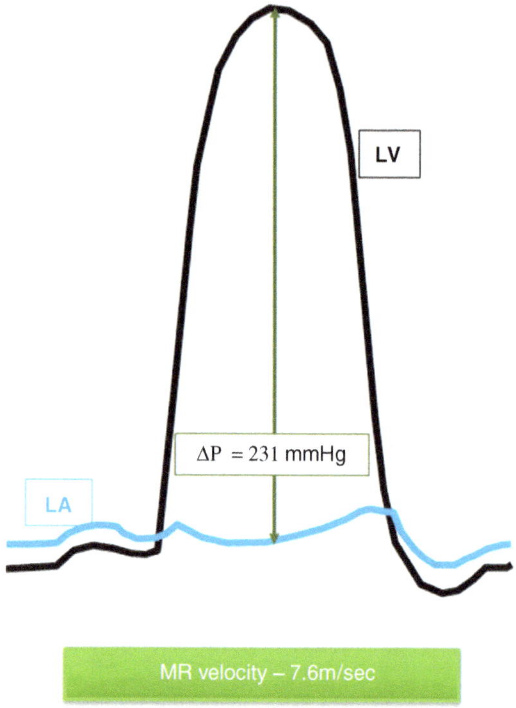

Fig. 7.11 **High MR velocity**. The measured peak mitral regurgitation velocity (7.6 m/s) implies a systolic pressure gradient between the left ventricle and left atrium of 231 mmHg. Assuming normal left atrial pressure (~10 mmHg), the peak left ventricular systolic pressure is estimated to be 241 mmHg. *LA* left atrium, *LV* left ventricle, *MR* mitral regurgitation

  - Driving pressure for MR—systolic gradient between LV and LA
  - Under normal conditions, LV systolic pressure = aortic systolic pressure (~110 mmHg)
  - Normal left atrial pressure ~ 10 mmHg
  - ΔP (LV-LA) ~100 mmHg → 4 V^2 = 100 → V = 5 m/s

- In the case shown V = 7.6 m/s → ΔP (LV-LA) = 4 × 7.6^2 = 231 mmHg (Fig. 7.11)
  - LV peak systolic pressure = ΔP (LV-LA) + LA pressure
  - Assuming normal LA pressure (10 mmHg) → LV peak systolic pressure = 241 mmHg
- LV systolic pressure may be elevated and EQUAL to aortic systolic pressure (Fig. 7.12, left panel) or may be elevated and HIGHER than aortic systolic pressure (Fig. 7.12, right panel)
  - Patient's blood pressure (left arm) at the time of the echo was 165/88 → A gradient of 241–165 = 76 mmHg exists between the LV and the aorta (Fig. 7.13).

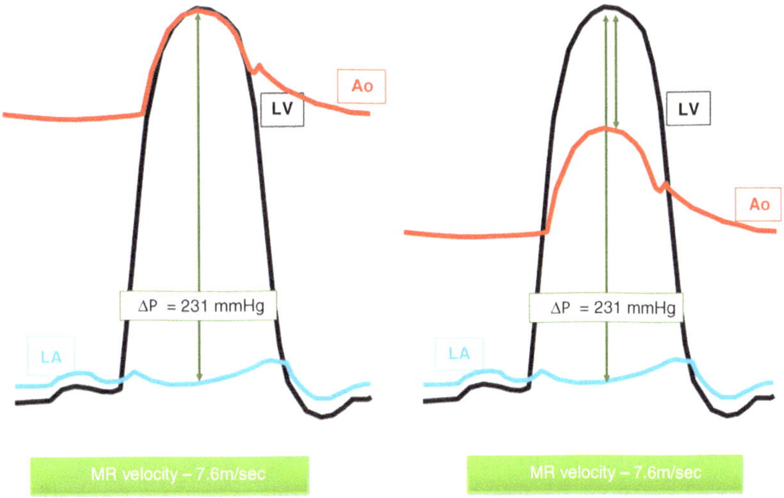

Fig. 7.12 Possible explanations for elevated left ventricular systolic pressure. Left panel—LV systolic pressure may be elevated and EQUAL to aortic systolic pressure. Right panel—Left ventricular systolic pressure elevated and HIGHER than aortic systolic pressure, meaning there is a systolic gradient between the left ventricle and the aorta

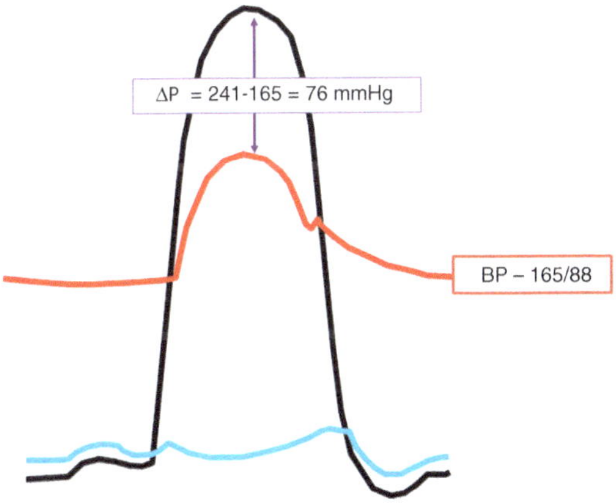

Fig. 7.13 **Calculated gradient between the left ventricle and the aorta**. Patient's blood pressure at the time of the exam was 165/88. The difference between the left ventricular systolic pressure (241 mmHg) and the aortic systolic pressure is thus 241–165 = 76 mmHg. *BP* blood pressure, Δ*P* pressure gradient

- Possible sites for gradient between LV and aorta:
  – Intra-cardiac: aortic valve, LVOT
  – Extra-cardiac: supravalvular aortic stenosis, coarctation, subclavian stenosis
- Patient did not have aortic valvular, subvalvular or supravalvular obstruction (Fig. 7.14)
- Vascular study showed significant obstruction of left subclavian artery (Fig. 7.15)

Teaching points:

- Flow velocity is determined by the pressure gradient driving the flow
- Abnormally high or low pressure gradients between intra-cardiac chambers need to be explained
- Important to use all available clinical information to help reach accurate conclusion (e.g. blood pressure at the time of the echocardiogram)

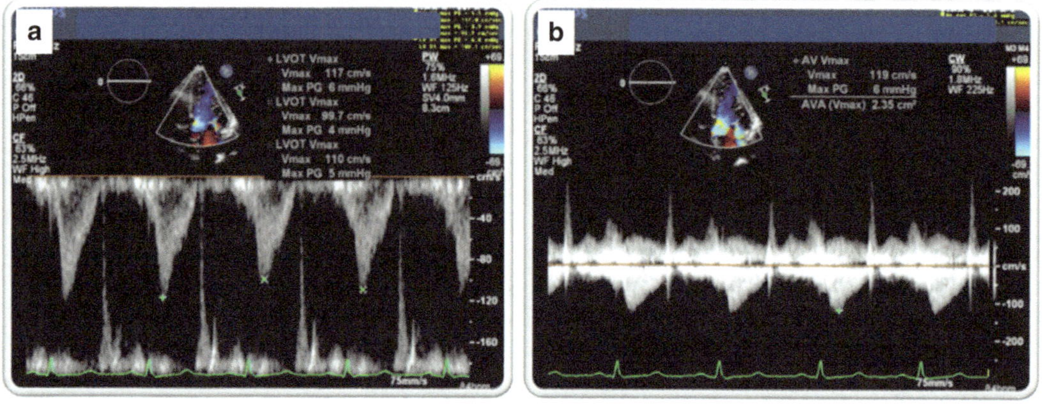

Fig. 7.14 **Spectral Doppler across LVOT and Aortic Valve**. (**a**) Pulsed wave spectral Doppler across the left ventricular outflow tract (LVOT) showing normal velocity (V_{max} = 1.1 m/s) (**b**) Continuous wave spectral Doppler across the aortic valve showing normal velocity (V_{max} = 1.2 m/s); these Doppler tracings rule out an intra-cardiac gradient between the left ventricle and the aorta

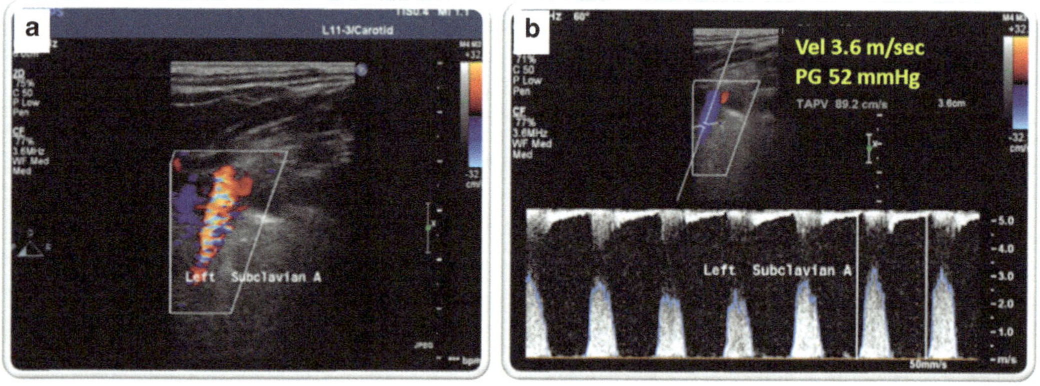

Fig. 7.15 **Left subclavian artery Doppler study**. (**a**) Color Doppler image of left subclavian artery showing turbulent flow (**b**) Spectral tracing of the subclavian artery shows elevated systolic velocity, at least 3.6 m/s, corresponding to a pressure gradient of at least 52 mmHg. Note: important to remember that a gradient between the left ventricle and the aorta can arise anywhere along the path between the left ventricle and the site of the aortic pressure measurement (i.e. may not be intra-cardiac)

Further Reading

Currie PJ, Seward JB, Chan KL, et al. Continuous wave Doppler determination of right ventricular pressure: a simultaneous Doppler-catheterization study in 127 patients. J Am Coll Cardiol. 1985;6(4):750–6. https://doi.org/10.1016/s0735-1097(85)80477-0.

Edelman SK, editor. Understanding ultrasound physics: fundamentals and exam review. second ed. Woodlands, TX: ESP; 1994.

Nagueh SF, Smiseth OA, Appleton CP, et al. Recommendations for the evaluation of left ventricular diastolic function by echocardiography: an update from the American Society of Echocardiography and the European Association of Cardiovascular Imaging. J Am Soc Echocardiogr. 2016;29(4):277–314. https://doi.org/10.1016/j.echo.2016.01.011.

Oh JK, Hatle L, Tajik AJ, Little WC. Diastolic heart failure can be diagnosed by comprehensive two-dimensional and Doppler echocardiography. J Am Coll Cardiol. 2006;47(3):500–6. https://doi.org/10.1016/j.jacc.2005.09.032.

Quiñones MA, Otto CM, Stoddard M, Waggoner A, Zoghbi WA, Doppler Quantification Task Force of the Nomenclature and Standards Committee of the American Society of Echocardiography. Recommendations for quantification of Doppler echocardiography: a report from the Doppler Quantification Task Force of the Nomenclature and Standards Committee of the American Society of Echocardiography. J Am Soc Echocardiogr. 2002;15(2):167–84. https://doi.org/10.1067/mje.2002.120202.

8 Aortic Valve

Learning Objectives

- To learn the causes, evaluation, and management of aortic stenosis
- To learn the causes, evaluation, and management of aortic insufficiency
- To learn the causes, evaluation, and management of congenital diseases of the aortic valve

General Characteristics of the Normal Aortic Valve (AV)

- The aortic valve area (AVA) is approximately 3–4 cm^2
  - Flow across AV should be laminar, without restriction or turbulence
- The AV is composed of 3 cusps (Left Coronary Cusp–LCC, Right-RCC, non–NCC) and 3 commissures (Fig. 8.1)
  - The left anterior descending (LAD) coronary artery originates from the LCC and the right coronary artery (RCA) from the RCC (unless anomalous coronaries)
  - NCC is always adjacent to the interatrial septum
  - On PSAX view at the basal level, all 3 cusps should be visualized
  - On PLAX view, most commonly the RCC and NCC are visualized
  - Nodules of Arrantius—small fibrous nodules at the center of the free margin of the cusp

    Normally a benign finding, but hypertrophy or excessive thickening of the nodules can cause aortic insufficiency

8.1 Aortic Stenosis (AS)

8.1.1 Etiology

- Calcific Degeneration
  - An active process of calcification, inflammation, and atherosclerosis
  - Mild calcification – a few areas of dense echogenic areas with little acoustic shadowing
  - Moderate/Severe – many areas of density with severe shadowing
- Congenital
  - Any congenitally abnormal valve is more prone to damage and stenosis
  - Bicuspid AV – the most common
  - Unicuspid AV
  - Quadricuspid AV – more commonly causes AI
- Rheumatic
  - Inflammatory disease of the AV that results in:

    Commissural fusion

    Thickened leaflets

    Systolic Doming
  - In patients with rheumatic MS, 90-100% will have some AV involvement (usually AI)

T. Rambhatla, G. Perk, *The Echocardiography Companion*,
https://doi.org/10.1007/978-3-030-47041-8_8

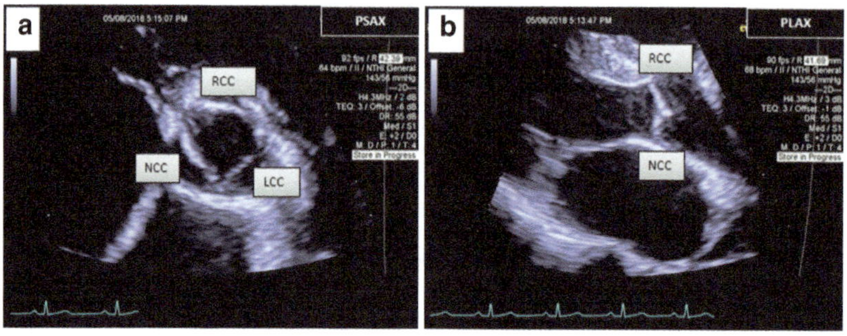

Fig. 8.1 **Normal aortic valve anatomy**. (**a**) Parasternal short axis view showing all three cusps. (**b**) Parasternal long axis view—In this view, the right coronary cusp is seen anteriorly and most commonly, the non-coronary cusp is seen next to the left atrium. Note: in some cases the left coronary cusp is visualized next to the left atrium. *LCC* left coronary cusp, *NCC* non-coronary cusp, *RCC* right coronary cusp

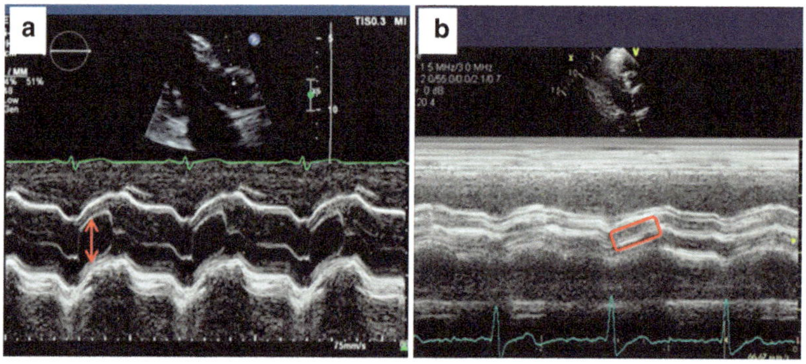

Fig. 8.2 **Aortic valve M-mode**. (**a**) Normal valve with wide systolic opening of both leaflets (red arrow). (**b**) Thickened, calcific aortic valve with minimal opening during systole, suggestive of severe aortic stenosis

- Other
  - Radiation induced – continuous fibrosis and severe calcification of the leaflets, aorto-mitral continuity, and anterior MV (posterior MV leaflet usually spared)
  - Mucopolysacharidoses/Lysosomal storage disease

8.1.2 Echocardiographic Assessment

Anatomic Assessment

1. M-Mode: provides a visual assessment of AV opening (Fig. 8.2)
2. 2D imaging: for basic anatomy (number of cusps, degree of calcification)
3. Planimetry for AVA measurement
   - AV orifice is visualized en-face from short axis view (either TTE or TEE)
     Note—SAX planimetry is only validated in senile calcific AS and not in congenital bicuspid aortic valve (likely due to doming of leaflet cusps)
   - 3D guided measurement is preferred—to ensure that the measurement is done at the leaflets tips (the narrowest part of the AV orifice) and not more proximal, where the orifice is wider

Doppler Assessment

1. Jet contour
   - Early peaking jet in mild AS vs. late peaking jet in more severe AS (Fig. 8.3)
2. Maximum Velocity(V_{max})
   - Note: Velocity may be underestimated if the angle of incidence between Doppler beam and aortic blood flow is suboptimal, however velocity can never be overestimated
     - Important to use multiple probe positions to find the position that aligns the Doppler beam as parallel as possible with the blood flow direction
   - Views to use:
     - Apical five chamber, suprasternal notch long axis view- parallel to the trachea, *right parasternal*, and subcostal.
     - Elderly patients and patients with acute angulation of aortic root frequently have V_{max} at right parasternal window
3. Peak and mean pressure gradient (mmHg)
   - The AV Peak gradient (PG) is calculated using the simplified Bernoulli equation

$$PG = 4V_{max}^2$$

     - This formula assumes that the LVOT velocity is negligible (<1.5 m/s)
   - If LVOT V_{max} > $1.5_{m/s}$ → use the modified Bernoulli equation.

$$PG = 4\left(AV\,V_{max}^2 - LVOT\,V_{max}^2\right)$$

     - High LVOT velocities can be seen in high output states (i.e. anemia, AI)
4. AVA calculation by continuity equation: (Fig. 8.4)

$$AVA = \frac{\pi LVOTr^2 \times LVOT_{VTI}}{AV_{VTI}}$$

LVOTr – radius of the LVOT $\left(\frac{measured\ LVOT\ diameter}{2}\right)$

   - This calculation is based on the continuity principle: flow (or stroke volume) proximal to a valve is equal to the flow through that valve
   - Pitfalls:
     - LVOT diameter—should be measured in PLAX in early to mid-systole; inner edge to inner edge; typically 1–2 mm proximal (more ventricular) to the annular plane (in general within 5 mm of the annular plane)
       Small errors in LVOT D measurement get squared and can lead to gross errors in AVA calculation
       Even accurate measurement can lead to errors due to the assumption that the LVOT is a circle when often it is not
     - LVOT VTI—PW sample volume should be placed 5 mm proximal to the AV
       Placing the cursor too close to the AV, within the area of flow convergence, can lead to a falsely elevated LVOT VTI and an overestimated AVA
     - AV VTI—Similar to AV V_{max}, must obtain largest VTI by measuring from different angles to ensure ultrasound beam most parallel to flow

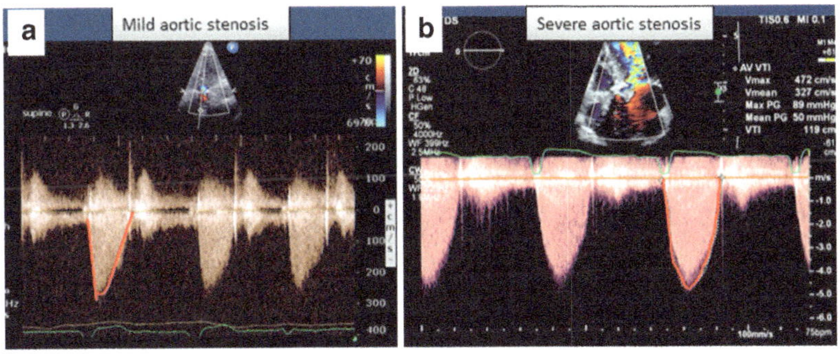

Fig. 8.3 Continuous wave Doppler in aortic stenosis. Continuous wave Doppler of the aortic valve from the apical five-chamber view. (**a**) Mild aortic stenosis, early peaking jet contour, maximum velocity 2.6 m/s. (**b**) Severe aortic stenosis, late peaking jet contour, maximum velocity 4.7 m/s

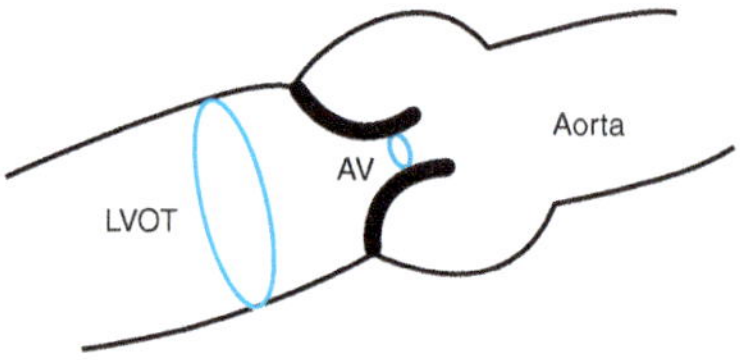

Fig. 8.4 **Continuity equation for aortic valve area calculation.** Aortic valve area calculation using the continuity equation is based on the principle that flow proximal to the valve is equal to the flow across the valve; i.e. flow across the left ventricular outflow tract = flow across the aortic valve. Cross sectional area of the LVOT is calculated based on diameter measurement on the PLAX view; LVOT VTI is measured on apical views; aortic VTI is measured where the maximum velocity is recorded. *AV* aortic valve, *AVA* aortic valve area, *LVOT* left ventricular outflow tract, *SV* stroke volume, *VTI* velocity time integral

If the largest VTI is not used AVA will be overestimated

- Modified continuity equation

$$\text{AVA} = \frac{\pi LVOTr^2 \times LVOT\ Vmax}{AV\,V\,\text{max}}$$

  - Instead of using the VTI, the Vmax can be used because the flow velocity profile is similar through the LVOT and the AV; V_{max} and VTI correlate.

5. Dimensionless Index (DI)
   - DI is also based on continuity principle

$$\text{DI} = \frac{LVOT_{VTI}}{AV_{VTI}} \text{ or } \frac{LVOT\,V_{\text{max}}}{AV\,V_{\text{max}}}$$

   - DI avoids the common errors related to LVOT diameter measurements seen with AVA
   - DI is useful in assessing Low Flow-Low Gradient (LFLG) AS

8.1.3 Diagnostic Criteria

	AVA (cm^2)	AVA indexed (cm^2/m^2)	Mean gradient (mmHg)	Velocity (m/s)	Dimensionless index
Mild	>1.5	>0.85	<20	<3	>0.5
Moderate	1–1.5	0.60–0.85	20–40	3–4	0.25–0.5
Severe	<1	<0.6	>40	>4	<0.25

Echo vs. Cath Hemodynamics (Fig. 8.5)

- Catheterization may be needed when echo evaluation remains non-diagnostic or with discrepant data
- Cath pullback provides a peak LV to peak aorta (P2P) gradient
  - Important to remember—P2P gradient is a measurement that uses two pressures that do not occur at the same time; LV pressure peaks earlier (in severe AS) than the aortic pressure
- Maximal instantaneous gradient (MIG), obtained by Doppler echo, is the highest gradient that the LV experiences
  - Calculation of P2P gradient by echo:

    Mitral regurgitation (MR) peak velocity is measured (allows calculation of systolic gradient between the left ventricle and the left atrium) → estimate of systolic ventricular pressure

    Systolic blood pressure (SBP) is the systolic aortic pressure

    $P2P = 4 \times (MR_{peak\ V})^2 - SBP$
  - MIG can predict P2P (rough estimate, not for accurate assessment)

    $P2P \cong 70\% \times MIG$

    Mean gradient $\cong 60\% \times MIG$
  - The MIG is always greater than P2P gradient but can overestimate gradients (in high CO states or due to the pressure recovery phenomenon)
- Cath calculation of AVA via Hakki (and Gorlin) equation

$$\text{AVA}\left(\text{cm}^2\right) = \frac{Cardiac\ Output\left({}^{lit}\!/_{\text{min}}\right)}{\sqrt{p2pgradient}}$$

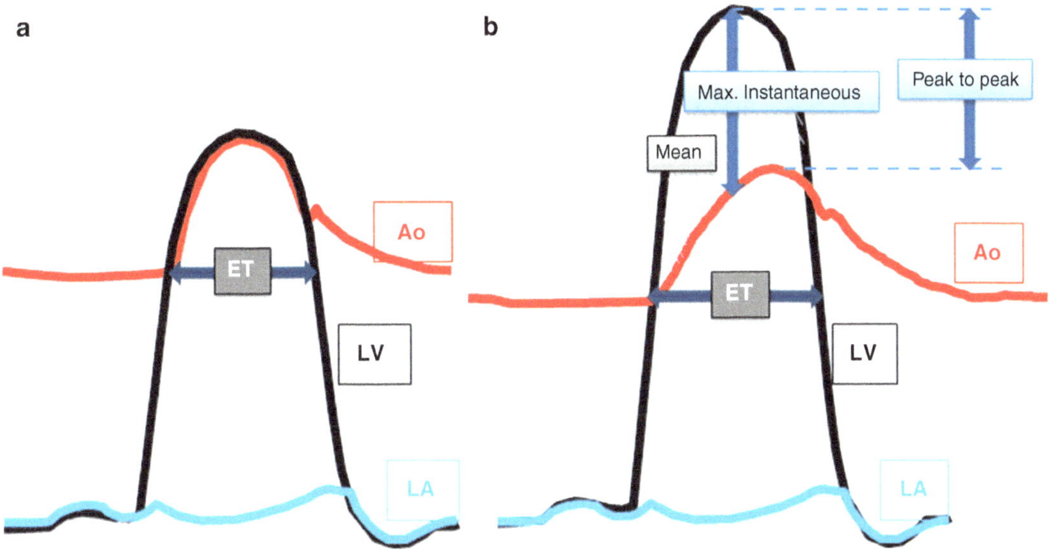

Fig. 8.5 **Comparing peak-to-peak and maximal instantaneous gradient**. Pressure curves of (**a**) normal physiology and (**b**) severe aortic stenosis. In aortic stenosis, there is a systolic gradient between the LV pressure and the aortic pressure. Important to note the difference between the Doppler derived maximal instantaneous gradient (measured on the continuous wave Doppler spectral tracing) and pullback derived peak-to-peak gradient. The maximal instantaneous gradient is higher than peak-to-peak gradient

Evaluation of Serial Stenoses

- Subvalvular, supravalvular, or valvular stenosis can all cause high velocity measurements by CW Doppler
- Patients can have more than one of these through the LV-LVOT-AV tract
  Note: High velocity by CW across LVOT/AV does not always mean aortic stenosis
- TEE may be necessary if serial stenoses are suspected, if it is unclear where the stenosis is, or for accurate planimetry of the AV

8.1.4 Discordance Between Calculated AVA and Measured Pressure Gradients (Fig. 8.6)

Severe gradients and AVA ≥1 cm^2 or low gradients and AVA <1 cm^2

1. Errors in measurement, Doppler placement, or calculations—which can result in an incorrectly small AVA or underestimation of gradients
2. Psuedo-Severe AS
   - Moderate AS with decreased EF and reduced stroke volume → weakened left ventricle incapable of opening a moderately stenotic AV → limiting AVA to <1cm^2; in this case, at normal flow conditions the AVA is >1 cm^2
3. Low flow-low gradient (LFLG) severe AS
   - True severe AS with systolic dysfunction and decreased EF causing low flow across the AV. The low flow state does not allow for generating high gradients across the valve; in this case, even at normal flow conditions the AVA is <1 cm^2
   - The cardiomyopathy can have contractile reserve (CR) meaning stroke volume can increase by ≥20% in response to an inotrope, or no CR
     - Patients without CR are at high risk for surgery (22% higher mortality in postoperative period than patients with CR) however in the long run, they benefit from surgery (65% 5-year survival with surgery vs. 11% survival without surgery)
     - Operative risk with TAVR is much less; ~4.3% mortality

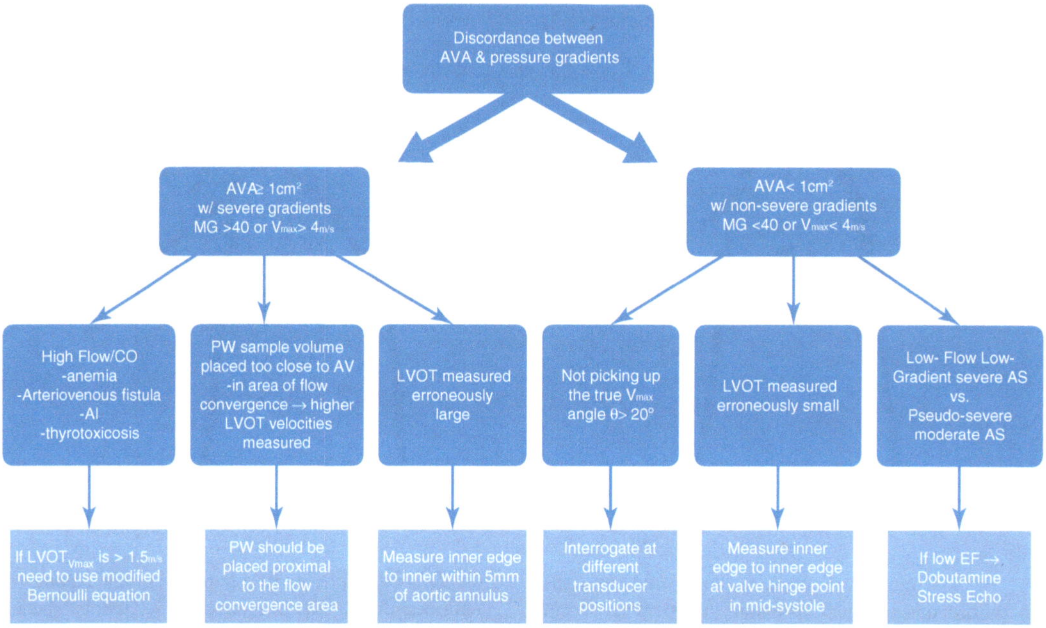

Fig. 8.6 **Algorithm for evaluation of discordant valve area and gradients**. *AS* aortic stenosis, *AI* aortic insufficiency, *AVA* aortic valve area, *CO* cardiac output, *EF* ejection fraction, *LVOT* left ventricular outflow tract, *MG* mean gradient, *PW* pulse wave Doppler, *SV* stroke volume

4. Paradoxical LFLG severe AS
   - True severe AS with normal EF but low flow (stroke volume index [SVi] < 35 cc/m^2) despite preserved EF, producing low gradients; must be due to conditions other than elevated BP and SBP must be <140 mmHg.
     - Can be seen in LVH with small cavity size, high afterload states, or low forward flow e.g. severe MR or TR
     - Occurs in up to 35% of severe AS patients
- Patients with paradoxical LFLG severe AS have better outcomes with surgery than with medical therapy alone

Differentiating among the 3 truly discordant scenarios

- Correlate with physical exam
  - Findings suggestive of milder forms of AS
    Early peaking murmur
    Loud A2
    Strong and early peripheral pulses
    If these findings are present and AVA calculation is severe → suspect overestimation of AS severity by echo (valve area calculated erroneously small)
- Dobutamine Stress Echo (DSE)—used to distinguish pseudo-severe AS from true severe LFLG AS as well as determine presence of CR (Fig. 8.7)
  - Important to verify coronary anatomy before DSE; known left main disease is a contraindication to DSE
  - Parameters to obtain: CR, AVA, mean PG, DI
- CT AV calcium score (AoV Ca)
  - Threshold value of 1651 Agatson units—82% sensitivity and 88% specificity for detecting severe AS, in patients with normal or reduced EF (≤40%)
  - Gender specific threshold—1200au for women and 2000au for men—independently associated with mortality

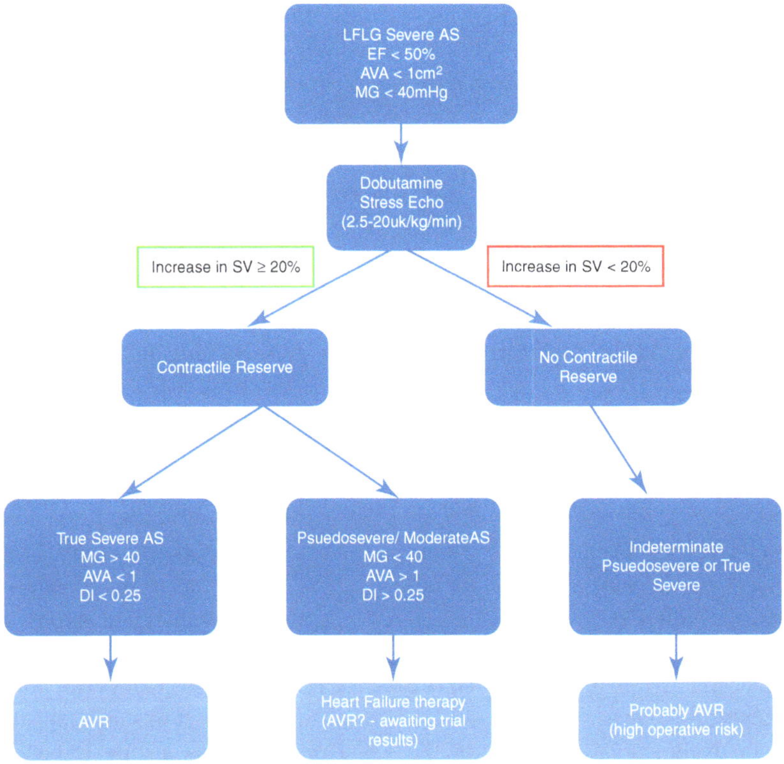

Fig. 8.7 **Dobutamine stress echo for aortic stenosis**. *AS* aortic stenosis, *AVA* aortic valve area, *DI* dimensionless index, *EF* ejection fraction, *LFLG* low flow low gradient, *MG* mean gradient, *SV* stroke volume

- Z_{va} index (valvuloarterial impedance)
  - Marker of global hemodynamic load on the LV
  - Measured by the ratio of total afterload on the LV (valvular and arterial) divided by stroke volume index

$$Z_{va}\frac{LVSP}{SVi}=\frac{SBP+MG}{Svi}$$

    LVSP—LV systolic pressure, SBP—systolic blood pressure, MG—mean gradient, SVi—stoke volume index
  - Z_{va} > 3.5—correlates with reduced maximum exercise capacity and increased mortality
- AVA_{proj}—projected aortic valve area
  - Estimation of "potential" aortic valve area in normal flow state; occasionally, even with Dobutamine stress echo, despite increase in stroke volume, normal flow is not reached
  - $AVA_{proj} = AVA_{rest} + VC \times (250\text{-}Q_{rest})$
    250—standard flow rate (250 mL/s), Q_{rest}—flow rate across the valve at rest (calculated from stroke volume and ejection time), VC—valve compliance (slope of the rise of the AVA in response to increased flow during a DSE
  - $AVA_{proj} \leq 1.0$ cm² or indexed $AVA_{proj} \leq 0.55$ cm² = Severe AS
    83–91% accurate for differentiating true severe AS from pseudo-severe AS

8.1.5 Compensatory Mechanisms-Adverse Consequences on the Heart

- Left ventricular concentric hypertrophy and pressure overload
  - LVH is a compensatory mechanism to help generate pressures that can overcome the increased afterload on the LV. Increased wall thickness leads to a decrease in wall tension (or afterload) on the heart muscle based on LaPlace's Law

    $$\text{Laplace law}: \\ \text{Wall Tension}(\text{afterload}) = \frac{Pressure \times Radius}{Wall\ thickness}$$

  - Degree of LVH has been shown to be an independent predictor of all-cause mortality in patients with AS
- Supply-demand mismatch ischemia
  - LV wall becomes too thick for adequate blood supply
  - → diastolic dysfunction/decreased systolic function can ultimately lead to wall thinning and LV dilation (end stage)
  - → arrhythmias
- Aortic Aneurysm—post-stenotic dilation of ascending aorta due to turbulent flow
  Note: Different mechanism than when seen with bicuspid aortic valve

8.1.6 Surveillance and Follow-up

- Patients can be asymptomatic with severe AS but once symptoms develop—high mortality rate without intervention. Symptoms and associated average survival are:
  - Angina—5 years
  - Syncope—3 years
  - CHF—1–2 years
- Asymptomatic patients
  - Mild AS: TTE every 3–5 years
  - Moderate AS: TTE every 1–2 years
  - Severe AS: TTE every 6–12 months
    50–66% develop symptoms within 2–5 years
  - Exercise stress test may be used for further evaluation of asymptomatic patients in order to:
    Confirm lack of symptoms
    Assess vital signs in response to exercise
    Assess for ability to augment EF with exercise
    Assess for a significant increase in gradients
  - Optimal timing of surgery in asymptomatic patients with severe AS is controversial
    If the patient is truly asymptomatic → TTE every 6–12 months—surveillance for surgical indications like development of LV dilation/dysfunction
- TTE indicated at any AS grade—with any change in symptoms/clinical status
- Exercise stress testing is contraindicated in symptomatic patients.

8.1.7 Management

Medical Treatment

- No medical therapy has been shown to halt AS progression or decrease mortality
  - Statins, antihypertensive drugs, and drugs targeting calcium metabolism have been tested but failed to show benefit

Surgical AV Replacement (SAVR)

- Indications:
  - Moderate AS—when another cardiac surgery needs to be performed
    Note: this indication may change in the future when TAVR procedures gain broader indications

- Asymptomatic severe AS and
  - EF < 50%
  - Another cardiac surgery needs to be performed
  - SAVR considered if very severe AS
    - V_{max} > 4.5 m/s or mean gradient > 50 mmHg + low surgical risk
    - (in these cases—rate of symptoms onset is 50% at 2 years; lower mortality rate observed with early surgery)
  - Exercise stress test showing decreased exercise tolerance or fall in SBP
- Any symptomatic patients with severe AS, regardless of LV size and function

Transcatheter AV Replacement (TAVR)

- TAVR has gained increasing acceptance as a treatment option for patients with severe aortic stenosis
- Several percutaneous valves have been developed; the two most commonly used types of TAVR valves are shown in Fig. 8.8
- Currently TAVR is indicated or considered for:
  - Severe symptomatic AS with prohibitive surgical risk

    Note: patients MUST have expected survival of >12 months and quality of life expected to improve
  - Severe symptomatic AS, high surgical risk, AND transfemoral approach feasible
  - Severe symptomatic AS, intermediate surgical risk, transfemoral approach feasible and no high risk features
  - Severe symptomatic AS, low surgical risk, transfemoral approach feasible, trileaflet aortic valve, age > 65 and no high risk features
- Proper patient selection is crucial for the success of the procedure
- Absolut contra-indications to TAVR include:
  - Patient too sick
  - Anatomic issues:
    - Native aortic annulus size too small or too big for current available valves
    - Coronary height inadequate → high risk of coronary obstruction
  - Active endocarditis
  - Concomitant other valve disease treatable only by surgery

Valve	Sapien	Medtronic Evolut
	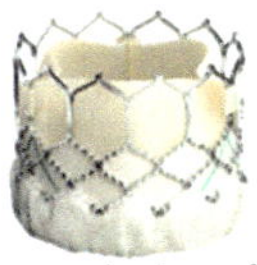 Reproduced with permission of Edwards Lifesciences LLC, Irvine, CA.	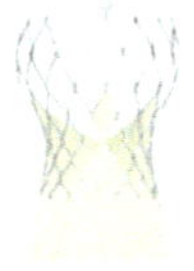 Reproduced with permission of Medtronic, Inc
Approach	Transfemoral preferred Alternate approaches can be used	Transfemoral preferred Alternate approaches can be used
Implant technique	Balloon Expandable Rapid pacing required	Self Expandable Often no rapid pacing needed Before full deployment, valve can be recaptured and repositioned

Fig. 8.8 **Comparing the currently available transcatheter aortic valves**

- Relative contra-indications to TAVR include:
  - Recent MI/significant untreated CAD (especially if requires CABG)
  - Recent hemodynamic/respiratory instability
  - Hypertrophic cardiomyopathy ± LVOT obstruction; risk of post-procedure severe LVOT obstruction
  - Severe pulmonary HTN/RV dysfunction
  - Contraindication to anticoagulation
  - Increased risk of annular rupture
  - Access site considerations/peripheral vascular disease

Balloon Aortic Valvuloplasty (BAV)

- There are no data to suggest improved longevity with BAV; some patients report improvement in symptoms
- Only considered as:
  - Bridge to surgery in hemodynamically unstable patient
  - Possible temporary role in managing severely symptomatic patients who are not candidates for immediate SAVR or TAVR (i.e. patients in refractory cardiogenic shock as a bridge to AVR)
  - Palliation in patients with prohibitive risk for TAVR or SAVR

8.1.8 Differential Diagnosis for Increased Gradients Across LVOT/AV Not Due to the AV

(1) Supravalvular stenosis
- Narrowing starting at sinotubular junction, just above sinus of Valsalva
  - 71% are seen in Williams-Beuren syndrome
    - Deletion mutation in chromosome 7, elastin gene mutation.
    - Characteristics: elfin facies, outgoing personality, mild to moderate intellectual disability, connective tissue abnormalities
    - Cardiac manifestations: 50% supravalvular stenosis, 30% peripheral pulmonary artery stenosis, 20% have both, 50% have bicuspid aortic valve
- Echo findings:
  - CW through AV—mid systolic peaking, parabolic shaped jet (appears like AS jet)
  - Additional findings:
    - Can create preferential high velocity jet into right innominate artery (due to Coanda effect) → higher BP in right arm then left arm.

(2) Dynamic subvalvular left ventricular outflow tract obstruction
- Due to systolic anterior motion (SAM) of the mitral valve
  - Classically—in hypertrophic cardiomyopathy with asymmetric septal hypertrophy
  - Can also be see in:
    - Hypercontractile LV
    - Hypertensive heart disease
    - Apical/mid LV infarct
    - Takotsubo Cardiomyopathy
    - Reduced LV chamber size
    - Post mitral valve repair
- Echo findings
  - M mode of AV –mid-systolic closure
  - 2D—anterior leaflet of mitral valve moves into the LVOT during systole
  - CW through AV- late peaking jet contour (Fig. 8.9)

(3) Fixed subvalvular obstruction—subaortic membrane
- Account for 8–20% of LVOT obstructions (more common than supravalvular membrane)
- Etiology:
  - Isolated fibrous membrane—90%
    - Membranous or muscular circumferential growth in the LVOT
    - Can adhere to AV, MV or both
    - Associated with: PDA, PV stenosis, aortic coarctation, VSD
  - Tunnel like muscular narrowing of LVOT—10%
  - Annular aortic hypoplasia or post-VSD repair—1-3%

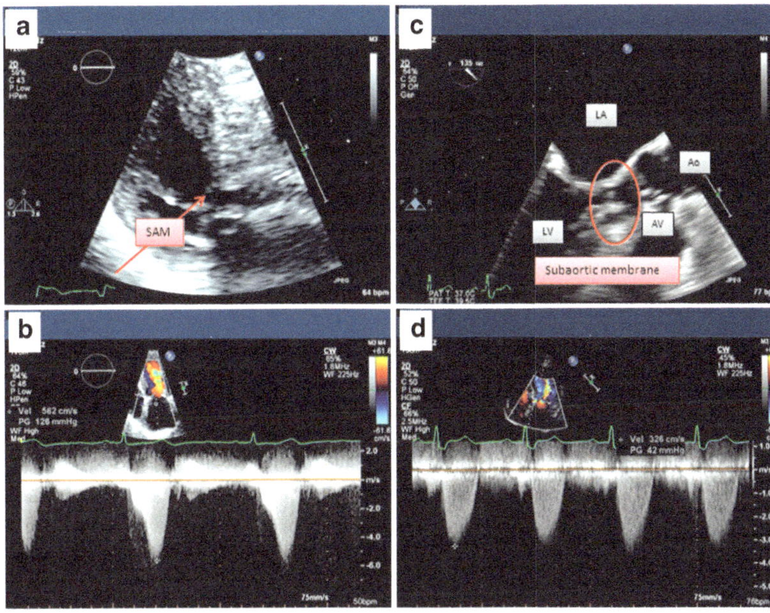

Fig. 8.9 **Dynamic vs. fixed LVOT obstruction.** (**a**) Systolic frame from parasternal long axis view showing systolic anterior motion of the mitral valve; the anterior mitral valve leaflet reaches the interventricular septum, creating obstruction to flow. (**b**) Spectral Doppler showing the pressure at the LVOT; obstruction develops during systole causing the gradient to peak late, creating a dagger shaped jet. (**c**) Sub-aortic membrane causing fixed LVOT obstruction. (**d**) Spectral Doppler tracing; the obstruction is present from onset of systole causing mid-systolic peaking, parabolic shaped jet (similar to aortic stenosis). *Ao* aorta, *AV* aortic valve, *LA* left atrium, *LV* left ventricle, *SAM* systolic anterior motion

- Echo findings:
  - Turbulent flow is seen below AV plane suggesting subvalvular stenosis
  - Mid systolic peaking, parabolic shaped jet which appears like AS jet (Fig. 8.9)
  - Patients often develop aortic insufficiency; progressive AV damage and scarring develops due to turbulent flow proximal to the valve
- Indications/considerations for surgical intervention:
  - Peak gradient >50 mmHg, mean > 30 mmHg
    Note: intervention indicated at lower gradients with progressive AI and LV dysfunction (LVESD ≥ 50 mm or EF < 55%)
  - Peak/mean gradient less <50/30 mmHg and ≥ 1 of the following:
    Female who wants to become pregnant
    LVH present
    Plans for strenuous competitive sports
  - Moderate AI
    Note: mild obstruction with mild AI—class III indication for intervention
- The surgical technique requires access through AV to cut out the membrane
  - If even mild AS is present—the AV should be excised to allow complete removal of the membrane (making AVR necessary)
- Follow-up surveillance is required because recurrence can occur after resection

(4) In addition to echocardiographic evaluation, physical examination can help differentiate a fixed obstruction from a dynamic LVOT

Murmur maneuver	Aortic stenosis	Supra/ subvalvular fixed stenosis	Dynamic LVOT obstruction
Decrease preload (Valsalva)	↓	↓	↑
Increase afterload (handgrip/ phenylephrine)	↓	↓	↓↓
Post PVC (increase inotropy)	↑	↑	↑↑↑

8.2 Aortic Insufficiency (AI)

8.2.1 Etiology

AI can be caused by:

- Aortic root pathology
- Primary valve pathology
- Secondary valve pathology

Aortic root pathology (57%)	Primary valve pathology (43%)	Secondary valve pathology (<1%)
HTN (most common cause) Aneurysm Dissection (10%) Marfan's disease (6%) Takayasu arteritis Loeys-Dietz syndrome Aortitis SOV aneurysm	Idiopathic (34%) Rheumatic fever Bicuspid AV Quadricuspid AV Infective endocarditis Cusp prolapse (RCC most common) Ankylosing spondylitis Other autoimmune disease/arteritis Anorectic drugs (fenfluramine-phentermine)	Subavalvular membrane Outlet VSD

8.2.2 Echocardiographic Assessment (Fig. 8.10)

Anatomic Assessment:

1. M mode
   - Aortic valve:
     - Premature opening—due to higher LVEDP resulting in earlier elevation of ventricular pressure above aortic pressure
   - Mitral Valve:
     - Fluttering of anterior leaflet due to regurgitant jet directed towards MV (not correlated with severity of AI)
     - Concave shape of anterior MV leaflet
       MV unable to open fully because of regurgitant jet (correlates with "Austin-flint" murmur of functional MS)
     - Early closure of MV (seen in acute severe AI)
2. Color M-mode
   - Assess AI duration in diastole
     Presence of diastolic MR (seen in severe AI)—sign of LVEDP higher than LA pressure
3. Baseline anatomy of aortic valve—presence of valve prolapse, calcifications, vegetations.

Color and Spectral Doppler Assessment:

1. AI jet width to LVOT height ratio—best on PLAX view
2. AI jet vena contracta—best on PLAX view
3. AI Jet area: LVOT area ratio—best on PSAX view. Apical five chamber view may overestimate jet area because AI jet seen after it has already widened
4. Effective regurgitant orifice area (EROA) of AI jet
   - Calculated EROA based on continuity equation and proximal isovelocity surface area (PISA) method:
   - Flow at the outer shell of PISA is equal to flow at the regurgitant orifice (EROA)

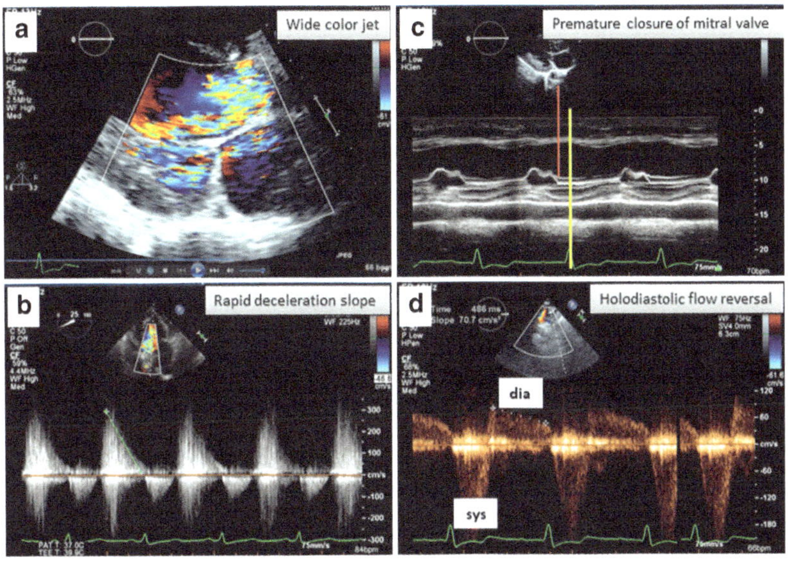

Fig. 8.10 **Severe aortic regurgitation**. (**a**) Parasternal long axis view color image showing wide color jet of AR occupying more than 65% of the left ventricular outflow tract (**b**) Continuous wave tracing of the AR jet showing rapid deceleration, due to rapid decay of pressure difference between the aorta and the left ventricle. (**c**) In acute severe AR, the LV diastolic pressure increases so rapidly that the mitral valve closes prematurely; the yellow straight line shows the timing of the QRS, the mitral valve closure point (red line) occurs significantly earlier. (**d**) Holodiastolic flow reversal in the descending aorta indicates at least moderate aortic insufficiency. *Sys* normal forward systolic flow, *dia* diastolic flow

- $2\pi r^2 \times$ Aliasing Velocity = EROA × peak AI velocity,
  r – PISA shell radius

$$\text{EROA} = \frac{2\pi r^2 \times \textit{Aliasing Velocity}}{\textit{Peak AI velocity.}}$$

  Note: peak AI velocity is influenced by the trans-aortic driving pressure; the higher the aortic pressure or lower the LVEDP → higher peak AI velocity

5. Regurgitation volume (RV)/fraction (RF) with CW Doppler
   - RV = EROA × AI VTI
     Proportional to EROA + driving pressure and driving time; influenced heavily by HR and diastolic blood pressure (DBP)
   - RV can also by calculated by comparing flow across two different valves (assuming only AI present, no MR)
     $\text{LVOT}_{\text{SV}} = \text{Effective SV} + \text{RV}$
     $\text{LVOT}_{\text{SV}} = \text{LVOT}_{\text{area}} \times \text{LVOT}_{\text{VTI}}$
     $\text{Effective}_{\text{SV}}$ = inflow volume across the mitral valve
     $\text{Effective SV} = \text{MV}_{\text{annulus area}} \times \text{MV}_{\text{VTI at annular level}}$
     $\text{RV} = (\text{LVOT}_{\text{area}} \times \text{LVOT}_{\text{VTI}}) - (\text{MV}_{\text{annulus area}} \times \text{MV}_{\text{VTI at annulus}})$

$$\text{Regurgitant fraction} = \frac{RV}{\text{LVOT}_{\text{SV}}}$$

6. Deceleration time (DT) and pressure half time (PHT) by CW Doppler
   - Time of AI jet deceleration correlates with the gradient between diastolic aortic pressure (DBP) and LVEDP.
   - In principle, as AI severity increases, DBP decreases faster and LVEDP increases faster → Ao to LV gradient dissipates faster → shorter DT and PHT
   - Both parameters are highly affected by compliance of the LV and the LV filling pressures, which limit accuracy in predicting AI severity
     – In chronic AI, LV compliance can initially increase → smaller increase in LVEDP.
     – Eventually compliance decreases and LVEDP increases → shorter DT and PHT even if the severity of AI has remained the same

Table 8.1 Echocardiographic criteria for aortic insufficiency severity

	Mild	Moderate	Severe[a]
Jet width (relative to LVOT)	<25%	25–65%	≥65%
Jet area (in LVOT)	<5%	5–59%	≥60%
Vena contracta	<3 mm	3–6 mm	>6 mm
Regurgitant volume	<30 cc	30–59 cc	≥60 cc
Regurgitant fraction	<30%	30–49%	≥50%
EROA	<0.1cm^2	0.1–0.29 cm^2	≥0.3 cm^2
Abdominal Ao flow reversal	Brief	Intermediate	Holodiastolic
PHT[b]	>500 ms	250–500 ms	<250 ms
DT[b]	>1800 ms	800–1800 ms	<800 ms
Slope[b]	<250 cm/s^2	250–400 cm/s^2	>400 cm/s^2

Ao aorta, *DT* deceleration time, *ERO* effective regurgitation orifice area, *PHT* pressure half time
[a]Severe AI also requires evidence of LV dilation
[b]These parameters are no longer in the guidelines; however, they are still often used as supportive data

    - Compliant LV and low LVEDP → long DT → possible underestimation of AI severity
    - Noncompliant LV and high LVEDP → short DT → possible overestimation of AI severity
  - These parameters are more accurate in acute AI than in chronic AI
7. Flow reversal in aorta by pulsed wave (PW) Doppler
  - Holodiastolic flow reversal in abdominal aorta—very specific for severe AI
  - Holodiastolic flow reversal in the descending aorta indicates ≥ moderate AI
  - Diastolic flow reversal velocity > 20 cm/s—consistent with severe AI

8.2.3 Diagnostic Criteria (Table 8.1)

Acute vs. Chronic Severe AI

- Chronic AI allows enough time for compensatory changes of the LV:
  - Increased compliance of LV ($C = \Delta V/\Delta P$)
    Increases in LV volume result in smaller increases in LV pressure thus mitigating increased diastolic pressures of the LV
  - LV dilation
    Allows acceptance of increased blood volume and produces increased SV → adequate forward flow and perfusion to the periphery initially maintained
- Acute AI → sudden increase in LV volume on an unprepared LV that has not had time to develop compensatory mechanism
  - → dramatic rise in LVEDP—can almost equal aortic DBP
  - Echocardiographic features seen in acute severe AI (may be seen in some cases of chronic severe AI, however, only if there is a significantly elevated LVEDP)
    Short deceleration time
    Premature MV closure (MV normally closes 40 ms after onset of QRS)
    Diastolic MR; seen with premature closure of the MV; the diastolic MR has low velocity (typically <2 m/s)

8.2.4 Compensatory Mechanisms-Adverse Consequences on the Heart

Tachycardia	Faster HR → Shorter diastole → less time for regurgitation of blood back into LV Note: AI can present with paradoxical angina (chest pain worse with bradycardia); prolonged diastole → longer AI time → lower end diastolic coronary perfusion pressure
Lower DBP & Premature opening of AV	Aortic regurgitation → lower aortic DBP → LV pressure rises above aortic pressure earlier → AV opens earlier → longer systole → longer ejection time
Premature closure of Mitral valve	Rapid increase in LV diastolic pressure → mitral valve closes early (sign of hemodynamically significant AI)

Eccentric hypertrophy/LV dilation	Volume overload → eccentric LV dilation which permits the LV to accommodate more volume with less dramatic increase in pressure (compliance increased)
Atrial fibrillation	A fib is often tolerated better in AI than in AS—shorter diastole and loss of the a-kick has less of a negative hemodynamic effect

8.2.5 Surveillance and Follow-up

Asymptomatic Patients:
- Mild—TTE every 3–5 years
- Moderate—TTE every 1–2 years
- Severe AI—TTE every 6–12 months

TTE is performed to assess for left ventricular dimensions and function.

8.2.6 Management

Medical Treatment
- Treatment of HTN (SBP > 140 mmHg) with calcium channel blockers, ACE inhibitors, or AR blockers
- Treatment with ACEI/ARBs or BBs for severe AI with symptoms or LV dysfunction in patients not eligible for surgery
- Vasodialators—have not been shown to alter the natural history of asymptomatic chronic severe AI—not routinely recommended for patients with normal LV function
  - They do improve hemodynamics and forward cardiac output and can be helpful in decreasing symptoms in patients at high risk for surgery.

Surgical Aortic Valve Replacement

(1) Indications:
- Moderate AI undergoing other Cardiac Surgery
- Asymptomatic severe AI
  - EF < 50%
  - If other cardiac surgery is required
  - EF > 50% and either
    LV dilatation with ESd > 50 mm
    LV dilatation with EDd > 65 mm + low surgical risk
- Symptomatic patients with severe AI, regardless of LV size and function

(2) TAVR has not had good outcomes for pure native AI without concomitant AS—a calcified stenotic valve is needed for the TAVR valve to stay in place. However, newer generations of TAVR valves have been tested and are showing better results.

8.3 Congenital Variants

8.3.1 Bicuspid AV

General Characteristics

- Occurs in 1–2% of general population
- Can be familial (20–30% of other family members will also have a bicuspid aortic valve)
  Note: class I recommendation for screening first degree family members.
- Different forms based on which 2 of the 3 cusps are fused together
- A visible fibrous ridge at the fusion line of the 2 fused cusps is called a raphe
- Two anatomical forms:
  - Asymmetric cusps—with a raphe (95%)
    LCC-RCC—70–85%
    RCC-NCC—15–30%
    LCC-NCC—<5%
  - Symmetric cusps—without a raphe (5%)
    Equal sized LCC and RCC

Echocardiographic Assessment

- M-mode—eccentric closure line of AV
- 2D imaging—the number of commissures and cusps should be assessed during systole (Fig. 8.11a)
  (In diastole a raphe may falsely appear to separate the cusps while the valve is closed)
- TEE more sensitive than TTE for diagnosis of bicuspid aortic valve (TEE sensitivity 92%, specificity 96%)

Clinical Manifestations

- Early onset aortic stenosis (AS) and/or aortic insufficiency (AI)
  - Aortic stenosis:
    - Most common complication
    - Most commonly presents in adulthood (from premature calcification of aortic valve)
    - Gradually progressive disease
    - Only 15% of adults 50 years of age have a normally functioning valve
  - Aortic insufficiency
    - Less common as compared to AS
    - Generally, occurs in younger patients as compared to AS
- Increased risk for infective endocarditis (IE)
- Associated anomalies

Aortic enlargement	• 50% develop aortic disease, 20% develop aortic aneurysm • Aneurysm most common in aortic root and tubular ascending aorta • Aortic disease is due to co-existing genetic abnormalities of the connective tissue
Coarctation of aorta	• 5–10% of patient with bicuspid aortic valve have coarctation • 50% of patients with coarctation have bicuspid aortic valve • Patients with a coarctation—10% have intracranial berry aneurysms
Turner syndrome	• 8% have aortic coarctation • 10–20% have bicuspid aortic valve • High risk of aortic dissection
Shone complex	• Subaortic stenosis, aortic coarctation, supravalvular mitral valve ring, parachute mitral valve, and bicuspid aortic valve

Surveillance and Follow-up

- For aortic valve—TTE according to AS/AI surveillance recommendations
- For aorta—Serial aortic imaging required, regardless of severity of aortic valve disease
  - For aortic root <4 cm—TTE every 2 years
  - For aortic root >4.5 cm—yearly imaging (echo, CMR, or CT)

Management

Medical Treatment

- Prevention of progression of aortic aneurysm—blood pressure control, beta blockers

Aortic Valve Replacement (SAVR)

- Bicuspid aortic valve stenosis is responsible for >50% of AV replacement (AVR) in Europe & US in patients ≤50 years old
- Indications:
  - Severe AI or severe AS—similar indications as in tricuspid AV
  - Note—if other indication for open heart surgery, AVR recommended/considered for:
    - Moderate bicuspid AS
    - Mild bicuspid AS, if the valve is calcified

Other Options

- AV repair
  - Tricuspid AV repair is not generally done because of suboptimal results; AV repair of bicuspid aortic valve has shown promising results; largely dependent on cusp anatomy
- Bicuspid AV and TAVR
  - Bicuspid AV patients have generally been excluded from TAVR trials; when attempted, lower device success rates noted likely due to larger annulus sizes, asymmetric leaflet or raphe calcification that could increase PVL, concomitant aortopathy, and the younger age of patients.
  - Recently MDCT has been used for classification of bicuspid valves according to the calcification distribution, allowing for identification of patients that may have more favorable outcomes with TAVR

Aortic Root Surgery

- 20% of patients requiring AVR for bicuspid aortic valve disease require concomitant aortic surgery
- Indications for root repair:
  - Asymptomatic—when aortic root >5.5 cm
  - Risk factors for dissection—when aortic root >5.0 cm (e.g. family history or rate of increase in root diameter > 0.5 cm/yr.)
  - If AVR needed for AS or AI—when aortic root >4.5 cm

- Valve sparing aortic root repair
  - Suitable for younger patients, minimal calcification, up to mild AI, near normal leaflets

8.3.2 Quadricuspid AV

General Characteristics

- Rare; 0.013–0.043% of the population

Echocardiographic Assessment:
(Fig. 8.11b)

Most common form—three large equally sized cusps and one small cusp

Clinical Manifestations

- 40% develop AI, generally does not cause AS
- 10% of patients have associated anomalous coronary anatomy
- Generally not associated with other congenital heart disease

Surveillance and Follow-up

- Same recommendations as for AI with tricuspid aortic valve

Treatment

- Same recommendations as for AI with tricuspid aortic valve

8.3.3 Unicuspid AV

General Characteristics

- Rare; 0.02% of the population
- 2 forms of unicuspid AV:
  - Unicomissural/eccentric (more common)
  - Acommisural/central

Echocardiographic Assessment
Number of commissures should be assessed when valve is open, during systole

Clinical Manifestations

- Early onset aortic stenosis (can present in children)
- Minimal calcification is needed to develop AS (unlike the senile calcific form of AS)
- Aorta dilatation (see bicuspid AV aboves)

Surveillance and Follow-up

- Same as for bicuspid aortic valve

Treatment

- When seen in children, BAV may be considered if aortic stenosis is severe, as an alternative to surgery
- In adults, surgical AVR is required when valve disease is severe

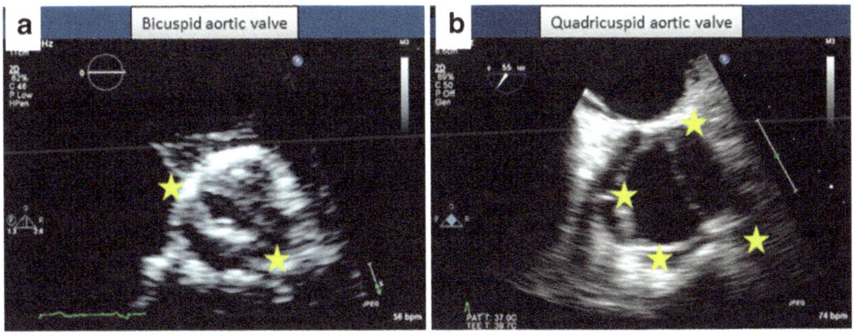

Fig. 8.11 **Congenitally abnormal aortic valve.** Systolic frames from parasternal short axis and TEE of (**a**) Bicuspid aortic valve, (**b**) Quadricuspid aortic valve. Note: evaluation should be carried out during systole and the number of commissures (yellow asterisk) should be evaluated to determine the anatomy of the valve

Further Reading

Blais C, Burwash IG, Mundigler G, et al. Projected valve area at normal flow rate improves the assessment of stenosis severity in patients with low-flow, low-gradient aortic stenosis: the multicenter TOPAS (Truly or Pseudo-Severe Aortic Stenosis) study. Circulation. 2006;113(5):711–21. https://doi.org/10.1161/CIRCULATIONAHA.105.557678.

Briand M, Dumesnil JG, Kadem L, et al. Reduced systemic arterial compliance impacts significantly on left ventricular afterload and function in aortic stenosis: implications for diagnosis and treatment. J Am Coll Cardiol. 2005;46(2):291–8. https://doi.org/10.1016/j.jacc.2004.10.081.

Clavel MA, Pibarot P, Messika-Zeitoun D, et al. Impact of aortic valve calcification, as measured by MDCT, on survival in patients with aortic stenosis: results of an international registry study. J Am Coll Cardiol. 2014;64(12):1202–13. https://doi.org/10.1016/j.jacc.2014.05.066.

Hachicha Z, Dumesnil JG, Pibarot P. Usefulness of the valvuloarterial impedance to predict adverse outcome in asymptomatic aortic stenosis. J Am Coll Cardiol. 2009;54(11):1003–11. https://doi.org/10.1016/j.jacc.2009.04.079.

Nishimura RA, Otto CM, Bonow RO, et al. AHA/ACC guideline for the management of patients with valvular heart disease: a report of the American College of Cardiology/American Heart Association Task Force on Practice Guidelines [published correction appears in J Thorac Cardiovasc Surg. 2014 Oct 21;64(16):1763. Dosage error in article text]. J Thorac Cardiovasc Surg. 2014;148(1):e1–e132. https://doi.org/10.1016/j.jtcvs.2014.05.014.

Nishimura RA, Otto CM, Bonow RO, et al. 2017 AHA/ACC Focused Update of the 2014 AHA/ACC Guideline for the Management of Patients With Valvular Heart Disease: A Report of the American College of Cardiology/American Heart Association Task Force on Clinical Practice Guidelines. Circulation. 2017;135(25):e1159–95. https://doi.org/10.1161/CIR.0000000000000503.

Quiñones MA, Otto CM, Stoddard M, Waggoner A, Zoghbi WA. Doppler Quantification Task Force of the Nomenclature and Standards Committee of the American Society of Echocardiography. Recommendations for quantification of Doppler echocardiography: a report from the Doppler Quantification Task Force of the Nomenclature and Standards Committee of the American Society of Echocardiography. J Am Soc Echocardiogr. 2002;15(2):167–84. https://doi.org/10.1067/mje.2002.120202.

Thaden JJ, Nkomo VT, Lee KJ, Oh JK. Doppler imaging in aortic stenosis: the importance of the nonapical imaging windows to determine severity in a contemporary cohort. J Am Soc Echocardiogr. 2015;28(7):780–5. https://doi.org/10.1016/j.echo.2015.02.016.

9 Mitral Valve

Learning Objectives

- To learn the causes, evaluation, and management of mitral stenosis
- To learn the causes, evaluation, and management of mitral insufficiency

General Characteristics of the Normal Mitral Valve (MV)

- The mitral valve complex includes the leaflets, commissures, annulus, chordae tendinae, papillary muscles and the underlying ventricular myocardium.
- Annular diameter ~3 cm; normal mitral valve area—4–6 cm^2
- Leaflet tissue is redundant with an area of ~10–12 cm^2 (50% greater than annular area)
- This is further increased in degenerative mitral valve disease/mitral valve prolapse/HCM
- Annulus
  - The MV annulus is 'Saddle Shaped' (Fig. 9.1) with the peaks of the saddle being anterior-posterior, and the troughs at the medial and lateral commissures.
  - Important to remember for diagnosing prolapse; diagnosis should be made on TTE on PLAX view (or possibly apical three chamber view). Apical four chamber view can overestimate prolapse
- Leaflets and scallops (Fig. 9.2)
  - The anterior mitral leaflet is longer (20–24 mm) than the posterior leaflet (10–14 mm)
  - The posterior leaflet, however, has longer attachments to the annulus
  - The overall size (surface area) of both leaflets is very similar
  - The posterior leaflet has anatomical scallops; the anterior leaflet segments are numbered according to the corresponding posterior leaflet scallops
  - Scallops are numbered from anterior/lateral edge at the LAA (1) to medial edge (3)

T. Rambhatla, G. Perk, *The Echocardiography Companion*,
https://doi.org/10.1007/978-3-030-47041-8_9

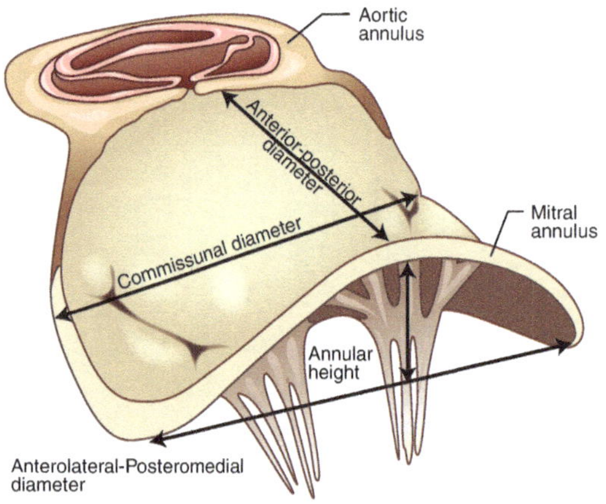

Fig. 9.1 Saddle shaped mitral annulus. The mitral annuls is saddle shaped; the anterior and posterior aspects of the mitral valve are higher than the medial and lateral commissures. Note: Due to this inherent "dip" of the annulus, mitral valve prolapse should be diagnosed based on parasternal long axis view (as opposed to the apical four chamber view)

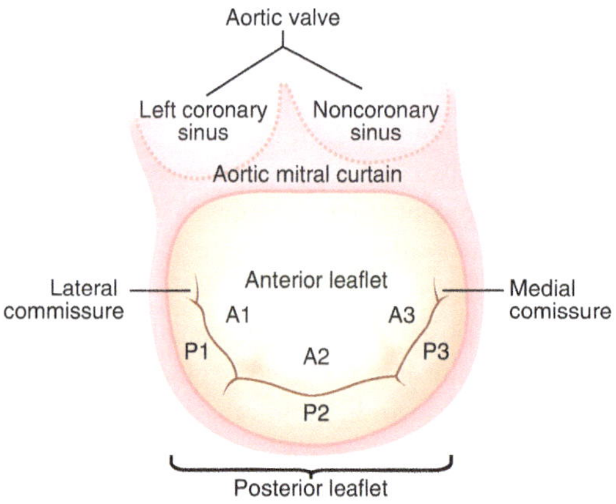

Fig. 9.2 Mitral valve leaflets and scallops. Mitral valve in the "surgical view"; the valve is visualized from the atrial perspective, aorta at 12 o'clock position, lateral commissure and left atrial appendage at 9 o'clock, and the posterior/medial commissure and tricuspid valve at 3 o'clock. The posterior leaflet has three scallops—P1 most lateral, P2 central, and P3 medial. The anterior leaflet area (not true scallops) is termed according to the corresponding posterior scallop.

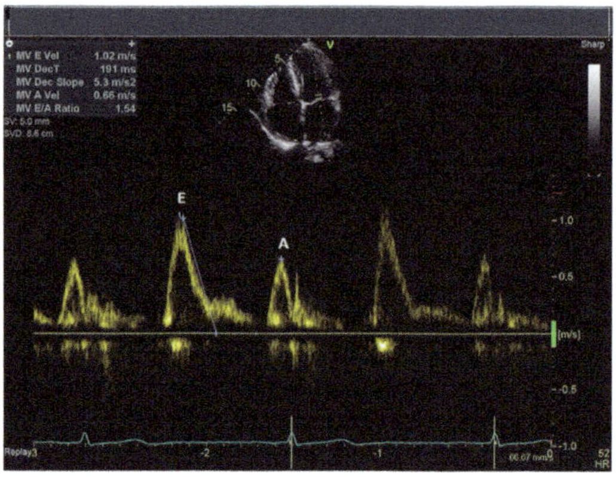

Fig. 9.3 Normal mitral inflow. Normal mitral valve inflow pattern assessed with pulse wave Doppler in the apical four chamber view. The sample volume is placed at the mitral leaflet tips. Early diastolic filling (E) and late atrial contraction (A) are normally seen

- Mitral inflow/LA emptying velocity and pattern: (Fig. 9.3)
  - Normal parameters: E velocity <1 m/s, deceleration time (DT) 160–200 ms, E:A 0.8–1.5
  - Faster E velocities, DT < 160 ms, or E:A > 1.5 can be suggestive of elevated LAP or severe MR; DT > 200 ms can be suggestive of abnormal relaxation or mitral stenosis

9.1 Mitral Stenosis (MS)

9.1.1 Etiology

- Rheumatic
  - Commissural fusion creating "fish mouth" appearance of the mitral valve
  - Decreased leaflet mobility with leaflet thickening, fibrosis and calcification
  - Sub-valvular thickening, chordal shortening and fusion

- Most patients have co-existent aortic regurgitation
- Degenerative/mitral annular calcification (MAC)
  - Fibrosis and calcification of the mitral annulus; leaflet tips commonly spared
  - More commonly causes MR than MS
  - Risk factors include HTN, DM, hyperlipidemia, known CAD/PVD. Early onset MAC may be seen in chronic kidney disease, connective tissue disease
- Congenital
  - Parachute mitral valve
    Single papillary muscle connects to both leaflets - a large (parachute like) anterior leaflet and a small posterior leaflet
  - Double orifice mitral valve
    In the en face view, similar appearance to post Alfieri stitch or post clip repair
- Radiation
  - Typically, fibrosis and calcification of anterior annulus and aorta-mitral curtain
  - The posterior annulus and leaflet tips are commonly spared
- Medications
  - Anorexigens (fenflurane), Ergotamine, SSRIs, Dopamine agonists (pergolide), and MDMA

9.1.2 Echocardiographic Assessment

Anatomic Assessment

1. M-mode of AV (Fig. 9.4)
   - MS results in loss of rapid filling of LV ➔ blunted slope of posterior movement of the aortic root after mitral valve opening
   - Assessment of S2-OS (opening snap) interval (i.e. IVRT)
     - S2-OS interval can be measured on AV M-mode as the interval between aortic valve closure (S2) and beginning of the posterior movement of the aortic root (OS)
       Shortens with: increasing LA pressure and worsening severity of MS
       Lengthens with: delayed relaxation

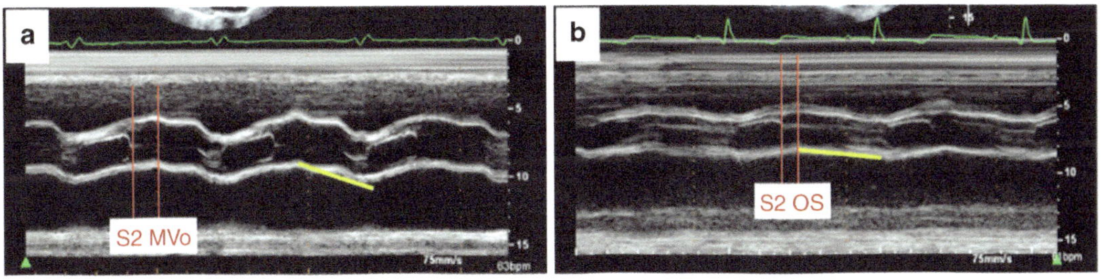

Fig. 9.4 Aortic valve M-mode in mitral stenosis. (**a**) Normal aortic valve m-mode in the presence of normal mitral valve; rapid early diastolic filling leads to a decrease in left atrial volume and a posterior movement of the adjacent aortic root (yellow line). In addition, the interval between the closure of the aortic valve (S_2) and mitral valve opening (MVo) can be easily seen and measured. (**b**) Aortic valve m-mode in mitral stenosis; loss of rapid early diastolic filling with persistently elevated left atrial volume and pressure causes blunting of the early diastolic posterior movement of the aortic root. In addition, with worsening mitral stenosis and increasing left atrial pressure, mitral valve opening happens earlier, shortening the S2-opening snap (OS) interval. *MVo* mitral valve opening, *OS* opening snap

2. M-mode of MV (Fig. 9.5)
   - Reduced E-F slope
   - Thickened leaflets
   - Reduced/absent A kick even in normal sinus rhythm (see below)
   - Paradoxical diastolic anterior movement of posterior mitral leaflet (in rheumatic MS)
3. 2D imaging
   - In rheumatic disease - commissural fusion and progressive fibrosis and calcification of leaflets cause the typical diastolic doming ("hockey stick deformity") (Fig. 9.6)
   - In degenerative disease—calcification and fibrosis extend from the annulus towards the leaflets
4. Planimetry
   - The mitral valve is funnel shaped with smallest orifice at the tip of the "cone"
   - Planimetry must be performed at the tips of leaflets, to avoid overestimating mitral valve area (MVA)
   - Biplane view and 3D imaging are essential for proper location of planimetry plane
   - With severe annular calcifications, accuracy reduced

Doppler Assessment

1. Mitral inflow pattern
   - Increased peak E Velocity
     - Reflective of increased early diastolic transmitral gradient (not necessarily the severity of MS)
     - Can also be seen in MR, VSD, high output states
   - Absent diastasis—continuous flow throughout diastole (Fig. 9.7)

     Note: in patients in sinus rhythm, despite A wave on mitral inflow Doppler tracing, M mode may not show an A wave; due to persistent gradient between LA and LV, mitral leaflets are open to maximal excursion throughout diastole. However, the Doppler tracing shows the increased flow that occurs with atrial contraction.
2. Mean mitral inflow gradient
   - MV inflow VTI (by CW Doppler) measures mean gradient across mitral valve throughout diastole

     Note: mean gradient is highly dependent on heart rate; tachycardia shortens diastole and filling time, causing an increase in mean gradient; bradycardia allows more time to empty LA, lowering the mean gradient.

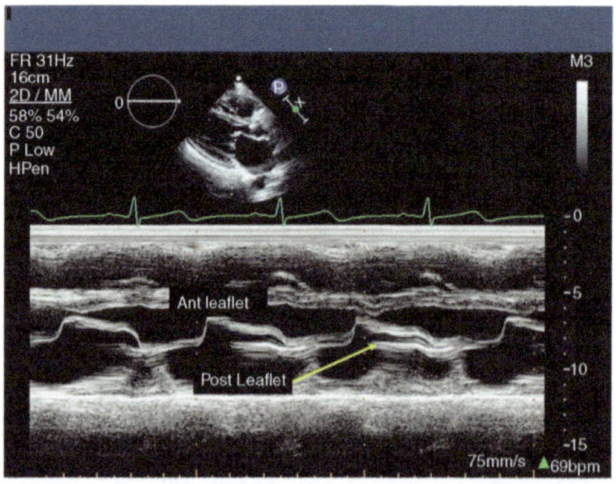

Fig. 9.5 Mitral valve M-mode in rheumatic mitral stenosis. M-mode of the mitral valve in rheumatic mitral stenosis showing thickened leaflets with flattening of the E-F slope and absent A wave (even in sinus rhythm). Due to commissural fusion, the posterior leaflet moves anteriorly with anterior leaflet during diastole.

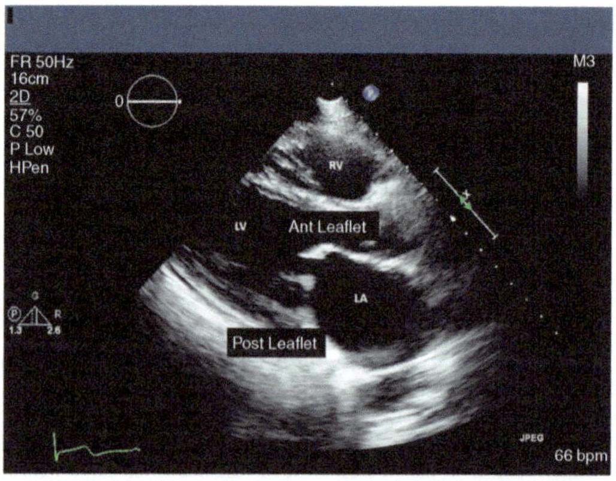

Fig. 9.6 PLAX view of mitral valve in rheumatic mitral stenosis. Parasternal long axis image in rheumatic mitral stenosis with thickened leaflets and typical doming of the mitral leaflets ("hockey stick" appearance) caused by commissural fusion and progressive fibrosis and calcification.

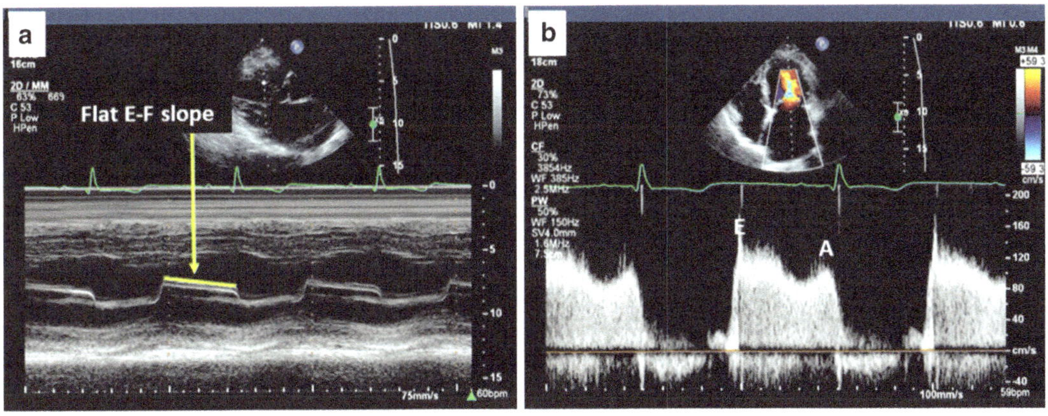

Fig. 9.7 **Mitral valve imaging in mitral stenosis.** (**a**) Mitral valve m mode in mitral stenosis showing flat E-F slope and loss of atrial contraction motion (A wave) of the mitral leaflets. (**b**) Continuous wave (CW) Doppler across the mitral valve showing increased peak E velocity, absent diastasis, and high mean left atrial pressure. Note that despite normal sinus rhythm (as evidence by the CW tracing clearly showing A wave), the m-mode tracing does not have the corresponding A wave; the persistent gradient between the LA and LV throughout diastole does not allow for the normal partial closure of the mitral valve seen during diastasis, however flow does increase as the atrium contracts

3. Pressure half-time (PHT)
   - The time it takes for the pressure gradient between LA and LV to decrease to half its initial value; depends on the rate of decline of the pressure difference across the MV during diastole
     Note: this is NOT the time it takes velocity to decline to half of its initial value (but rather the time it takes for the velocity to decline to $\frac{V1}{\sqrt{2}}$)
   - Normal PHT—65–80 ms
   - In patients with isolated rheumatic mitral stenosis MVA is calculated by
     $$\text{MVA} = \frac{220}{PHT}$$
   - More severe MS ➔ longer PHT
     – Conditions that decrease the LA-LV pressure gradient cause the PHT to shorten ➔ overestimation of MVA by this formula.
       ASD with left to right shunt (left atrium empties into the LV as well as into RA ➔ LA pressure drops faster)
       Severe AI (aortic regurgitant volume increasing LVEDP ➔ quick equalization of pressures between LA and LV)
   - MVA by pressure half time has been validated in rheumatic MS patients without coexisting heart disease—should not be used for MVA calculations in other conditions. Changes in diastolic function can effect PHT and cause over/underestimation of MVA.
     Note: immediately following mitral balloon valvuloplasty, acute alterations in flow, LA compliance & interatrial flow (through transseptal puncture site) change the rate of LA-LA pressure equilibration
4. PISA method—proximal isovelocity surface area (Fig. 9.8)
   - Based on the continuity principle; flow proximal to the valve equals the flow at the valve
   - The flow proximal to the valve is calculated by measuring the PISA radius at a known aliasing velocity
   - Flow at the PISA shell (mitral inflow) is calculated as
     $$\text{Mitral inflow} = 2\pi r^2 \times \frac{\theta}{180} \times V_{\text{alias}}$$
     r—PISA radius, θ—angle between mitral leaflets during diastole, V_{alias}—aliasing velocity
   - Flow at the PISA shell equals the flow through the mitral valve
   - Mitral valve area calculated as:
     $$\text{MVA} = \frac{2\pi r^2 \times V_{\text{alias}} \times \frac{\theta}{180}}{MV_{max}}$$

- There are many pitfalls (technical as well as physiological) for using PISA method for MVA calculation; not commonly used

5. MVA calculation by continuity equation

$$\text{MVA} = \frac{\pi LVOTr^2 \times LVOT\,VTI}{MV\,VTI}$$

LVOTr —radius of the LVOT, MV VTI—from CW Doppler across MV inflow.

This calculation is based on the continuity principle: in the absence of significant regurgitant lesions or shunts, flow (or stroke volume) throughout the heart is constant.

$$\text{LVOT}_{\text{area}} \times \text{LVOT VTI} = \text{MVA} \times \text{MV VTI}$$

9.1.3 Diagnostic Criteria (Table 9.1)

9.1.4 Compensatory Mechanisms-Adverse Consequences on the Heart

- Increased LA size
  - Atrial fibrillation—40% of patients with severe MS develop AF
  - LA thrombus

    44% LA, 66% LAA

    Patients may present with embolic complication (e.g. stroke/TIA) even in normal sinus rhythm.
- Pulmonary hypertension (venous)
- Tachycardia

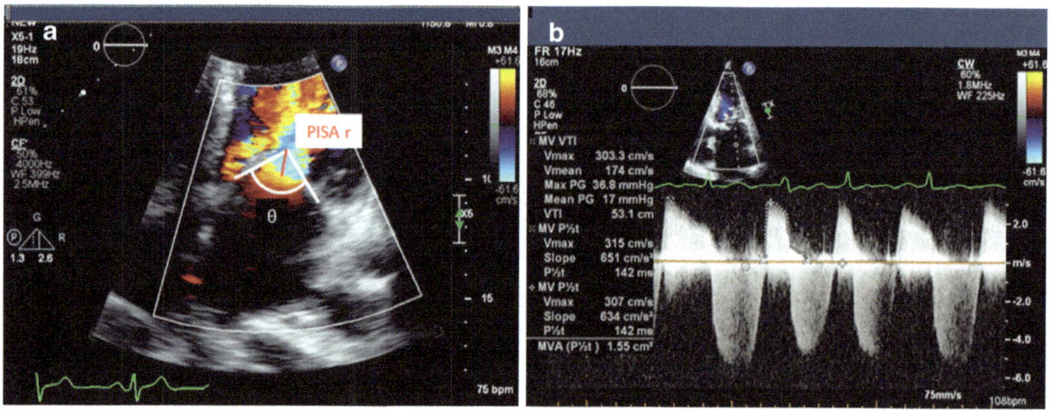

Fig. 9.8 **PISA method for MVA calculation in mitral stenosis.** (**a**) The proximal isovelocity surface area (PISA) is identified by the area where diastolic flow convergence proximal to the valve can be seen. The distance between the PISA border and the mitral valve opening is measured (r). The angel between the opened mitral leaflets (θ) should be measured. (**b**) Mitral valve VTI is traced from the continuous wave spectral Doppler across the mitral inflow. Mitral valve area is calculated by:

$$\text{MVA} = \frac{2\pi r^2 \times V_{\text{alias}} \times \dfrac{\theta}{180}}{MV_{max}}$$

MV mitral valve, MVA mitral valve area, V_{alias} aliasing velocity

Table 9.1 Echocardiographic criteria for rheumatic mitral stenosis severity

	Anatomy	Mean gradient (mmHg)	Mitral valve area (MVA) (cm²)	Diastolic pressure half time (ms)	Additional features
Mild/moderate (progressive)	Mild valve doming during diastole	<5	>1.5	<150	Mild LA enlargement Normal rest PASP
Severe	Commissural fusion, diastolic doming	5–10 Very severe: >10	<1.5 Very severe: <1.0	≥150 Very severe: ≥220 ms	Severe LA enlargement PASP > 30 mmHg

9.1.5 Surveillance and Follow-Up

- TTE with any change of symptoms
- TTE every 3–5 years for MVA > 1.5 cm^2, 1–2 years for MVA 1–1.5 cm^2, yearly for MVA < 1 cm^2
- Exercise stress test for further evaluation in patients with:
  - Known MS, intermediate gradient across MV, and unclear origin of symptoms;
  - If mean gradient increases to >15 mmHg or PA systolic pressure increases to > 60 mmHg ➔ symptoms probably due to MS

9.1.6 Management

Medical Treatment

- Heart rate control is recommended in patients with MS and atrial fibrillation or in sinus rhythm if symptomatic with exercise
- Anticoagulation with a vitamin K antagonists in patients with MS and AF, prior embolic event, or LA thrombus

Percutaneous Mitral Balloon Commissurotomy (PMBC) or Surgical MV Replacement

- PMBC is recommended over surgery in patients with favorable valve morphology in the absence of contraindications; otherwise surgical intervention with mitral valve replacement (MVR) should be performed
- Indications:
  - Asymptomatic patients
    PMBC—Very severe MS
    PMBC—severe MS + new onset Atrial fibrillation
  - Symptomatic patients
    PMBC—severe MS
    MVR—severe MS, if undergoing concomitant other cardiac surgery
    MVR—severe MS, severely symptomatic class III/IV + not high risk for surgery + not candidates for PMBC or failed previous PMBC
    MVA > 1.5 cm^2 if there is hemodynamically significant findings during exercise
- Contraindications to PMBC:
  - More than moderate MR
  - Presence of LA or LAA thrombus
  - TEE must be performed to assess the severity of MR and exclude LA thrombus
- Anatomy and suitability for PMBC—Wilkins/Abascal score used (Table 9.2).
  - Favorable anatomy: score <8 and no significant commissural calcifications

9.1.7 Rare conditions Mimicking Mitral Stenosis

- Cor-Triatriatum sinister
  - LAA is part of distal/lower chamber

Table 9.2 Wilkins Abascal score for percutaneous mitral balloon commissurotomy*

Points	Leaflet mobility	Valve thickness	Subvalvular thickening	Valvular calcification
1	Highly mobile with little restriction	Normal (4–5 mm)	Minimal chordal thickening	a single area of calcification
2	Decreased mobility in mid-portion and base of leaflets	Mid-leaflet/marginal thickening	Chordal thickening 1/3 length	Confined to leaflet margins
3	Forward movement of valve leaflets in diastole	Total leaflet thickening (5–8 mm)	Chordal thickening 2/3 length	Up to mid-leaflet
4	No or minimal forward movement of leaflets in diastole	Severe thickening (≥8 mm)	Complete chordal thickening to papillary muscle	Throughout most of the valve leaflets

*Note: Score is typically calculated based on TTE imaging

- Supravalvular mitral ring
  - LAA part of basal/upper PV chamber
- Chordal shortening/fusion

9.2 Mitral Regurgitation (MR)

9.2.1 Etiology

Mitral regurgitation can be caused by abnormality of any of the components of the mitral valve apparatus (leaflets, commissures, annulus, chordae tendinae, papillary muscles and the underlying ventricular myocardium).

Common classifications include:

- Primary vs. secondary MR (Tables 9.3 and 9.4)
- Carpentier classification (Table 9.5, Fig. 9.9).

Table 9.3 Etiology of primary MR—intrinsic abnormality of the mitral valve leaflets

Etiology	Details	Jet direction
Myxomatous degeneration	Spectrum of severity and types of myxomatous changes: **Fibroelastic deficiency (FED):** Generally focal/segmental pathology, thin leaflets **Forme fruste:** intermediate form of a disease, refers to myxomatous degeneration/thickening of more than one leaflet but overall valve size normal **Barlow's disease**: Diffuse involvement, thickened leaflets **Mitral valve prolapse (MVP)**: can result from FED or Barlow's disease. P2 prolapse most common. Can progress with chordal rupture and flail segment.	Eccentric jet Directed opposite of prolapsed/flail segment
Degenerative—annular calcification (MAC) and thickening	Calcification occurs at annulus level, with relative sparing of commissures, aorto-mitral continuity, leaflet tips, and subvalvular apparatus. Common with aging Risk factors—same as for CAD/atherosclerosis Premature MAC seen in HCM, ESRD, connective tissue disease	Central or directed to either side
Inflammatory	**Rheumatic:** thickening/fusion and later calcifications of subvalvular apparatus and commissures. 40% have combined MS and MR **Collagen vascular disease:** noninfectious/marantic endocarditis **Radiation:** thickening and calcification of valve leaflet, typically anterior > posterior	Central or directed to either side
Infectious	Vegetations, aneurysm formation, leaflet dissection and/or perforation Anterior MV leaflet endocarditis can complicate AV endocarditis with aortic regurgitation (jet lesion)	Variable
Congenital	Cleft MV (associated with primum ASD, often anterior MV leaflet) Parachute mitral valve	Towards affected leaflet

Table 9.4 Etiology of secondary MR—abnormal MV function due to LA and/or LV remodeling

Etiology	Details	Jet direction
Ischemic	**Adverse LV remodeling**: Apical displacement of the leaflets (most often the posterior leaflet) causes tethering/tenting and restricted mobility resulting in incomplete mitral valve closure. **Intraventricular dyssynchrony**: Segmental wall motion abnormalities or LBBB can cause displacement of the leaflets with incomplete closure of the valve. **Ruptured papillary muscle**: can be seen with acute MI; more prevalent in inferior MI and rupture of posterior papillary muscle due to the single blood supply (PDA) of the posterior papillary muscle	Towards the tethered leaflet
Functional	Annular dilatation with decreased coaptation zone. Can be caused by LV or LA dilatation.	Central
Systolic anterior motion of the mitral valve (SAM)	Can be seen in: HOCM, HTN with localized septal hypertrophy, hyperdynamic LV function, and small cavity size with volume depletion. Presence of MAC (particularly at the posterior annulus) increases the likelihood of SAM and MR	Typically—perpendicular jet to the LVOT turbulent jet)

Table 9.5 Carpentier Classification of MR (Fig. 9.9)

	Type I	Type II	Type IIIa	Type IIIb
Leaflet motion	Normal	Increased	Restricted opening and closing (in systole and diastole)	Restricted closing (systole only)
Etiology	Leaflet perforation or annular dilatation	Myxomatous degeneration (most common, 20–40% of all MR)	Rheumatic	Functional or ischemic
Pathology	Endocarditis Dilated cardiomyopathy	Leaflet prolapse Chordal/papillary muscle rupture	Commissural fusion Leaflet thickening or calcification Chordal fusion	Chordal thickening/shortening PM apically displaced Leaflet tenting

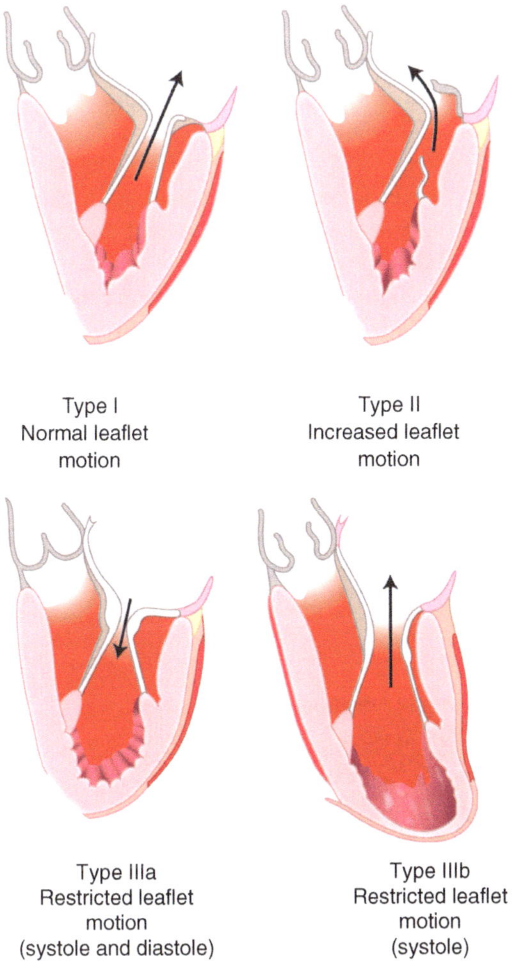

Fig. 9.9 Carpentier classification of mitral regurgitation. The Carpentier classification is one of the ways to define mitral regurgitation mechanism; it is based on leaflet anatomy and motion.

9.2.2 Echocardiographic Assessment

Anatomic Assessment

1. M-mode of the mitral valve—helpful in certain pathologies, e.g. mitral valve prolapse (Fig. 9.10) and systolic anterior motion (Fig. 9.11).
2. 2D imaging: baseline anatomy of mitral valve—presence of leaflet abnormalities (e.g. valve prolapse), coaptation depth, annular size, presence of calcifications, vegetations, tears, etc.

Doppler Assessment

1. Jet contour
    - Functional MR: early rounded jet contour, severity is greater earlier in systole, may end early (before end systole)
    - SAM with dynamic left ventricular outflow obstruction: intermediate peaking jet contour, the worse the obstruction, the earlier the MR
    - MVP: late systolic MR, small measured VTI
    - Acute severe MR: dense, triangular shaped/early peaking
2. Jet area—good for "eyeballing" and MR exclusion, but should not be used as the sole method for quantification due to many pitfalls
    - Eccentric jet hugging the LA wall (Coanda effect)
    - Large, dilated LA (jet will occupy a smaller percentage of the LA area)

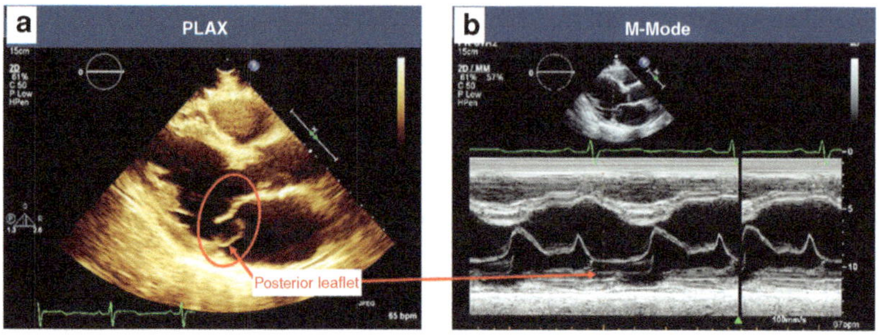

Fig. 9.10 **Mitral valve prolapse.** (**a**) Systolic frame from a parasternal long axis (PLAX) view of the mitral valve showing posterior leaflet prolapse. (**b**) M-mode image showing the systolic posterior bowing of the mitral leaflet

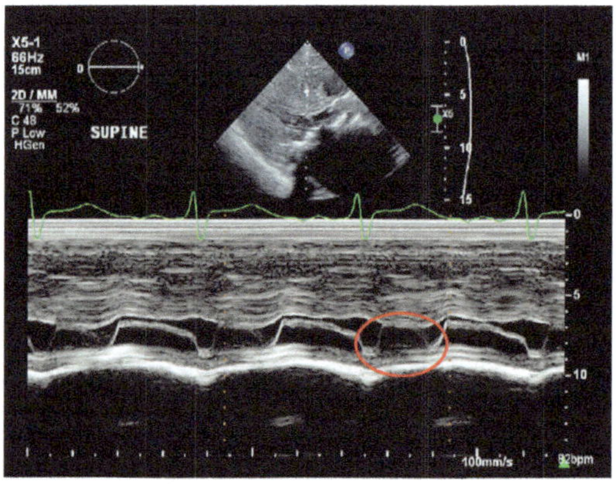

Fig. 9.11 **Mitral valve M-mode with systolic anterior motion.** M-mode image showing systolic anterior motion of the mitral valve (red circle). Note: important to pay attention to the timing of the finding; the diastolic motion of the mitral leaflet towards the septum is normal

- Poorly compliant LA
- Technical considerations like color gain, filter setting, frame rate
- Hemodynamic state: HTN, hypotension or volume status can change appearance of MR jet

  Note: sedation during TEE or general anesthesia for open heart surgery can change hemodynamic conditions and appearance of MR

3. Vena contracta (VC)—surrogate for measurement of the effective regurgitant orifice area.
   - VC width—measured on PLAX view, at the narrowest part of the jet
4. Direct measurement of EROA—utilizing 3D multiplanar reconstruction, direct planimetry of the EROA area can be performed. Only the area of the aliased signal (highest velocities) should be measured. (Fig. 9.12)

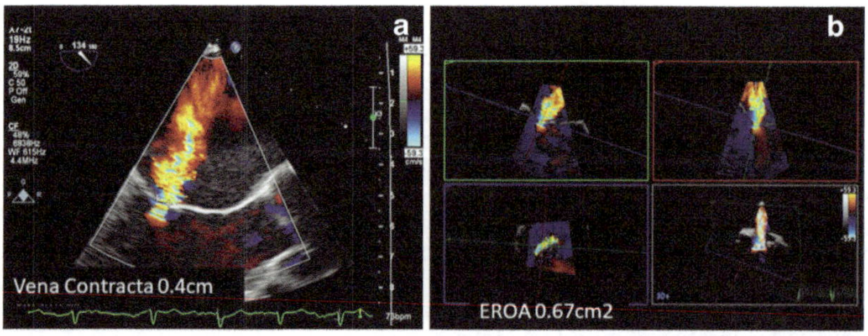

Fig. 9.12 **3D Based direct planimetry of MR EROA.** (**a**) Transesophageal image, from the mid-esophageal LVOT view, with measurement of mitral regurgitation vena contracta. In 2D imaging, the vena contracta is used as a surrogate for EROA and should be measured at the narrowest portion of the jet. (**b**) 3D multiplanar reconstruction with direct planimetry of the effective regurgitant orifice area (EROA)

5. Proximal isovelocity surface area (PISA) (Fig. 9.13)
   - Calculation of the effective regurgitant orifice area (EROA) based on continuity principle
   - Flow at the outer shell of PISA is equal to flow at the regurgitant orifice

$$2\pi r^2 \times V_{alias} = EROA \times MR\ V_{max}$$

$$EROA = \frac{2\pi r^2 \times V_{alias}}{MR\,Vmax}$$

   - EROA × MR VTI = MR regurgitant volume (RV)
   - Under normal hemodynamic conditions, MR velocity is approximately 5–6 m/s (which correlates with SBP in the range of 110–144 mmHg) allowing shortcuts for MR severity calculations

Shortcuts for quick estimation of ERO and MR severity	
Aliasing velocity set to 40 cm/s and MR Vmax ~5 m/s	**EROA** $\cong \frac{r2}{2}$
Aliasing velocity set to 30 cm/s and MR Vmax ~5 m/s and PISA r = 1 cm	**EROA > 0.4 cm²**

EROA-effective regurgitation orifice area, r-PISA radius

Note: High velocity MR (Vmax > 6m/s) can be seen when LV systolic pressure is high; examples include:
   - Hypertension
   - Aortic stenosis
   - LVOT obstruction
   - Aortic coarctation
   - Subclavian stenosis

Note: in mitral valve prolapse with end-systolic MR, calculated EROA will not represent true MR severity since the MR duration is short; Regurgitant volume must be calculated (utilizing MR VTI) in order to properly categorize MR severity.

6. Volumetric calculations - RV can also by calculated by comparing flow across two different valves (assuming only MR present, no AI or any shunt)

Inflow volume across the mitral valve = Effective SV + RV

Inflow volume across the mitral valve = $MV_{\text{annulus area}} \times MV_{\text{VTI at annular level}}$

Effective SV = $LVOT_{SV}$

LVOT SV = $LVOT_{area} \times LVOT_{VTI}$

RV = $(MV_{\text{annulus area}} \times MV_{\text{VTI at annulus}}) - (LVOT_{area} \times LVOT_{VTI})$

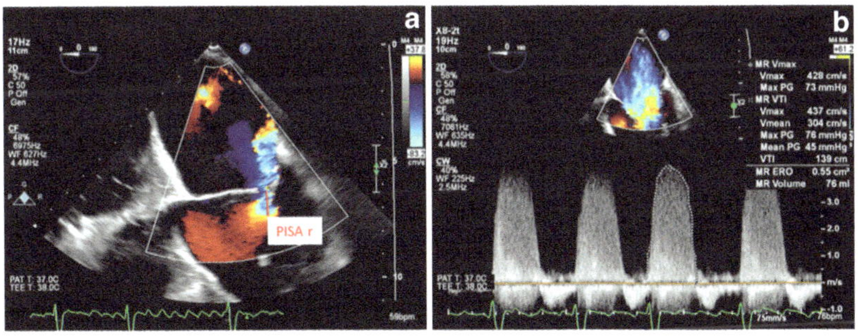

Fig. 9.13 PISA method for EROA calculation in mitral regurgitation. Proximal isovelocity surface area (PISA) calculation of mitral regurgitation is based on the continuity principle; the flow at the outermost shell of the PISA (proximal to the valve) is equal to the flow at the regurgitant orifice. As blood flow converges to the regurgitant orifice, the velocity increases and isovelocity hemispheric shells form. (**a**) The surface area of the PISA hemisphere is calculated using the measured radius (r) and formula for hemisphere surface area calculation (=$2\pi r^2$). The velocity at the outer edge of the PISA is the aliasing velocity (V_{alias}); thus the flow at the PISA shell is calculated as: $2\pi r^2 \times V_{alias}$. (**b**) The velocity at the effective regurgitant orifice area (EROA) is the maximal velocity of the regurgitation jet (as the EROA is smallest orifice though which the jet passes). Using continuity principle, the EROA can be calculated by: $EROA = \frac{2\pi r^2 \times V_{alias}}{MR\,Vmax}$

Supportive Findings:

1. Moderate to severe LA enlargement
2. Pulmonary hypertension (at rest or with exercise)
3. Systolic reversal of flow in pulmonary veins
4. Tall mitral E wave (> 1.2m/sec)
5. Eccentric jet extending to posterior wall
6. Coanda effect

9.2.3 Diagnostic Criteria (Table 9.6)

9.2.4 Compensatory Mechanisms-Adverse Consequences on the Heart

- Pulmonary edema
  - Pulmonary edema severity correlates with increased left atrial pressure
  - Worse in smaller noncompliant left atrium—seen in acute severe MR
- LV and LA dilatation
  - Increased chamber size and compliance allows more regurgitant blood to be accepted without increasing left atrial pressure

9.2.5 Surveillance and Follow-Up

Asymptomatic Patients

- Mild MR—Undetermined if routine surveillance at ≥3 year intervals is appropriate; Inappropriate at <3 year intervals
- Moderate to severe MR—appropriate to perform TTE at ≥1 year intervals
- TTE is indicated with any change of symptoms or new onset atrial fibrillation

9.2.6 Management

Medical Treatment

- Acute severe MR
  - Vasodilators/afterload reduction to increase forward cardiac output and decrease LV to LA regurgitation
  - Titratable medications preferred (IV nitroprusside or nicardipine); often limited by low BP
  - Intra-aortic balloon pump can be very helpful as a temporizing measure
- Vasodilator therapy is *not* indicated for asymptomatic normotensive patients with chronic primary MR and normal LV function

Surgical Treatment for Chronic Primary MR

- MV repair is recommended over valve replacement when surgery is indicated.
  - Shown to have improved LV function and survival when performed at experienced centers
  - MV replacement should not be done for isolated severe primary MR limited to less than one half of posterior leaflet unless repair has been attempted and was unsuccessful
- Severe MR in asymptomatic patients with:
  - LV dysfunction (EF 30–60% or LVESD ≥ 40 mm)
  - Undergoing cardiac surgery for other indications
  - Repair may be considered if LV function is preserved and likelihood of successful durable repair is >95% with expected mortality of <1% at a center of excellence

Table 9.6 Echocardiographic criteria for MR severity

	Anatomy	Vena contracta (mm)	Regurgitation volume/fraction (cc)/(%)	EROA (cm^2)	Jet area/LA (%)
Mild/moderate (progressive)	Normal coaptation	<7	<60/50	<0.4	<40
Severe	Loss of coaptation/ flail gap	≥7	≥60/50	≥0.4	≥40

  - Repair may be considered if MV is non rheumatic, LV function is preserved, high likelihood of successful repair + either new onset atrial fibrillation or resting pulmonary hypertension (estimated PA systolic pressure > 50 mmHg)
- Severe MR in symptomatic patients
  - EF > 30%—MV intervention recommended
  - EF ≤ 30%—MV intervention may be considered
- Moderate MR
  - If undergoing cardiac surgery for other indications

9.2.7 MR Management in Special Scenarios

HCM/SAM

- Important to remember—the "common" treatments for MR and heart failure (e.g. afterload reduction, inotropic support) worsen SAM, LVOT obstruction and MR severity.
- "ASH crash" may develop: hypercontractility ➔ worse SAM ➔ worse MR ➔ decreased chamber size ➔ further increase in outflow obstruction ➔ further worsening of MR.

Medical Management

- Must maintain filled heart—IV fluids
- Decrease contractility—beta blockers, calcium channel blockers, disopyramide
- In clinically unstable and hypotensive patients—IV phenylephrine (increase afterload and decrease LVOT obstruction to break the ASH crash cycle)

Invasive Therapies

- Septal reduction therapy
  - Eligible patients: symptomatic with NYHA III or IV, provoked or resting gradient ≥ 50 mmHg, anterior septal thickness > 16 mm
  - Surgical myectomy or alcohol septal ablation are currently available treatment options for patients meeting criteria for non-pharmacologic intervention
  - Factors influencing the decision between these options include anatomical considerations, comorbidities, concomitant cardiac problems, local expertise and patient preference
- Mitral valve intervention
  - Mitral valve repair can be done along with septal myectomy, particularly if the anterior leaflet is elongated or if concomitant primary mitral valve pathology present
  - Mitral valve replacement as the primary mode of treatment is rarely done
- Dual chamber pacemaker
  - Patients with PPM previously implanted for other indications may undergo a trial of RV apical pacing
  - Currently, PPM implantation for LVOT/MR relief is not recommended when other forms of therapy are available.

Note About Diastolic MR (Fig. 9.14)

- Occurs when the LV diastolic pressure exceeds left atrial pressure causing premature closure of mitral valve
- Mitral valve closes before the QRS ➔ MR occurs in late diastole
  - It is usually a low velocity MR jet (<2 m/s) as left ventricular pressure is not yet high (since left ventricular systole did not start yet)
- Can be seen with:
  - Acute severe AI, severe diastolic dysfunction
  - AV disassociation, significant first degree AV block, PVCs

    Following atrial contraction, atrial relaxation starts ➔ left atrial pressure drops below left ventricular pressure (due to AV block, LV systole is delayed) ➔ MR occurs down the pressure gradient.
- Diastolic MR is NOT a volume overload phenomenon; it is a marker of altered diastolic hemodynamics.

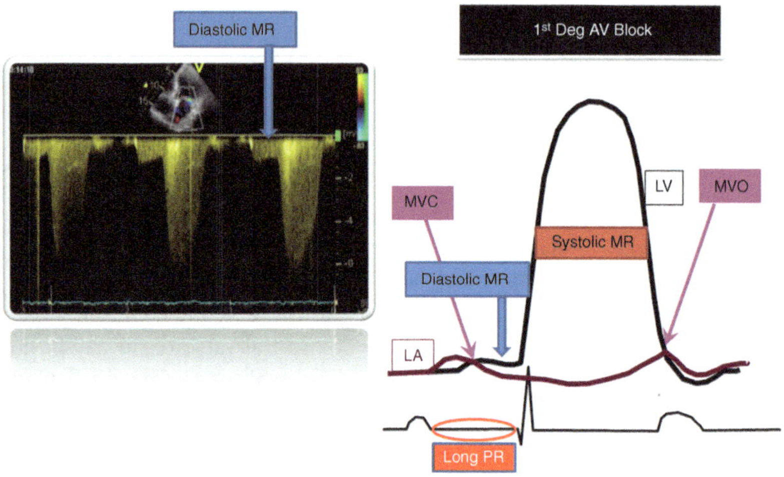

Fig. 9.14 **Diastolic mitral regurgitation.** (**a**) Spectral tracing showing diastolic mitral regurgitation. Diastolic MR occurs when left ventricular diastolic pressure exceeds left atrial pressure, resulting in premature closure of the mitral valve and a low velocity regurgitation jet (usually less than 2 m/s). This can be seen with severely elevated left ventricular diastolic pressure (e.g. acute severe AI) or with conduction system disease; first degree AV block (shown by diagram)—left atrial pressure drops following the atrial contraction, however due to the prolonged AV delay ventricular systole starts late, such that left atrial pressure drops even below LV pressure before ventricular contraction begins

Further Reading

Nishimura RA, Otto CM, Bonow RO, et al. 2014 AHA/ACC guideline for the management of patients with valvular heart disease: a report of the American College of Cardiology/American Heart Association Task Force on Practice Guidelines [published correction appears in J Thorac Cardiovasc Surg. 2014 Oct 21;64(16):1763. Dosage error in article text]. J Thorac Cardiovasc Surg. 2014;148(1):e1–e132. https://doi.org/10.1016/j.jtcvs.2014.05.014.

Nishimura RA, Otto CM, Bonow RO, et al. 2017 AHA/ACC focused update of the 2014 AHA/ACC Guideline for the management of patients with valvular heart disease: a report of the American College of Cardiology/American Heart Association Task Force on Clinical Practice Guidelines. Circulation. 2017;135(25):e1159–95. https://doi.org/10.1161/CIR.0000000000000503.

Zoghbi WA, Adams D, Bonow RO, et al. Recommendations for noninvasive evaluation of native valvular regurgitation: a report from the American Society of Echocardiography developed in collaboration with the society for cardiovascular magnetic resonance. J Am Soc Echocardiogr. 2017;30(4):303–71. https://doi.org/10.1016/j.echo.2017.01.007.

10 Tricuspid and Pulmonic Valves

Learning Objectives

- To learn the causes, evaluation, and management of tricuspid regurgitation and stenosis
- To learn the causes, evaluation, and management of pulmonic insufficiency and stenosis

TRICUSPID VALVE

General Characteristics of the Normal Tricuspid Valve (TV)

- The tricuspid valve complex includes the fibrous annulus, leaflets, cords and papillary muscles (generally 2 or 3 papillary muscles).
- The tricuspid valve is apically displaced
  - Apical displacement of the TV (relative to the MV) is one of the characteristics that help identify the TV and hence the morphologic right ventricle (atrio-ventricular valves follow the "anatomic" ventricle)
  - The relative apical displacement of the TV creates the "atrio-ventricular" septum, separating the left ventricle and the right atrium (Fig. 10.1)
- The TV is the largest valve; annular diameter between 2.5–4 cm, valve orifice area of 7–9 cm^2
- Leaflets
  - Classically composed of three leaflets: sepal, anterior, and posterior. However number of leaflets may vary

    Posterior leaflet may be divided into two (appearance of 4-leaflet valve)

    Separation between anterior and posterior leaflet may be difficult to discern (appearance of a 2-leaflet valve)

    Echocardiographic identification of the different leaflets is a matter of great debate in the echocardiographsy literature.

    Ideally, leaflets should be identified by an en-face view of the valve;

    Note: on TEE, transgastric view at 0–30° angle often allows en-face view of the TV
  - The leaflet tissue is generally redundant with an area that is greater than the annular area
- Tricuspid inflow/RA emptying velocity and pattern
  - The TV inflow pattern resembles mitral inflow pattern (E and A waves)
  - Velocities generally slightly lower than MV inflow velocities, as TV is larger.

10.1 Tricuspid Stenosis (TS)

10.1.1 Etiology

- Uncommon in adult population
- Rheumatic:
  - Generally accompanies rheumatic mitral stenosis
  - Hemodynamically significant TS only occurs in 5% of rheumatic heart disease

T. Rambhatla, G. Perk, *The Echocardiography Companion*,
https://doi.org/10.1007/978-3-030-47041-8_10

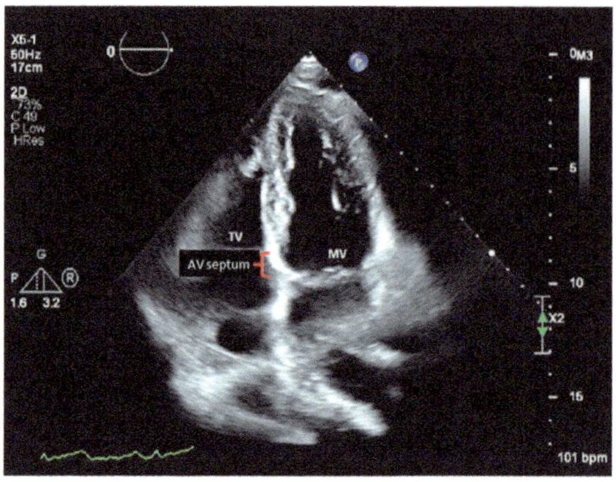

Fig. 10.1 **Apical displacement of the tricuspid valve.** The normal tricuspid (TV) valve is slightly more apically displaced than the mitral valve (MV), creating the atrioventricular septum (AV septum), which separates the left ventricle and the right atrium

- Other causes: congenital (e.g. TV atresia), Lupus valvulitis, infective endocarditis, endomyocardial fibrosis, carcinoid heart disease, RA tumors or clots protruding into the TV orifice (can cause TV obstruction mimicking TV stenosis), pacemaker leads.

10.1.2 Echocardiographic Assessment

Anatomic Assessment

- Thickened/shortened/calcified leaflets with restricted motion
- In rheumatic disease—diastolic doming of the leaflets

Doppler Assessment

- Tricuspid Inflow CW
  - Tricuspid inflow gradient varies with heart rate, stroke volume, respiratory cycle phase
  - Generally, severe TS is associated with mean gradient >5–10 mmHg at heart rate of 70/min
- Pressure Half-time (PHT)
  - Pressure half time > 190 msec is consistent with severe TS
  - Tricuspid valve area (TVA) may be calculated as:

$$\text{TVA}\left(\text{cm}^2\right) = \frac{190}{PHT}$$

10.1.3 Diagnostic Criteria

	Tricuspid valve area (cm^2)	Pressure half-time (msec)
Severe TS	<1	>190

10.1.4 Surveillance and Follow-Up

Asymptomatic Patients

- Mild TS—Undetermined if routine surveillance at ≥3 year intervals is appropriate; Inappropriate at <3 year intervals
- Moderate to severe TS—appropriate to perform TTE at ≥1 year intervals
- TTE is indicated with any change of symptoms or new onset atrial fibrillation

10.1.5 Management

Medical Treatment

- Diuretics can relieve symptoms of right sided congestion (LE edema, hepatic congestion) but at the risk of causing a low flow state to the left side

Invasive Treatment

- Options include: surgical TV repair/replacement or percutaneous balloon valvuloplasty
- Indications:
  - Symptomatic severe TS
  - Patient with severe TS undergoing left heart surgery
- Choice of procedure:
  - Overall greater experience with valve repair/replacement
  - Many patients with severe TS have concomitant TR, making balloon valvuloplasty less preferable
  - Assessment of surgical risk
  - Tumors, masses, vegetations, thrombi—are all contraindications to balloon valvuloplasty.

10.1.6 Differential Diagnosis

Cor Triatratum Dexter (very rare).

10.2 Tricuspid Regurgitation (TR)

10.2.1 Etiology

Primary TR	Secondary TR
Acquired diseases: Degenerative/ Myxomatous TV Rheumatic disease Endocarditis Trauma Carcinoid Iatrogenic (PPM/ICD leads, RV biopsy) *Congenital*: Ebstein's anolmaly Repaired tetralogy of Fallot L Transposition of the great vessels Others	Left heart disease (valvular disease or LV dysfunction) Right ventricle disease (volume overload, cardiomyopathy) Right atrium disease (atrial fibrillation) Pulmonary hypertension

- Trace to mild tricuspid regurgitation is seen in majority of normal individuals
- Tricuspid regurgitation can be caused by abnormality of any of the components of the tricuspid valve apparatus (leaflets, commissures, annulus, chordae tendinae, papillary muscles and underlying ventricular myocardium)
- The most common etiology for TR is secondary (functional) TR from annular dilatation

10.2.2 Echocardiographic Assessment

Anatomic Assessment

1. 2D imaging
   - Baseline anatomy of tricuspid valve—presence of leaflet abnormalities (e.g. valve prolapse), coaptation depth, annular size, presence of calcifications, vegetations, tears, PM/ICD wires.
     Note: annular dilation defined as annular diameter ≥ 4 cm (or ≥ 2.1 cm/m^2) on apical four chamber view.

Doppler Assessment

1. Jet contour (Fig. 10.2)
   - TR jet is usually holosystolic, parabolic and round in shape.
   - May become midsystolic and eccentric in case of pinched leaflet due to device wire
   - In severe TR with non-coapting leaflets, jet becomes triangular with low velocity (essentially equilibration of RV/RA pressures).
     Note: RVSP cannot be accurately assessed since modified Bernoulli equation is not validated for non-restrictive flow
2. Jet density
3. Jet area
   - Obtained on apical 4-chamber view, RV inflow view or subcostal view
   - Eccentric jets may be underestimated
4. Vena Contracta
   - Obtained on apical 4-chmaber view or RV inflow view
   - 3D based direct measurement of EROA can also be utilized
5. PISA radius for calculation of effective regurgitant orifice area (EROA)
   - Generally obtained on apical 4-chamber view
   - Same principles as for MR PISA assessment apply for TR assessment
6. Systolic flow reversal in hepatic veins

- TR is load dependent and respiratory cycle dependent
  - Regurgitant volume increases with volume overload, and decreases with volume depletion
  - Inspiration increases venous return ➔ increases TR regurgitant volume
- Best to reach euvolemia before diagnosing severe TR

10.2.3 Diagnostic Criteria (Table 10.1)

10.2.4 Surveillance and Follow-Up

Asymptomatic Patients

- Mild TR - Undetermined if routine surveillance at ≥3 year intervals is appropriate; Inappropriate at <3 year intervals
- Moderate to severe TR - appropriate to perform TTE at ≥1 year intervals
- TTE is indicated with any change of symptoms or new onset atrial fibrillation

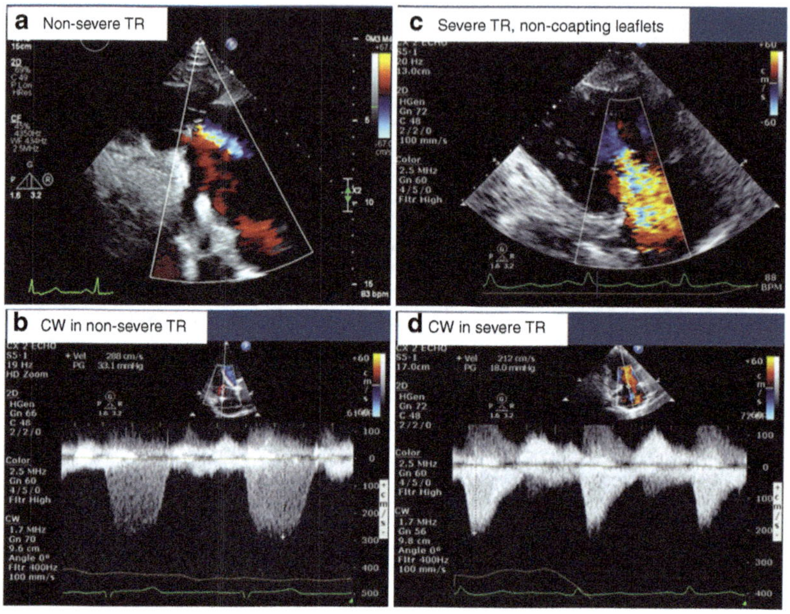

Fig. 10.2 Tricuspid regurgitation jet contour. (**a**) Systolic frame from RV inflow color view, showing mild tricuspid regurgitation (TR). The vena contracta and jet area are small. (**b**) Continuous wave (CW) Doppler showing parabolic shaped jet. (**c**) Systolic frame from RV inflow color view showing torrential TR. The 2D images from this patient showed non-coapting TV leaflets. The color jet has a very wide vena contracta and large jet area. (**d**) Continuous wave Doppler shows a dense jet with triangular, early peaking contour due to rapid equalization of pressures between the right ventricle and right atrium

Table 10.1 Echocardiographic criteria for TR severity

	Mild	Moderate	Severe
Anatomy	Normal	Mild-moderate annular dilation. Moderate thickening, or distortions	Annular dilation ≥4.0 cm (or 2.1 cm/m^2) Marked leaflet tethering Flail or grossly distorted leaflets
CW Jet	Faint	Dense	Dense
CW Shape	Parabolic	Variable	Triangular, early peaking
Color Jet area	<5 cm^2	5–10 cm^2	>10.0 cm^2
Vena contracta	<0.3 cm	0.3–0.69 cm	>0.70 cm
PISA radius	≤0.5 cm	0.6–0.9 cm	>0.9 cm
EROA	<0.2 cm^2	0.2–0.39 cm^2	≥0.4 cm^2
Regurgitant volune	<30 mL	30–44 mL	≥45 mL
IVC	Normal	Mildly dilated (2.1–2.5 cm)	Dilated >2.5 cm
Hepatic vein flow	Systolic dominance	Systolic blunting	Systolic reversal
Tricuspid inflow	A-wave dominant	Variable	Inflow E wave > 1 m/s
RA/RV size	Usually normal	Normal or mildly dilated	Usually dilated

10.2.5 Management

Medical Treatment
- Diuretics
- Pulmonary vasodilators

Surgical Treatment Recommended
- Severe TR, if already undergoing left sided valve surgery

Surgical Treatment Considered
- Mild, moderate or greater functional TR if undergoing left sided surgery and either TV annulus dilation or prior evidence of right heart failure
- Severe TR, symptomatic and unresponsive to medical therapy
- Severe TR, asymptomatic or minimally symptomatic with RV dilation or systolic dysfunction
- Moderate functional TR and pulmonary hypertension, if undergoing left heart surgery

Transcatheter Interventions
- Currently still experimental and done only in the context of clinical trails

PULMONIC VALVE

General Characteristics of the Normal Pulmonic Valve (PV)

- Similar to the aortic valve, the PV is tri-leaflet valve with no anatomic annulus, or chordal attachments.
- The PV is the most anterior valve; its opening is directed towards the left shoulder; often better evaluated with TTE than TEE

10.3 Pulmonic Stenosis (PS)

10.3.1 Etiology

Pulmonic stenosis is a rare finding in adults

- Most common etiology for PS: residual congenital defect either after corrective surgery or without intervention.
- Tumors or vegetations
- Carcinoid disease: most commonly combination of PS and pulmonic regurgitation (PR)
- Extrinsic compression of the RVOT/proximal PA causing functional PS

  Note: although PS is rare, it is important to always make sure no PS present (with CW Doppler across RVOT/PV); this confirms the assumption that RV systolic pressure equals PA systolic pressure allowing estimation PA systolic pressure from TR gradient (see Chap. 7).

10.3.2 Echocardiographic Assessment

Anatomic Assessment
1. M-mode
   - Exaggerated a-wave can be seen in PS complicated by RVH, RV diastolic dysfunction and elevation of RVEDP (Fig. 10.3)
   - Systolic doming of PV can be seen in congenital PS (even with mild stenosis)
2. 2D imaging
   - Assessment of valve anatomy (e.g. systolic doming of leaflets, dysplastic leaflets)
   - Right ventricular hypertrophy
     - RVH: thickness > 5 mm
   - Post stenotic dilatation of PA

Doppler Assessment
1. Color aliasing distal to the PV
2. Maximum velocity/peak pressure gradient
   - Views to use:
     - Usually maximum velocity obtained by CW from the PSAX
     - Modified five chamber view
     - In children and some adults—subcostal view
     - If subvalvular stenosis present (e.g. in certain congenital diseases)—must account for the subvalvular velocity when calculating peak gradient
3. Prominent A reversal in hepatic vein flow (correlates with exaggerated a wave on m-mode)
4. Elevated RV systolic pressure as estimated from peak TR velocity

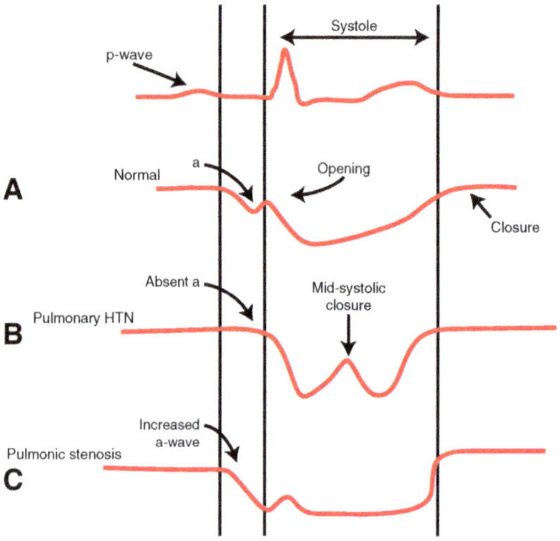

Fig. 10.3 **Pulmonic valve M-mode.** Diagram of normal pulmonic valve M-mode, and changes that occur with pulmonary hypertension or pulmonic valve stenosis. (**a**) Normal valve tracing shows posterior motion of the pulmonic valve leaflet during atrial contraction, caused by corresponding increase in right ventricular (RV) pressure. (**b**) In pulmonary hypertension, no posterior motion of the leaflet is noted at end diastole as the atrial kick does not generate enough pressure within the right ventricle to overcome pulmonary artery diastolic pressure. Pulmonary hypertension also causes midsystolic partial closure of the pulmonic valve until late systole when the right ventricular pressure rises again as contraction continues. (**c**) In pulmonic stenosis, right ventricular diastolic pressure is elevated due to chronic pressure overload; atrial contraction further increases this pressure, which is not opposed by pulmonary artery pressures; this results in exaggerated premature posterior motion of the pulmonic valve

10.3.3 Diagnostic Criteria

	Velocity (m/s)	Peak gradient (mmHg)
Mild/moderate	<4	≤64
Severe	>4	>64

Supportive signs of hemodynamic significance:

- RVH
- Post stenotic dilatation of main PA

10.3.4 Management

Medical Treatment

- No medical therapy has been shown to halt PS progression or decrease mortality

Invasive Treatment

- Options include: Balloon valvuloplasty or surgical PV replacement
  Note—when intervention is required and anatomy suitable—balloon valvuloplasty is the preferred treatment option
- Indications for balloon valvotomy:
  - Asymptomatic
    Peak Gradient > 60 mmHg or mean > 40 mmHg and less than moderate PI
    Domed PV or dysplastic PV
  - Symptomatic
    Peak gradient > 50 mmHg or mean > 30 mmHg and less then moderate PI
    Domed PV or Dysplastic PV
- Indications for surgical pulmonic valve replacement:
  - Severe PS + either:
    Dysplastic PV, hypoplastic PV annulus, severe PI, infundibular/supravalvular PS

10.3.5 Differential Diagnosis

- Supravalvular pulmonic stenosis
  - Isolated area of narrowing at a main pulmonary artery or multiple areas of narrowing including at branches
  - RV pressure overload can be diagnosed by echo or catheterization
  - CT can localize the area of narrowing
  - Can occur in association with other congenital defects
- Subvalvular (infundibular) pulmonic stenosis
  - Primary fibromuscular thickening at the RVOT is rare; can be discrete or extensive
  - Secondary narrowing of the RVOT (due to RVH) is more common. If due to PS—typically regresses after correction of valvular lesion.
  - RVOT obstruction is a key feature in Tetralogy of Fallot
  - High subvalvular velocity over time can cause PV damage with secondary pulmonic regurgitation
  - In general, no post stenotic dilatation of PA is seen with subvalvular PS

10.4 Pulmonic Insufficiency (PI)

10.4.1 Etiology

Primary PI	Secondary PI
Acquired diseases: • Rheumatic disease • Endocarditis • Carcinoid Congenital disease Following surgical correction of congenital cardiac disease	Pulmonary artery dilatation from: • Pulmonary hypertension • Marfan's syndrome • Idiopathic PA dilation

- Trace to mild pulmonic insufficiency is seen in many normal individuals
- PI can be due to primary leaflet abnormalities or secondary to annular dilatation

10.4.2 Echocardiographic Assessment

Anatomic Assessment

1. 2D imaging: baseline anatomy of pulmonic valve—presence of leaflet abnormalities (e.g. flail, dysplastic cusps), mobility abnormalities, poor leaflet coaptation, vegetations.
2. Pulmonary artery size
3. Signs of hemodynamic effect of significant PI: RV dilatation, paradoxical septal motion with flattening of the septum (in diastole only or both systole and diastole)

Doppler Assessment

1. Jet width (relative to pulmonic valve annulus) and vena contracta
2. Jet density on CW Doppler
3. Jet deceleration slope
   - Steeper deceleration in more severe PI
4. Early termination of PI diastolic flow
   - PI envelope looks triangular due to rapid equilibration of PA and RV pressure
     Note: if RVEDP elevated from other causes, rapid equilibration of pressures can occur even without severe PI
5. Flow reversal in a branch PA
6. Increased forward flow across PV
   - Measured by PW Doppler VTI at RVOT compared to systemic flow
7. Regurgitant volume (RV) and fraction (RF)
   - Calculated by comparing flow in RVOT and LVOT (only if no shunts or AI)

10.4.3 Diagnostic Criteria

	Mild	Moderate	Severe
Jet size (at Nyquist limit 50–70 cm/s)	Thin, narrow	Intermediate	Broad Variable length
Jet width/ pulmonary annulus ratio			>0.7
Jet density/ contour	Faint	Dense	Dense/early termination
Deceleration time			<260 mSec
Pressure half time			<100 mSec
PI time/ diastole			<0.77
Flow reversal in branch PA			Prominent
Pulmonic systolic VTI	Slightly increased	Intermediate	Increased
RV size	Normal	Normal or dilated	Dilated

- Cardiac MRI is recommended to quantify PI and serially follow RV volume and function

10.4.4 Surveillance and Follow-Up

- Moderate or severe PI – TTE yearly, cardiac MRI periodically
- Earlier assessment for any change of symptoms

10.4.5 Management

Medical Treatment

- Asymptomatic, severe PI, normal RV—no treatment required
- Secondary PI—treatment of underlying cause
- Right heart failure with RV dysfunction (in patients who cannot undergo intervention)—medical therapy for right heart failure (e.g. diuretics, ACE inhibitors, digoxin) for symptoms control. No treatment has been shown to change prognosis of the disease.

Surgical Treatment

- Reserved for severe symptomatic PI

- Can be considered for asymptomatic patients with
  - RV dysfunction
  - Atrial/ventricular arrhythmias
  - Progressive TR
- Homograft is the valve of choice

Further Reading

Nishimura RA, Otto CM, Bonow RO, et al. 2014 AHA/ACC guideline for the management of patients with valvular heart disease: a report of the American College of Cardiology/American Heart Association Task Force on Practice Guidelines [published correction appears in J Thorac Cardiovasc Surg. 2014 Oct 21;64(16):1763. Dosage error in article text]. J Thorac Cardiovasc Surg. 2014;148(1):e1–e132. https://doi.org/10.1016/j.jtcvs.2014.05.014.

Nishimura RA, Otto CM, Bonow RO, et al. 2017 AHA/ACC focused update of the 2014 AHA/ACC Guideline for the management of patients with valvular heart disease: a report of the American College of Cardiology/American Heart Association task force on clinical practice guidelines. Circulation. 2017;135(25):e1159–95. https://doi.org/10.1161/CIR.0000000000000503.

Zoghbi WA, Adams D, Bonow RO, et al. Recommendations for noninvasive evaluation of native valvular regurgitation: a report from the American Society of Echocardiography developed in collaboration with the society for cardiovascular magnetic resonance. J Am Soc Echocardiogr. 2017;30(4):303–71. https://doi.org/10.1016/j.echo.2017.01.007.

Prosthetic Valves

11

Learning Objectives

- Recognize the various types of prosthetic valves and general principles of normal PHV function
- Learn the causes of prosthetic valve dysfunction, their echocardiographic evaluation and principles of management

General Considerations

1. Currently available prosthetic valves:
   (a) Surgically implanted valve
      - Mechanical valves:
        – Bi-leaflet and single tilting disc are currently used
        – Caged-ball valve has been discontinued however occasionally encountered on echo if implanted many years ago
      - Bioprosthetic valves
        – Stented valves
        – Stentless valves
        – Homografts and autografts (e.g. Ross procedure)
   (b) Percutaneous implanted valves
      - Balloon expandable valves (e.g. Edwards-Sapien valve)
      - Self expanding valves (e.g. Medtronic Evolut valve)
      - Likely more valve designs will become available to clinical use
2. Echocardiographic assessment PHVs is more demanding than native valves evaluation
3. Visualization may be compromised by artifacts
4. Discerning between normal and abnormal PHV may be difficult for several reasons:
   - All mechanical valves have some built-in regurgitation ("washing jets")
   - All PHVs have some degree of obstruction compared to native valves; normal PHV velocities are usually higher than native valves velocities

T. Rambhatla, G. Perk, *The Echocardiography Companion*,
https://doi.org/10.1007/978-3-030-47041-8_11

11.1 Echocardiographic Evaluation Post Valve Replacement

Follow up Echocardiogram

- Initial echo post op:
  - Purpose—"finger print" PHV so baseline hemodynamics are known
  - Should be done 2–6 weeks post operatively to allow for hemodynamic stabilization as well as chest wall edema to subside, pain to resolve etc.
  - Prosthetic valves often inherently have higher velocities due to smaller effective orifice area (EOA). During hospitalization and immediate post operative period, anemia or a hyper-adrenergic state can create even higher velocities and gradients
  - If patient is sent back to referring institution, initial post echo should be done pre-discharge
- Follow up echocardiograms:
  - Asymptomatic
    - For bioprosthetic valves—routine echo starting around 5 years post operatively
    - For mechanical valves—no routine echo indicated
  - Symptomatic
    - Follow up echo indicated for any change in symptoms, functional capacity, or new physical exam findings

11.2 Normal Echocardiographic Findings with PHV

- Physiologic regurgitation
  - There is a physiologic "signature" regurgitation seen in all mechanical prosthetic valves, due to the closing of leaflets, often producing a low velocity non turbulent jet, largest with bileaflet valve
  - Bioprosthetic valves may have just a central trace regurgitant jet
- Cavitation phenomenon ("bubbles")
  - Local pressure depression during the opening/closing of mechanical valves
  - Occurs with normally functioning valves, exact mechanism unknown, not artifact
- Pressure recovery phenomenon
  - Source of error with echo evaluation of PHV, usually seen with bi-leaflet mechanical valves
  - There can be a focal increase in velocity (often through the central orifice of bi-leaflet valves) which causes a local decrease in pressure
  - After exiting the valve, the velocity slows down and the pressure "recovers". However, since continuous wave Doppler records the highest pressure gradient along the path of the beam, the Doppler based gradient may be higher than that obtained by catheter based technique.
- Valve Size
  - The valve reference size is the outer ring diameter (not the annulus size, which is larger, and not the EOA which is smaller)

- Typical valve sizes range from 19 mm to 29 mm; expected EOA (cm^2) is larger as reference size increases
- Stented bioprosthetic valves generally have smaller EOA than stentless bioprosthetic valves
- Mechanical valves tend to have larger EOA compared to same size bioprosthetic valves

11.3 Anticoagulation Post Valve Replacement

Anticoagulation (AC) recommendation is with Coumadin; NOACs have not been tested yet.

	INR Goal	Antiplatelet
Aortic valve		
Mechanical	2.0–3.0	Asa 81 mg daily lifelong
+ risk factors for TE[a]	2.5–3.5[a]	
Bioprosthetic	Typically for first 2–3 months, INR goal 2–3	Asa 81 mg daily lifelong
TAVR	Often vendor/institution specific Trials ongoing comparing antiplatlet/anticoagulation strategies	
Mitral valve		
Mechanical	2.5–3.5	Asa 81 mg daily lifelong
+ risk factors for TE[a]	3.0–4.0[a]	
Bioprosthetic/MV repair	Typically first 2–3 month, INR goal 3	Asa 81 mg daily lifelong

TE Thromboembolism
[a]Risk factors—atrial fibrillation, previous episode of TE, low EF, hypercoagulable state

Bridging for Non-Cardiac Procedures

- Bridging AC is probably not required for modern bi-leaflet tiling disk mechanical AVs; in general, AC can be held for 3–4 days pre-procedure and restarted as soon as possible
- Bridging with heparin or LMWH is required pre- and post-procedure:
  - Non-modern bi-leaflet tilting disk mechanical AV
  - Mechanical MV
  - Right sided mechanical valve
  - Recent TE (within one year)
  - Previous TE while off AC
  - History of AF, EF < 30%, or hypercoagulable state

11.4 PHV Complications

- Obstruction/stenosis
  - Can occur either due to thrombus or pannus formation
  - Thrombus
    - More common in mechanical valves
    - Thrombosis of TV is 20× more common > MV 2× > AV
    - Onset may be acute or delayed
    - Physical Exam—change or loss of the mechanical click
    - Requires STAT diagnosis and treatment (heparin, possibly fibrinolytics, surgery)
    - Diagnosis with TEE (can be limited due to shadowing artifact) or fluoroscopy
  - Pannus: fibrous ingrowth at the suture ring caused by an Inflammatory host vs. valve reaction
    - Distinguished from thrombus by: smaller size, more dense and echogenic, less mobile
    - More common in AV > MV
    - Diagnosis with CT or TEE
- Thromboembolism
  - Most commonly due to inadequate anticoagulation of mechanical valves
  - Rare with bioprosthetic valves
- Structural valve deterioration (SVD)
  - Most frequent complication of bioprosthetic valves

  - Wear and tear damage, sheer stress, mechanical factors, and calcifications can cause either stenosis and/or regurgitation
  - More common in younger patients, those prone to calcification (renal failure, diabetes)
- Infective Endocarditis (IE)
  - Similar rates in mechanical and bioprosthetic valves
    - Mechanical valve IE is usually due to seeding of the sewing ring-annulus junction and may be complicated by paravalvular leak or paravalvular abscess (usually vegetations not attached to leaflet discs)
    - Bioprosthetic IE may have both valve vegetations and/or sewing ring vegetations
- Valve Dehiscence
  - Complication of prosthetic valve IE, often have PVL
  - If there is ≥40% dehiscence, a "rocking motion" of the valve can be seen (excursion >15° during cardiac cycle)
- Paravalvular abscess
  - Typically requires TEE for diagnosis
    - 2D: visualize thickening around the valve and adjacent tissues
    - Color Doppler: flow can be seen in and out of thickened area
  - Urgent CT surgery is commonly indicated
  - Aortic root abscess can cause conduction abnormalities, heart block
- Paravalvular Leak (PVL)
  - Regurgitation between the sewing ring and the annulus due to an incomplete seal
  - Early onset PVL—due to technical aspects of the surgical technique
  - Late onset PVL—due to suture dehiscence, suspect IE
  - Regurgitant jet is often eccentric and hard to diagnose; requires a high index of suspicion (i.e. audible murmur but no evidence on TTE, need TEE to diagnose)
  - Can cause hemolysis (due to sheer stress on RBC) and heart failure (may be worsened by hemolysis)
- LVOT obstruction
  - Can occur with high profile MV prosthesis
  - More common in smaller LV cavities (i.e. LVH, septal knuckle)
- Patient prosthetic mismatch (PPM)
  - Properly functioning valve without stenosis however too small for patient size, causes elevated gradients across the PHV
  - Diagnosed by EOA index < 0.85 cm^2/m^2 (EOAi = EOA/BSA)
    - Desirable EOAi > 0.85
    - Moderate PPM < 0.85
    - Severe PPM < 0.65

11.5 Prosthetic Aortic Valve Assessment

11.5.1 Prosthetic Aortic Valve: Increased Gradient

Increased gradients across a PHV can be due to:

1. Obstruction of the PHV (thrombosis, pannus, SVD, IE)
2. Increased flow through a normal PHV (high flow state, PHV regurgitation, PPM)

Effective orifice area of prosthetic heart valve

$$\text{EOA} = \frac{LVOT_{VTI} \times LVOT\ area}{PrV_{VTI}}$$

- Parameters to differentiate between various etiologies: (Fig. 11.1, Table 11.1)
  - Jet contour
  - Acceleration time (AT) through the AV
  - Dimensionless index (DI)

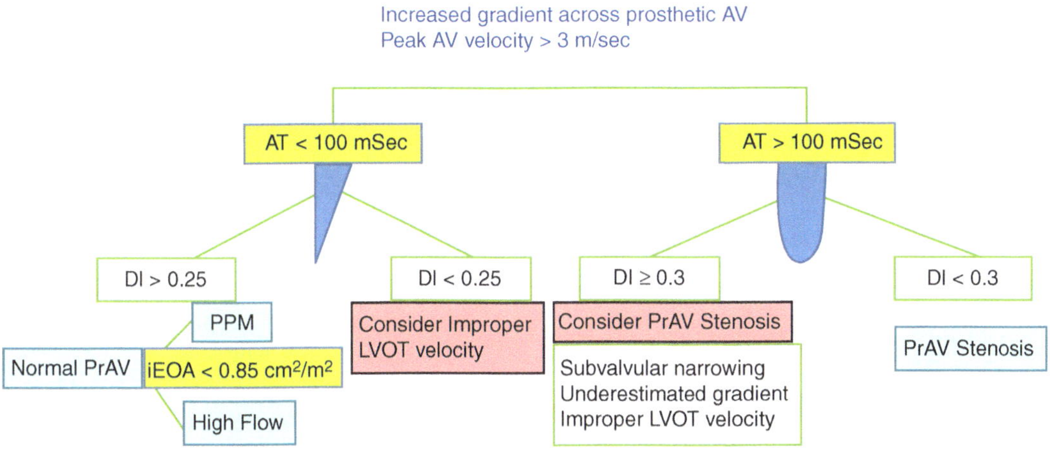

Fig. 11.1 Evaluation of Increased gradient across prosthetic aortic valve. *AT acceleration time, DI dimensionless index, iEOA indexed effective orifice area, LVOT left ventricular outflow tract, PrAV prosthetic aortic valve, PPM patient prosthesis mismatch*

Table 11.1 Echo parameters for prosthetic aortic valve stenosis

	Normal	Possible stenosis	Significant stenosis
Peak velocity (m/s)	<3	3–4	>4
Mean gradient (mmHg)	<20	20–35	>35
DI	≥0.30	0.29–0.25	<0.25
EOA (cm^2)	>1.2	0.8–1.2	<0.8
Jet contour	Triangular, early peaking	Triangular to intermediate	Rounded, symmetrical
AT (ms)	*<80*	*80–100*	*>100*

DI Dimensionless index, *EOA* effective orifice area, *AT* acceleration time

11.5.2 Prosthetic Aortic Valve: Regurgitation

Prosthetic valve regurgitation may be more challenging to image due to acoustic shadowing from the prosthesis

- Often requires both TTE and TEE with integrating off axis views, and Doppler parameters that are not influenced by acoustic shadowing (i.e. pressure half time, diastolic flow reversal, etc.)
- It is also crucial to differentiate transvalvular from paravalvular regurgitation – different complications and therapeutic options
  - On TTE, the PSAX view is helpful to localize and define extent of PVL

	Mild	Moderate	Severe
Jed width (%LVOT D)	≤25%	26–64%	≥65%
Jet density	Incomplete/ faint	Dense	Dense
RV (mL)	<30	30–59	≥60
Flow reversal in descAo	No/brief in early diastole	Intermediate	Holodiastolic
LVOT:RVOT flow	~ or ⇑	⇑⇑	⇑⇑⇑

11.6 Prosthetic Mitral Valve Assessment

Comprehensive assessment of prosthetic mitral valve (ProMV) requires both TTE (which is better for assessing LV function) and TEE (provides good visualization of the left atrium and regurgitation, but may be limited for the evaluation of the LV due to acoustic shadowing).

11.6.1 Prosthetic Mitral Valve: Increased Gradient

Increased gradients across ProMV may be due to same etiologies as seen in ProAV

1. Obstruction of the PHV (thrombosis, pannus, SVD, IE)
2. Increased flow through a normal PHV (high flow state, PHV regurgitation, PPM)

	Normal	Possible stenosis	Significant stenosis
Peak Velocity (m/s)	<1.9	1.9–2.5	≥2.5
Mean gradient (mmHg)	≤5	6–10	>10
PHT (mS)	<130	130–200	>200
EOA (cm²)	≥2.0	1–2	<1
VTI ProMV: LVOT	<2.2	2.2–2.5	>2.5

Note: EOA—must use the continuity equation for calculation (PHT method not accurate or validated in PHV)

- Parameters to differentiate between various etiologies: (Fig. 11.2)
  - Peak velocity in early diastole and mean MV gradient (with HR)
  - Pressure half time (cutoff for elevated: ≥ 130 ms)
  - VTI ratio

$$\text{ProMV VTI ratio} = \frac{MV\ inflow\ VTI}{LVOT\ outflow\ VTI}$$

    Note: Different than the AV VTI ratio (or DI) – which is the ratio of the flow proximal to the aortic valve and the flow at the valve (same valve)
    Cutoff for elevated: >2.2
  - In addition: pulmonary artery pressure, extent of regurgitation

11.6.2 Prosthetic Mitral Valve: Regurgitation

Detection and quantification of ProMR may be difficult with TTE, particularly with mechanical valves. May need high index of suspicion and indirect clues:

- Peak mitral inflow velocity ≥ 1.9 m/s, mean inflow gradient ≥5 mmHg, short PHT/DT
- Max TR jet velocity > 3 m/s
- Hyperdynamic LV with low LVOT SV
  - Elevated MV inflow VTI: LVOT VTI >2.2
  - 2D based stroke volume greater by >30% as compared to SV calculated by LVOT Doppler
- Large systolic flow convergence in LV towards MV prosthesis

TEE is much more sensitive and specific than TTE and allows for:

- Imaging the MV in multiple planes
- Differentiating physiologic from pathologic regurgitation
- Differentiating valvular vs. paravalvular regurgitation
- Identifying and localizing origin of a PVL

The most accurate assessment of ProMR severity is achieved by combining TTE and TEE parameters.

	Mild	Moderate	Severe
Vena contracta (cm)	<0.3	0.3–0.59	≥0.6
RV (mL)	<30	30–59	≥60
RF (%)	<30	30–49	≥50
EROA (cm²)	<0.20	0.20–0.49	≥0.50
Color jet area (%LA)	<20	20–39	≥40
Jet density/ contour	Faint/ parabolic	Dense/ parabolic	Dense/early peak triangular
PV flow	S > D	Systolic blunting	Systolic reversal

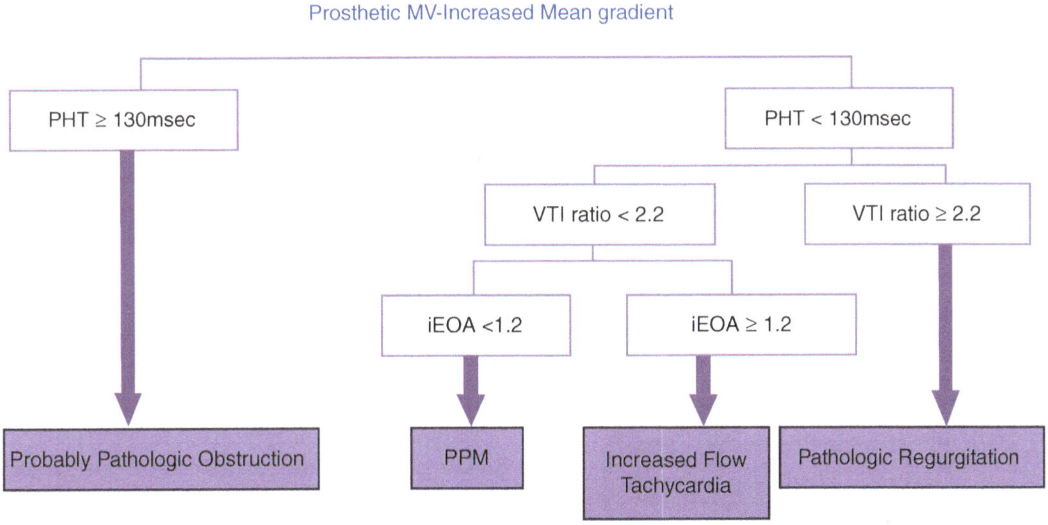

Fig. 11.2 Evaluation of increased gradient across prosthetic mitral valve. *iEOA indexed effective orifice area index, PHT pressure half time, VTI velocity time integral, PPM patient prosthesis mismatch*

11.7 Prosthetic Tricuspid Valve Assessment

- The anterior location of the TV generally allows for adequate visualization and assessment by TTE in the parasternal, apical, and subcostal views.
- When needed, additional imaging with TEE is also recommended.
  Note: due to respiratory variation, Doppler measurements should be averaged over 5 cardiac cycles

11.7.1 Prosthetic Tricuspid Valve: Increased Gradient

- Obstruction may be observed by:
  - 2D imaging—thickened restricted leaflets
  - color Doppler—narrowed and turbulent inflow
- ProV Tricuspid Stenosis is suggested with:
  - E inflow V_{max} > 1.7 m/s
  - Mean gradient ≥ 6 mmHg
  - PHT ≥ 230 ms

11.7.2 Prosthetic Tricuspid Valve: Regurgitation

	Mild	Moderate	Severe
Valve structure	Normal	Abnormal/dehisced	Abnormal/dehisced
Jet area (cm^2)	<5	5–10	>10
Vena contracta (cm)	Not defined	<0.7	≥0.7
Jet density/contour	Faint, parabolic	Dense, variable	Dense, early peak
Hepatic flow	Normal	Blunted	Holosystolic reversal
RA, RV, IVC	Normal	Dilated	Markedly dilated

11.8 Prosthetic Pulmonic Valve Assessment

- The PV can be visualized in the PSAX view at the basal (AV) level on TTE
- The pulmonary valve can be difficult to assess with either TTE and TEE because of its anterior/superior location; in addition, the eccentric shape of the RVOT makes diameter measurements difficult and inaccurate.

11.8.1 Prosthetic Pulmonic Valve: Increased Gradient

- ProPV stenosis does not have well defined criteria, but should be suspected when there is:
  - Peak velocity > 3 m/s (>2 m/s through a homograft)
  - Increasing peak velocity on serial studies
  - Cusp / leaflet thickening or immobility
  - Elevated RVSP or decreased RV systolic function

11.8.2 Prosthetic Pulmonic Valve: Regurgitation

	Mild	Moderate	Severe
Jet with (% PA)	≤25%	26–50%	>50%
Jet density	Faint	Dense	Dense
DT	Slow	Variable	Steep early termination of diastolic flow
PA flow reversal	None	Present	present
VTI RVOT: LVOT	~ or ⇑	⇑⇑	⇑⇑⇑

Significant ProPV regurgitation—evidence of RV volume overload:

- Dilated RV
- Paradoxical septal flattening

Further Reading

Singh M, Sporn ZA, Schaff HV, Pellikka PA. ACC/AHA versus ESC guidelines on prosthetic heart valve management: JACC Guideline comparison. J Am Coll Cardiol. 2019;73(13):1707–18. https://doi.org/10.1016/j.jacc.2019.01.038.

Zoghbi WA, Adams D, Bonow RO, et al. Recommendations for noninvasive evaluation of native valvular regurgitation: A report from the American Society of Echocardiography Developed in Collaboration with the Society for Cardiovascular Magnetic Resonance. J Am Soc Echocardiogr. 2017;30(4):303–71. https://doi.org/10.1016/j.echo.2017.01.007.

Cardiomyopathies

12

Learning Objectives

- To learn the causes, evaluation, and management of Hypertrophic Cardiomyopathy (HCM).
- To learn the causes, evaluation, and management of Restrictive Cardiomyopathy (RCM)
- To learn the causes and evaluation of Dilated Cardiomyopathy (DCM).
- Briefly review other miscellaneous cardiomyopathies.

General Indications for Echocardiography in Cardiomyopathies

- Initial evaluation of known or suspected cardiomyopathy (DMC, HCM, RCM)
- Re-evaluation of known cardiomyopathy with a change in clinical status, exam, or to guide medication/therapy changes
- Routine surveillance ≥1 year of known cardiomyopathy without change in status

12.1 Hypertrophic Cardiomyopathy (HCM)

12.1.1 Definition

Unexplained left ventricular hypertrophy (LVH) in a non-dilated ventricle without a history of hypertension or other cardiac or systemic disease that could cause the observed LVH

- Left ventricular wall thickness ≥ 15 mm is generally considered the cutoff
- Wall thickness 13–15 mm is referred to as borderline; may be diagnostic in patients with family member with HCM
- Note: genotype positive, phenotype negative (and phenotype borderline) HCM patients need to be followed closely with serial echocardiograms to assess for phenotypic presentation

12.1.2 Etiology

HCM is caused by gene mutations in the cardiac sarcomere

- >200 mutations in >10 genes have been identified to cause HCM
- Usually—autosomal dominant inheritance pattern

Electronic supplementary material The online version of this chapter (https://doi.org/10.1007/978-3-030-47041-8_12) contains supplementary material, which is available to authorized users.

T. Rambhatla, G. Perk, *The Echocardiography Companion*,
https://doi.org/10.1007/978-3-030-47041-8_12

12.1.3 HCM Mimics and Differential Diagnosis

- Systemic disorders that can present as HCM (5–10% of cases)
  - Friedrich's Ataxia—90% have cardiac involvement
  - Noonan's Syndrome—15–20% have cardiac involvement
  - Lysosomal Storage Diseases
    Danon disease
    Anderson-Fabry's disease
    Pompei's disease
- Infiltrative diseases: Amyloid, Sarcoid, Hemochromatosis
- Endomyocardial fibrosis (mimics apical HCM)
- Hypertensive cardiomyopathy
- Severe aortic stenosis
- Athlete's Heart
  - There are echocardiographic and clinical criteria to help make this very important distinction (Fig. 12.1)
  - Often requires further investigation (i.e.: MRI for scar/LGE, telemetry monitoring for NSVT, thorough family history, genetic testing etc.)
  - A helpful distinguishing criterion is the observed response to deconditioning
    Athletes heart should have a decrease in LV wall thickness after training cessation (<6 months) vs. no effect on patients with HCM
- Sigmoid septum or 'septal knuckle'-Isolated basal septal hypertrophy
  - Observed with increased frequency in elderly individuals; may occur as part of the cardiac remodeling associated with aging
  - HCM can still be diagnosed with this configuration, but is less commonly associated with a gene mutation
    Note: these age-related geometric changes with increased angulation between the aorta and LV cavity can result in provokable LVOT obstruction

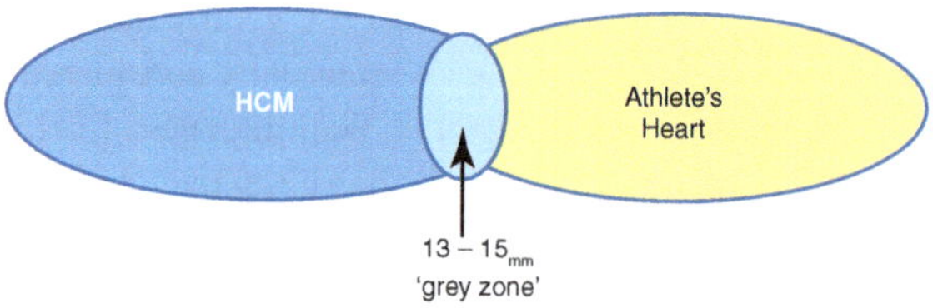

HCM	PARAMETER	ATHLETE'S HEART
>15mm	LV thickness	<13mm
Asymmetric / unusual	LVH pattern	Concentric
Reduced	LV cavity size	Increased
< 45mm	LVEDD	>55mm
Impaired relaxation	Diastolic function	Normal
Reduced	MV e'	Increased
Abnormal / bizarre QRS / T	ECG	Mostly normal

Fig. 12.1 **Hypertrophic cardiomyopathy vs. Athlete's heart**. *ECG electrocardiogram, HCM hypertrophic cardiomyopathy, LV left ventricle, LVH left ventricular hypertrophy, LVEDD left ventricular end diastolic dimension, MV mitral valve*

12.1.4 HCM Morphologic Variants (Fig. 12.2)

- Septal predominance HCM
  - Asymmetric hypertrophy most pronounced in the basal anteroseptal wall
  - Most common variant ~50% of HCM patients; low genetic prevalence ~10%
  - The variant most likely to have resting or provokable LVOT obstruction
- Reverse curve/mid ventricular HCM
  - Convex septal hypertrophy most pronounced in the mid-septal wall
  - 30% of HCM cases; high genetic prevalence ~80%
  - Often seen in younger patients and with RV involvement
  - Less likely to have a resting LVOT gradient; some may have provokable LVOT obstruction
  - May have a higher incidence of aneurysm formations, which carries a higher risk of ventricular arrhythmias and sudden cardiac death (SCD)
- Apical HCM (Fig. 12.3, Videos 12.1A and 12.1B)
  - 10% of HCM cases worldwide; 15–25% of cases in Japan, 3% of HCM cases in the United States
  - LVH $\geq$ 15 mm; most pronounced at the apical segments of the LV and true apex
  - Frequently missed on 2D echo alone; often requires contrast echo or cardiac MRI for diagnosis
  - ECG—large negative T waves across the precordium (seen in ~93% of cases); ECG manifestations may precede overt hypertrophy seen on echo
  - The apical variant was once believed to carry a lower mortality; outcomes however similar to classic HCM
- Neutral Septum
  - Symmetric hypertrophy of the basal, mid, and apical septum (concentric LVH)
  - 8% of cases

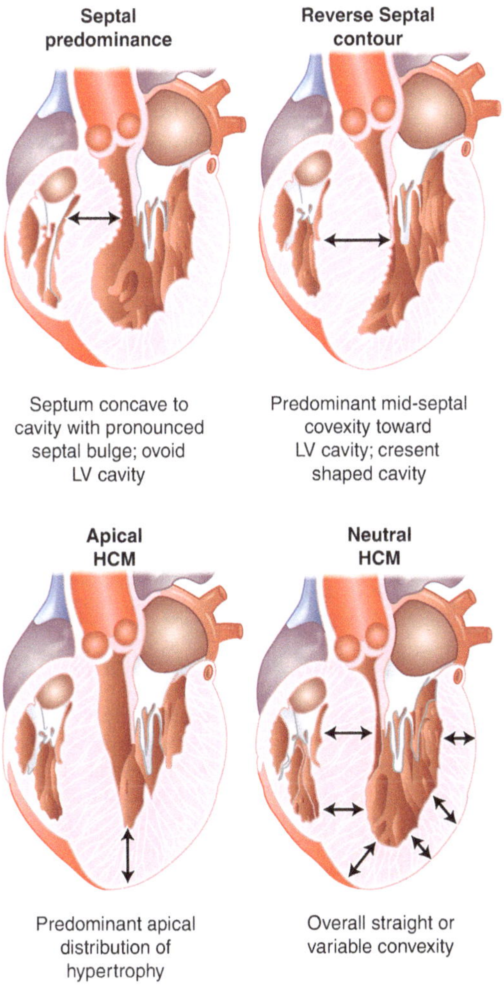

Fig. 12.2 **Morphologic variants of hypertrophic cardiomyopathy**

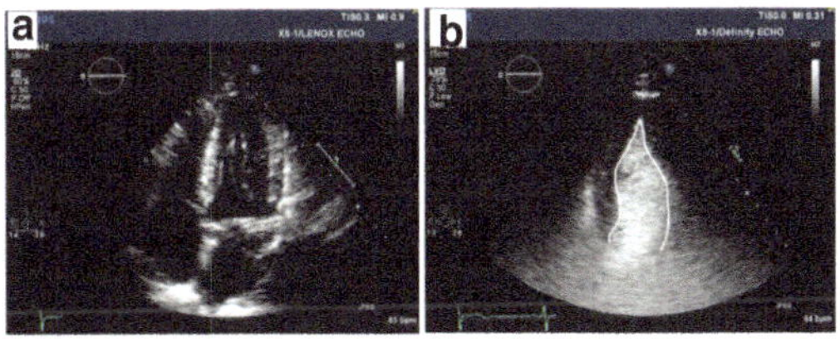

Fig. 12.3 **Apical hypertrophic cardiomyopathy**. (**a**) Systolic frame from 2D apical four chamber view (**b**) corresponding contrast enhanced image of apical hypertrophic cardiomyopathy (HCM). Note the typical "spade shaped" heart seen with contrast enhancement. In addition to clearly delineating the hypertrophic apical segments of the LV, contrast enhancement is important to rule out apical aneurysm, which are common with this variant (not present on this example)

12.1.5 Echocardiographic Assessment

Anatomic Assessment

1. M-Mode of AV (Fig. 12.4a)
   - With LVOT obstruction → mid-systolic closure of AV can be seen
   - Correlates with the palpable bisferiens pulse—rapid pulse upstroke from quick acceleration prior to development of LVOT obstruction, then loss of forward flow due to LVOT obstruction, followed by resumption of forward flow.
2. M-mode of MV (Fig. 12.4b)
   - Systolic anterior motion of the mitral valve (SAM) → allows assessment of degree and duration of leaflet-septal contact
3. 2D imaging:
   - LV wall thickness; septal hypertrophy relative to posterior wall; visualize apex

     Echo contrast should be used for apical variants and for diagnosis of apical aneurysms that may occur with all morphologic variants
   - LV volume and function assessment—typically LV systolic function is preserved; LV volumes may be low
   - Mitral Valve assessment

     Premature/increased mitral annular calcifications seen commonly

     Redundant/myxomatous/elongated MV leaflets are common

     Papillary muscle abnormalities

     Visualization of SAM of the anterior mitral leaflet

Doppler Assessment

1. LVOT Jet (Fig. 12.5)
   - Late peaking systolic jet (for high velocities, CW Doppler assessment necessary)

     LVOT gradient is dynamic—time required for enough pressure generation and LVOT narrowing to create the gradient → late peaking

     Careful attention required when imaging with Doppler to try and separate from MR jet and potential other systolic jets (e.g. AS, systolic cavity obliteration)

     If no resting SAM or LVOT obstruction → provoking maneuvers required (e.g. Valsalva)
2. MR Jet
   - Typically - MR in HCM is due to incomplete coaptation from SAM resulting in a posterolateraly directed jet

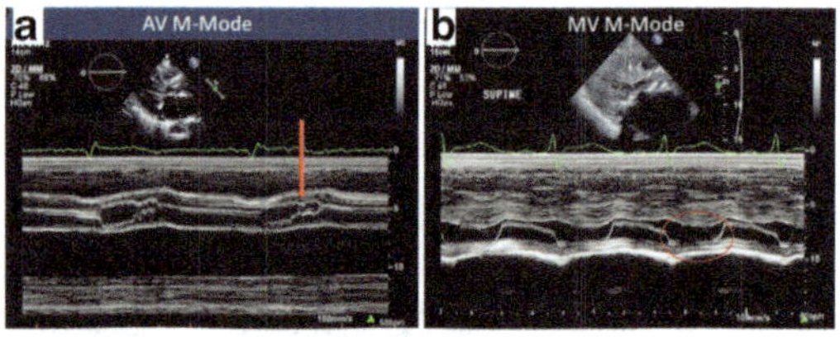

Fig. 12.4 **M Mode in hypertrophic obstructive cardiomyopathy**. (**a**) M-mode of the aortic valve shows mid-systolic partial closure of the valve (red arrow), secondary to left ventricular outflow tract (LVOT) obstruction. (**b**) M Mode of the mitral valve shows systolic anterior (SAM) motion of the mitral valve during mid-systole (red circle); note the extent of the SAM on this example—the anterior leaflet reaches all the way to the septum and maintains leaflet-septal contact for most of systole—these findings suggest hemodynamically significant LVOT obstruction

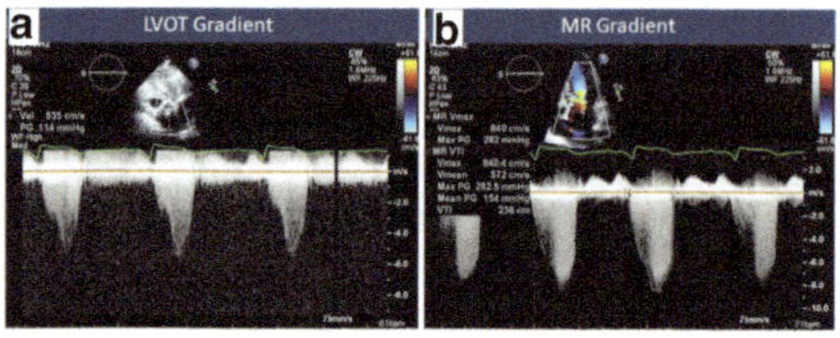

Fig. 12.5 **Spectral Doppler in hypertrophic obstructive cardiomyopathy**. (**a**) Continuous wave (CW) Doppler of dynamic LVOT obstruction showing the typical late-peaking contour. Peak velocity of 5.4 m/s corresponds to peak LVOT gradient of 114 mmHg. (**b**) CW of the corresponding mitral regurgitation (MR) jet. The MR jet contour has a more rounded appearance and peak velocity is higher (8.4 m/s). Note: MR jet velocity is ALWAYS higher than LVOT velocity as the gradient between LV and left atrium is higher than between LV and aorta

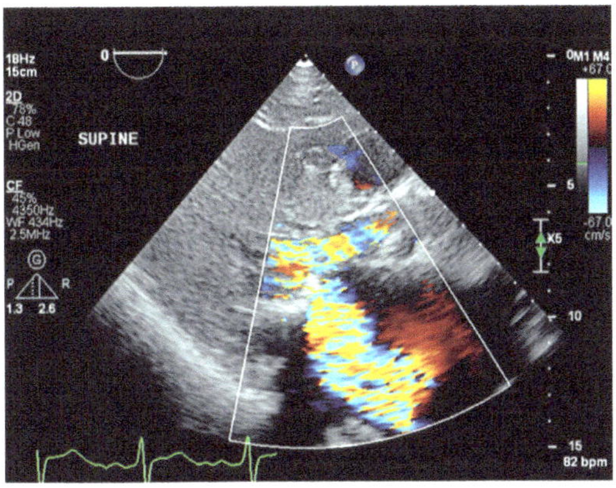

Fig. 12.6 **Crossed swords in hypertrophic obstructive cardiomyopathy**. The typical "crossed swords" appearance created by the turbulent LVOT color flow, which appears perpendicular to the posterolaterally directed mitral regurgitation jet

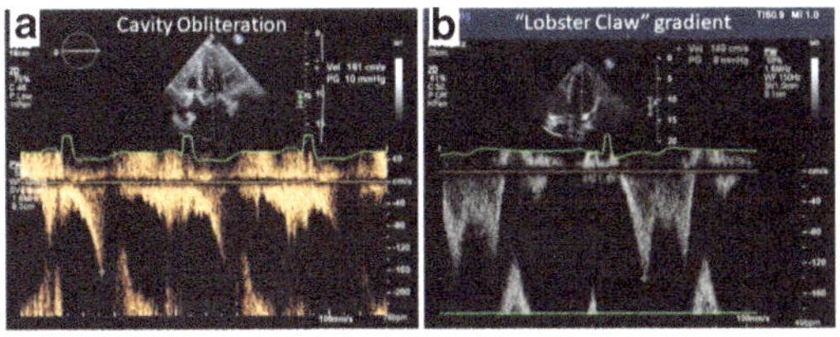

Fig. 12.7 **Mid cavity obliteration**. Mid-cavity systolic obstruction is typically seen with apical hypertrophic cardiomyopathy and produces a very late peaking, 'stalactite' jet contour. (**a**) The peak of the jet is even later than the typical left ventricular outflow tract obstruction. (**b**) Occasionally, with severe cavity obliteration, a 'lobster claw' jet contour occurs; short initial systolic forward flow → mid-systolic deceleration and blood trapping in the apex → early diastolic forward flow of the "trapped" volume

Note: direction of the jet is inadequate criteria by which to judge for presence or absence of intrinsic mitral valve disease

- Classic "crossed swords" can be seen—MR jet perpendicular to turbulent flow in LVOT (Fig. 12.6, Video 12.2)

3. Mid-cavity obstruction (Fig. 12.7)
   - Different than LVOT obstruction
   - Typically seen with apical HCM; can be seen with other variants as well
   - Occurs at the end of systole; produces very late peaking, 'stalactite' like jet (typically peak is later than in LVOT obstruction)
   - If severe obstruction/obliteration → short initial forward flow, mid-systolic decrease in ejection velocity, blood trapping in the apex, and forward flow of trapped blood during diastole ("lobster claw" configuration)

12.1.6 Pathophysiology of HCM, SAM, LVOTO, and MR

- LVOT obstruction develops as a result of systolic anterior motion of the mitral valve with mid-systolic leaflet-septum contact.
- The morphologic changes that predispose to SAM and LVOT obstruction include:
  - Septal hypertrophy with narrowed LVOT diameter and increased angulation, which changes the direction and velocity of blood flow through the LVOT
  - Apical displacement of the papillary muscles
  - Elongated anterior mitral valve leaflet
- High velocity blood enters the narrowed LVOT during systole
- Drag forces/Venturi effect act on the mitral valve leaflets causing movement of the leaflet into the LVOT → LVOT obstruction and often MR
- Severity of MR depends on various anatomic characteristics
  - For example: restricted posterior leaflet that cannot move anteriorly with the anterior leaflet results in more severe MR
  - In general there is a correlation between LVOT obstruction and MR severity.
- LVOT obstruction can develop under certain hemodynamic conditions, without underlying HCM:
  - Sigmoid septum ('septal knuckle'), HTN, severe AS – worsened by volume depletion or hypercontractility
  - Hypercontractile states (e.g. sepsis on vasopressors with B1 activity, during dobutamine stress echo)
  - Antero-apical MI with increased basal contractility
  - Takotsubo with hypercontractile basal segments
  - Post MV repair/replacement/TMVR

12.1.7 HCM Physiologic Variants: Obstructive and Non-Obstructive

Hemodynamic classification	Resting LVOT gradient	Provoked LVOT gradient
Basal obstructive	≥ 30 mmHg	↑↑ ≥30 mmHg
Labile (latent) obstructive	<30 mmHg	≥ 30 mmHg
Non-obstructive	<30 mmHg	<30 mmHg

- Apical HCM always causes non-obstructive HCM
- The morphologic variant most likely to produce obstructive HCM is septal predominance

12.1.8 Clinical Manifestations

Patients may present with:
- Clinical symptoms (see below)
- Asymptomatic (discovered during family screening)
- Murmur detected during routine examination
- Abnormal ECG on routine exam
  - Large voltage, often large Q waves in the lateral leads, tall R waves in V1–V2
  - Apical HCM—classic deep T wave inversions across entire pericardium

Common clinical symptoms:
- Dyspnea on exertion—can be due to:
  - Diastolic dysfunction
  - LVOT obstruction
  - Mitral regurgitation
  - Systolic dysfunction (in advanced cases)
- Chest pain—classic angina or atypical chest pain
  - Exertional chest pain can occur despite normal coronaries—due to:
    Increased oxygen demand (myocyte hypertrophy, increased muscle mass)
    Increased wall stress due to elevated diastolic pressures
    Microvascular disease
    Reduced vasodilator reserve
- Arrhythmias—may present with palpitations, pre/syncope, dyspnea
  - Ventricular arrhythmias—mechanisms:
    Ischemia induced
    Scar related—Progression of supply-demand mismatch → infarct/fibrosis → scar
  - Supraventricular arrhythmias
    20% of HCM patients develop AF, portends a worse prognosis compared to NSR (4× higher mortality rate)
    Tolerated very poorly hemodynamically (due to compromised diastolic function and significant hemodynamic sensitivity to losing atrial kick)
    There is also an increased incidence of WPW in HCM patients
- Syncope or pre-syncope—can occur due to:
  - Arrhythmias
  - LVOT obstruction
  - Exaggerated baroreflex with significant vasodilatation
    25% of HCM patients have autonomic dysfunction with abnormal nervous system response to exercise with vasodilation/bradycardia/LVOT obstruction

12.1.9 Management

Medical Therapies

- Avoid afterload reducing agents if possible
- Maintain adequate preload—avoid diuretics if possible
- Decrease contractility with negative inotropes—beta blockers, calcium channel blockers, Disopyramide
- Avoid ethanol—can increase LVOT gradient

Surgical Myectomy

- Indications:
  - Persistent symptoms despite maximal medical management (including heart failure with NYHA III/IV, chest pain, or syncope related to hemodynamic compromise from LVOT obstruction)
  - LVOT gradient ≥50 mmHg
  - Anterior septal thickness sufficient for safely performing the procedure (otherwise risk of post op VSD)
- Preoperative and intra-operative echo guidance is crucial:
  - Measuring and guiding to septal area with max thickness (note—surgical visualization may be limited as surgery performed through aortic valve)
  - Identification of MV abnormalities
  - Assessing results and elimination of LVOT obstruction.
- Occasionally mitral valve surgery is required in addition to myectomy (e.g. when septal thickness not excessive and elongated anterior leaflet is the main contributor to SAM and LVOT obstruction)

Alcohol Septal Ablation

- Less invasive treatment option for properly selected patients
- Procedure: injection of alcohol into septal perforator branch of the left anterior descending artery in attempt to create localized infarct at the base of the antero-septum
- Echo guidance is essential:
  - Once the septal perforator is cannulated, echo contrast is injected into the artery (utilizing a balloon catheter to prevent back flow of the echo contrast)
  - Distribution of echo contrast within the myocardium (visualized by continuous echocardiographic imaging) represents the territory to be infarcted once alcohol is injected.
  - Echo should confirm limited vascular distribution, at the area of maximal septal thickness, and no opacification of other area (e.g. right ventricle, extensive anterior wall distribution)
  - Post alcohol injection, echo confirms reduction in septal thickness, elimination of SAM and resolution of LVOT gradient
- Should not be done if septum >30 mm due to uncertain effectiveness
- Complicated by complete heart block in 10–25% of cases

Factors influencing the decision between surgical and catheter based treatment include anatomical considerations, comorbidities, concomitant cardiac problems, local expertise and patient preference.

ICD

- Prevention of SCD is an important aspect of treatment of patients with HCM
- Those patients with HCM who have not yet met criteria for an ICD, should be re-evaluated on a Q1–2 year basis for eligibility

Dual Chamber/Biventricular Pacing

- In general—no longer practiced
- Patients with PPM previously implanted for other indications may undergo a trial of RV apical pacing
- Currently, PPM implantation for LVOT obstruction/MR relief is not recommended when other forms of therapy are available
- At this time, insufficient data exists regarding the use of biventricular pacing for relief of LVOT obstruction

12.1.10 Screening

Serial echoes for clinically unaffected first degree relatives recommended

- Q12–18 months for children/adolescents/high risk families
- Q5 years for adults

12.2 Restrictive Cardiomyopathy (RCM)

12.2.1 Definition

A group of myocardial disorders with diastolic dysfunction resulting in restrictive filling, diastolic pressure overload, and severe biatrial enlargement; diastolic volumes are normal or reduced and systolic function is generally preserved.

12.2.2 Etiology

Primary RCM

- Idiopathic or Familial
- Age of onset 20–30 yrs. of age, present with congestion, embolic events, SCD
- Management is symptomatic relief of congestion
- Transplant is the only treatment, poor prognosis

Secondary RCM

Infiltrative Diseases
- Amyloid
  - The most common cause of RCM in the US
  - Four types:
    Senile—age related accumulation of Transthyretin protein
    AL—light chain protein accumulation (70% of cases do not have multiple myeloma)
    Familial/Genetic—Transthyretin mutation (treatment is liver transplantation)
    AA—secondary amyloid due to chronic inflammation and accumulation of acute phase proteins
- Sarcoid (more commonly causes DCM)
- Hemochromatosis (more commonly causes DCM)

Endomyocardial Fibrosis
- Tropical
  - Most common cause of RCM worldwide; endemic to tropical areas (central Africa, Brazil, India). Suspected etiology is infectious/environmental.
- Leofflers
  - Hypereosinophillic syndrome: >1500 Eosinophils >6 months (other causes for eosinophilia excluded)
- Echo findings—both can mimic apical HCM or apical thrombus (but do not have the associated wall motion abnormalities that are the usual risk factors for apical thrombi)
  - Can also have associated fibrosis of the RV and subvalvular apparatus (→ MR or TR)

Other Causes
- Storage Diseases
  - Fabry's Disease—"Binary appearance"
  - Danon's, Noonan's, Pompe's

- Radiation—post mediastinal radiation therapy
  - RV more involved than LV
  - Can also cause conduction abnormalities, premature CAD, valve disease, constrictive pericarditis

12.2.3 Clinical Manifestations

- Congestion/Heart Failure
  - In AL amyloidosis albumin may be low due to nephrotic syndrome, further worsening volume overload
- Exertional Syncope
  - Bad prognostic sign
- Pericardial disease
  - Less prone to tamponade, even with large effusions because of high ventricular stiffness and pressure

- Stroke and atrial fibrillation
  - Elevated cardiac pressures and severe biatrial enlargement and dysfunction → high rates of intracardiac thrombus formation
    Note: thrombi can form even in sinus rhythm
- Sudden cardiac death
- In cardiac amyloid, ICD does not improve survival—SCD often from PEA

12.2.4 Echocardiographic Assessment

Anatomic Assessment

1. Normal sized ventricles (wall thickness depends on etiology)
2. Generally Preserved EF (reduced EF may be seen at end stage)
3. Biatrial enlargement, often severe; atria can be larger than the ventricles
   - Amyloidosis (Fig. 12.8, Video 12.3)
     - Granular sparkly appearance (although not specific with harmonic imaging)
     - Thickened valves and interatrial septum
     - Small pericardial effusion
     - Strain imaging—basal segments effected with apical sparing ("cherry on top" pattern)

Doppler Assessment

1. Restrictive Filling Pattern

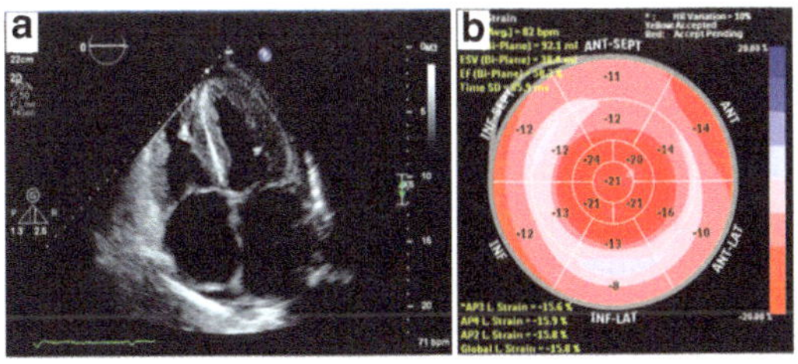

Fig. 12.8 **Cardiac amyloidosis.** (**a**) Apical four-chamber view showing bi-ventricular thickened, 'sparkly', granular myocardium, biatrial enlargement, thickened valves, and a small pericardial effusion. (**b**) Strain imaging typically shows diminished longitudinal strain with apical sparing ("cherry on top" pattern)

- Increased mitral E velocity—high atrial pressure
- Decreased A velocity—due to high ventricular end diastolic pressure, atrial contraction does not contribute much
- Markedly increased E/A ratio > 2.0
- Short deceleration time (DT < 160 ms)—rapid equilibration of pressures of LA/LV
- Decreased isovolumic relaxation time (IVRT < 70 ms)—MV opens early because of higher LAP
- Low TDI mitral e' velocities—myocardial relaxation is significantly impaired, out of proportion to observed ejection fraction
- Hepatic and pulmonary vein flow—systolic velocity is less than diastolic velocity (S < D)
- Increase in hepatic vein inspiratory diastolic flow reversal

2. Low TDI mitral S′ velocities (S′ < 5 cm/s, from the septal mitral annulus)
3. Patients often have pulmonary hypertension (PA systolic pressure estimated > 55 mmHg)

12.2.5 Management

- Cardiac medications are generally poorly tolerated in RCM
  - Restrictive filling with poorly compliant ventricle(s) → fixed stroke volume
  - Cannot be augmented with optimization of hemodynamic status without worsening filling pressures
  - Heart rate dependent to maintain cardiac output
  - Blood pressure very sensitive to changes in afterload → vasodilators—poorly tolerated → hypotension
  - Negative inotropes are poorly tolerated
  - Negative chronotropic agents like calcium channel blockers are contraindicated
    Note: in amyloidosis RCM → high risk for digoxin toxicity due to interaction with amyloid fibrils

- Diuretics may be used cautiously when needed
- High risk of thrombi formation—low threshold for anticoagulation and TEE if DCCV required

12.3 Dilated Cardiomyopathy (DCM)

12.3.1 Definition

Cardiomyopathy characterized by systolic dysfunction and LV dilatation in the absence of coronary artery disease or abnormal loading conditions (hypertensive/valvular).

12.3.2 Etiology

- 50% of cases of DCM are idiopathic
  - 25–35% of cases are genetic, over 60 genes have been causally linked to DCM
  - All patients should have a detailed family history of at least 3 generations
- Infectious
  - Viral (enterovirus, Coxsackie B, Echovirus, Adenovirus, HCV, HIV—10% of AIDS patients)
  - Chagas disease
- Toxic/metabolic
  - Alcohol—generally if consumption of >80 g of EtOH/day (~ 5–6 drinks per day) for >5 years
  - Chagas disease
  - Chemotherapy—anthracyclines (type I), Trastuzumab (type II)
  - High dose cyclophosphamide, taxos, 5-FU, interferon
  - Hypothyroidism or hyperthyroidism, Pheochromocytoma
- Inflammatory
  - Celiac disease, IBD, Whipple's disease
  - RA/SLE, Systemic Sclerosis, Mixed Connective Tissue Disease Churg Straus
  - Giant cell/Takayasu arteritis
- Hypersensitivity
  - Drugs—Sulfas, Cephalosporins, diuretics, digoxin, dobutamine, antidepressants
- Tachycardia or PVC mediated
  - With a heart rate >100–120 s for ~2 weeks or frequent PVCS (>10k in 24 h)
  - Often improves within 4 weeks after resolution of arrhythmias
- Endocrine
  - Diabetic cardiomyopathy
  - Obesity
  - Growth Hormone
- Iron overload/Hemochromatosis
  - Genetic (HFE mutation) or secondary to frequent blood transfusions
  - Diagnosis: serum ferritin > 200, transferrin saturation > 55%
  - 15% have cardiac involvement
  - Endomyocardial biopsy often not useful; deposits more commonly subepicardial than subendocardial
- Sarcoidosis
  - 5% of sarcoid patients have cardiac involvement
  - Unexplained conduction abnormalities or ventricular arrhythmias due to focal granuloma scarring
  - Initially may have focal wall motion abnormalities in non-coronary distribution → late stage can have global dilated CM
  - Cardiac MRI with gadolinium enhancement—diagnostic
- Peripartum
  - Development of HF and LV EF < 45% towards the end of pregnancy or within 5 months postpartum
  - Almost always globally reduced EF ± LV dilation
- Obstructive Sleep Apnea
  - Cor Pulmonale and RV involvement
  - Can also cause left sided DCM—suspected stress induced mechanism

- Nutritional
  - AIDS, anorexia, pregnancy, alcoholics
  - Thiamine (B1) deficiency—commonly seen in alcoholics
  - Selenium deficiency, carnitine deficiency, severe hypocalcemia
- Takotsubo—stress induced cardiomyopathy
- Dyssynchrony/LBBB
  - Dyssynchrony induced cardiomyopathy—usually seen with wide LBBB (>150 ms) or paced rhythm
  - May not respond well to guideline directed medical therapy (GDMT); early CRT may improve outcomes

12.3.3 Clinical Manifestations

- DCM presents with signs and symptoms of heart failure
- Timing and severity of symptoms depend on the individual etiology for DCM, as does the prognosis

12.3.4 Echocardiographic Assessment (Fig. 12.9, Videos 12.4A and 12.4B)

Anatomic Assessment

1. M-Mode of the mitral valve
   - Increased E-point septal separation
2. M-Mode of the LV
   - Increased end diastolic and end systolic diameter
3. 2D imaging
   - LV Dilatation—both end diastolic and end systolic volumes are increased
   - Sphericity Index—with worsening remodeling → progressive dilatation along the short axis (SAX) relative to the long axis (LAX) → ventricular cavity becomes less elliptical and more spherical → LAX:SAX ratio close to 1 (normally >1.5)
   - Enlargement of other cardiac chambers (LA, RV,RA) with disease progression
   - Decreased systolic function—often global
   - Important to exclude LV clot (contrast echo often required)

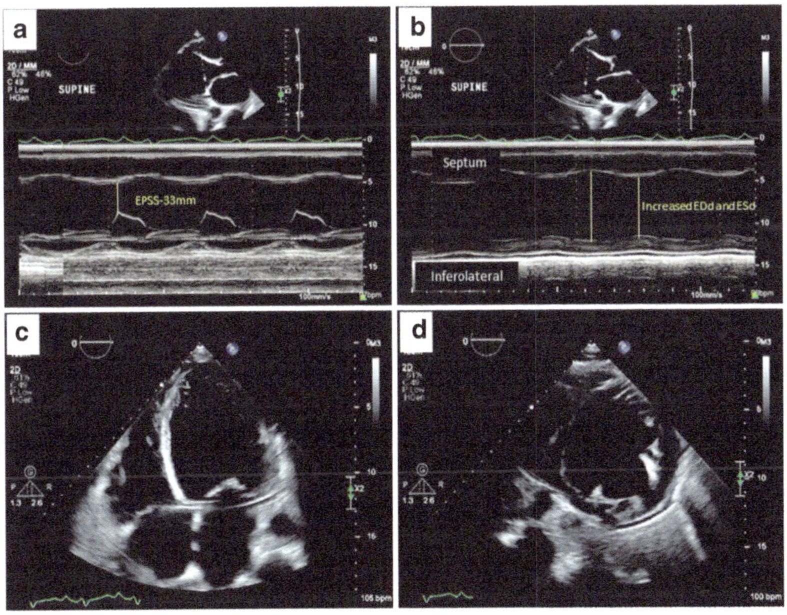

Fig. 12.9 **Dilated cardiomyopathy.** (**a**) M Mode at the mitral valve level showing increased E-point septal separation (EPSS) caused by decreased stroke volume and increased left ventricular volume. (**b**) M mode at the basal ventricular level showing increased end-diastolic (EDd) and end-systolic dimensions (ESd), as well as limited motion of the septum and inferolateral wall. (**c**, **d**) Apical four-chamber view and parasternal short axis view showing severely dilated left ventricle (and reduced ejection fraction)

Doppler Assessment

1. ↓S′ mitral annulus—systolic function impairment
2. Functional mitral regurgitation
3. Reduced dP/dT (measured on MR spectral Doppler tracing)
4. Dyssynchronous ventricular contraction

12.3.5 Management

- Similar to guideline directed medical therapy (GDMT) for heart failure with reduced ejection fraction (HFrEF)
- Mainstays of medical therapy include: beta blockers, ACE inhibitors, angiotensin receptor blockers, angiotensin receptor-neprilysin inhibitors, aldosterone antagonist
- Re-synchronization therapy/ICD when applicable.

12.4 Ventricular Non-Compaction

- Cardiomyopathy that occurs due to arrest of myocardial compaction during embryogenesis resulting in a noncompacted "spongy" myocardial layer
- Initially described as isolated left ventricular non compaction (IVNC), however, concurrent RV involvement can occur, or rarely isolated RV involvement

12.4.1 Clinical manifestations

- Heart failure
- Thromboembolism - higher chance of LV thrombus due to blood stasis in recesses
- Ventricular arrhythmias/sudden cardiac death

12.4.2 Echocardiographic Assessment

Anatomic Assessment

- Noncompacted myocardial layer has deep sinusoid with multiple trabeculations and intertrabecular recesses that communicate with ventricular cavity
- For diagnosis: ≥2:1 ratio of noncompacted to compacted myocardium during diastole
- By MRI—ratio of noncompacted to compacted myocardium ≥ 2.3:1
- Color Doppler and/or echo contrast should be used to better visualize recess depth

12.4.3 Management

Medical Management

- Same as DCM—GDMT for HFrEF
- Thromboembolism Prophylaxis
  - No official guideline recommendations
  - Some advocate for treatment with anticoagulation (or antiplatelet agents) for all patients with non-compaction and EF ≤ 40% for thromboembolism prevention

12.5 Right Sided Cardiomyopathies

12.5.1 Arrhythmogenic Right Ventricular Cardiomyopathy (ARVC)

- Abnormal desmosomal proteins lead to replacement of the RV myocardium with fatty and fibrous tissue → dilated and thin RV with reduced systolic function

Clinical Manifestations

- Palpitations
- Syncope
- Atypical chest pain
- Dyspnea/heart failure/right heart failure
- EKG abnormalities—Epsilon wave, prolonged S wave, or T wave inversions in V1–V3
- Ventricular Arrhythmias/sudden cardiac death
- Asymptomatic—diagnosed during family screening of affected family member

Echocardiographic Assessment

Anatomic Assessment

1. RV is dilated, thin, and has reduced EF

  - RVOT dilation ≥ 30 mm in PLAX or > 32 mm in PSAX
  - RV apical pouching—can develop RV free wall aneurysm
  - 'Triangle of dysplasia'—triangular area formed by the basal free wall, RV apex, and RVOT (inflow, apex, outflow)—affected first and the most dysplastic
2. Prominent RV trabeculation
3. Prominent RV moderator band that is hyperreflective

   Note: echocardiographic findings may be variable; other imaging modalities (e.g. cardiac MRI) typically required.

Management

- GDMT for heart failure symptoms
- Restriction of athletic activity:
  - Low intensity activity only
  - Avoid all competitive sports (risk of sudden cardiac death increased five fold)
- ICD for primary prevention and secondary prevention

12.5.2 Differential Diagnosis for Right Sided Cardiomyopathies

Carcinoid Heart Disease
(Fig. 12.10, Videos 12.5A and 12.5B)

- Occurs when a serotonin producing carcinoid tumor metastasizes to the liver
- Primarily affects the RV because serotonin is inactivated by the lungs
- Serotonin produces carcinoid plaques that lead to fibrosis and dysfunction of the valves that are exposed (usually the TV, occasionally PV).

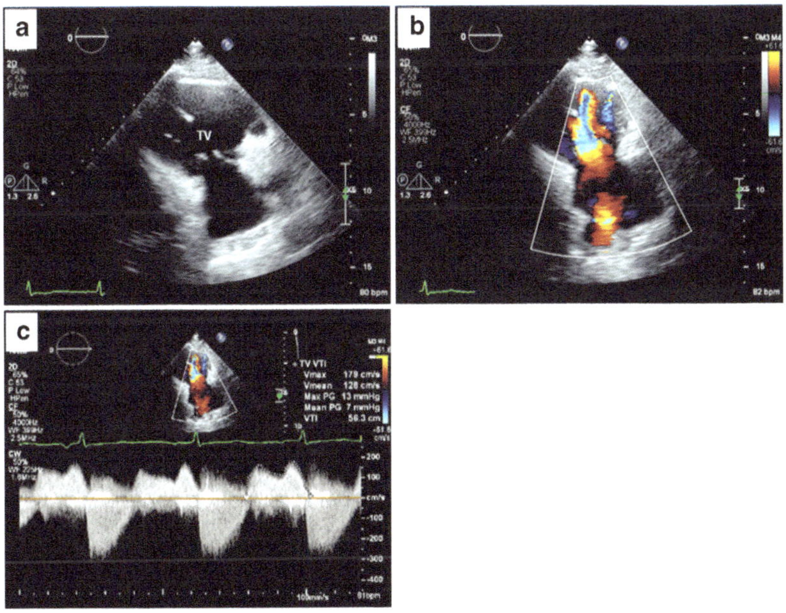

Fig. 12.10 **Carcinoid Heart Disease**. (**a**) RV inflow view showing thickened and restricted tricuspid valve (TV) leaflets. (**b**) Diastolic frame from RV inflow color view showing turbulent tricuspid inflow jet. (**c**) Continuous wave Doppler showing both severe tricuspid regurgitation (dense, early peaking, triangular jet contour) and significantly elevated inflow gradient

Echocardiographic Assessment

- Thickened and short/retracted valve leaflets with limited mobility and incomplete coaptation (usually TV; PV can be affected)
  Note: MV can be involved in the presence of a PFO/ASD with enough RV/RA pressure overload to cause right to left shunting; serotonin bypasses lungs (no inactivation)

Clinical Manifestations and Management

- Acute serotonin effects of wheezing, flushing, diarrhea; treatment with IV octreotide
- Symptoms of TR and right sided heart failure—valve replacement

Ebstein's Anomaly

- See Chap. 15—congenital heart disease.

Uhl's Syndrome

- Complete absence of RV myocardium
- RV endocardium and epicardium appose each other producing "parchment like RV wall"

Drugs

- Fenfluramine, Ergots

Further Reading

Authors/Task Force Members, Elliott PM, Anastasakis A, et al. 2014 ESC Guidelines on diagnosis and management of hypertrophic cardiomyopathy: the Task Force for the Diagnosis and Management of Hypertrophic Cardiomyopathy of the European Society of Cardiology (ESC). Eur Heart J. 2014;35(39):2733–79. https://doi.org/10.1093/eurheartj/ehu284.

Gersh BJ, Maron BJ, Bonow RO, et al. 2011 ACCF/AHA Guideline for the Diagnosis and Treatment of Hypertrophic Cardiomyopathy: a report of the American College of Cardiology Foundation/American Heart Association Task Force on Practice Guidelines. Developed in collaboration with the American Association for Thoracic Surgery, American Society of Echocardiography, American Society of Nuclear Cardiology, Heart Failure Society of America, Heart Rhythm Society, Society for Cardiovascular Angiography and Interventions, and Society of Thoracic Surgeons. J Am Coll Cardiol. 2011;58(25):e212–60. https://doi.org/10.1016/j.jacc.2011.06.011.

Japp AG, Gulati A, Cook SA, Cowie MR, Prasad SK. The diagnosis and evaluation of dilated cardiomyopathy. J Am Coll Cardiol. 2016;67(25):2996–3010. https://doi.org/10.1016/j.jacc.2016.03.590.

Pereira NL, Grogan M, Dec GW. Spectrum of restrictive and infiltrative cardiomyopathies: Part 1 of a 2-Part Series. J Am Coll Cardiol. 2018;71(10):1130–48. https://doi.org/10.1016/j.jacc.2018.01.016.

Pereira NL, Grogan M, Dec GW. Spectrum of restrictive and infiltrative cardiomyopathies: Part 2 of a 2-Part Series. J Am Coll Cardiol. 2018;71(10):1149–66. https://doi.org/10.1016/j.jacc.2018.01.017.

Pericardial Disease

13

Learning Objectives

- To learn the causes, evaluation, and management of acute pericarditis
- To learn the causes, evaluation, and management of pericardial effusion and cardiac tamponade
- To learn the causes, evaluation, and management of constrictive pericarditis
- Briefly review congenital abnormalities of the pericardium

13.1 General Characteristics of the Pericardium

13.1.1 Anatomy of the Pericardium

The pericardium is a double layered sac consisting of a fibrous and serous layer that encloses the heart and the proximal great vessels (aortic root, pulmonary artery, and pulmonary veins) (Fig. 13.1)

- Fibrous pericardium
  - The outer layer of the pericardium, composed of collagen fibers and short elastic fibrils; provides protection to the heart, and contacts directly with extracardiac (intrathoracic) structures:
    Superiorly w/the great vessels
    Anteriorly w/the sternum (via sternopericardial ligaments)
    Inferiorly w/the diaphragm (via central tendon of the diaphragm)
    Laterally w/the parietal pleura
    Posteriorly w/the main bronchi, esophagus, and descending thoracic aorta
- Serous Pericardium
  - The inner layer of the pericardium, composed of mesothelium which forms 2 layers (the parietal and visceral layers) separated by the pericardial space
  - The parietal pericardium—lines the fibrous pericardium
    Highly reflective echogenic linear structure seen on 2D imaging
    Electrically inert—inflammation of this layer does not cause pain
  - Pericardial space
    A physiologic small amount of fluid (<50 cc) is always present to reduce friction between the heart and the connected thoracic structures
  - Pericardial reflections—2 Areas where the visceral pericardium connects with parietal pericardium
    Transverse sinus—separates great arteries from PA and the SVC.
    Oblique sinus—behind the left atrium and bordered by the PVs and IVC
    - Excess fluid can accumulate in this area and cause LA compression and

Electronic Supplementary Material The online version of this chapter (https://doi.org/10.1007/978-3-030-47041-8_13) contains supplementary material, which is available to authorized users.

T. Rambhatla, G. Perk, *The Echocardiography Companion*,
https://doi.org/10.1007/978-3-030-47041-8_13

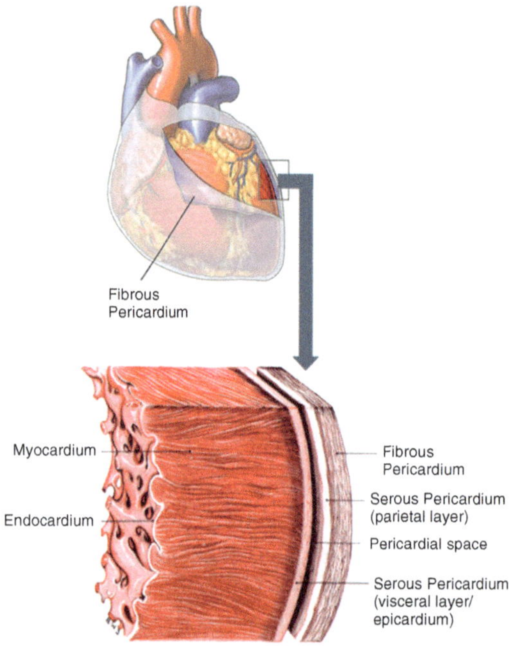

Fig. 13.1 **Pericardial anatomy**. The pericardium consists of two layers: the outer fibrous pericardium and the inner serous pericardium. The serous pericardium consists of an outer parietal pericardium, the pericardial cavity, and the inner visceral pericardium (also called the epicardium). Epicardial fat, nerve supply, and the coronary vasculature run between the myocardium and the visceral pericardium (the epicardium)

regional tamponade (can be seen post cardiac surgery or in supine patients)

- The visceral pericardium (epicardium)
  Electrically active—responsible for chest pain in pericardial inflammation
- Pericardial thickness:
  - Normal pericardial thickness is <3 mm; ≥3 mm is considered thickened
  - CT is the gold standard for diagnosing pericardial thickness
  - Limitations with echo
    Echo cannot distinguish parietal layer and visceral layer in the absence of an effusion that separates the layers
    Echo is not reliable to diagnose calcification of the pericardium (as can be seen in constrictive pericarditis) because the parietal layer is echogenic ➔ difficult to distinguish from calcification
    Echo cannot diagnose pericardial inflammation (requires MRI)

Note: 18% of constrictive pericarditis have normal pericardial thickness ➔ can only be diagnosed anatomically with CT or MRI imaging

13.1.2 Physiology of the Pericardium

Mechanical Effects of the Pericardium

- Separates the heart from other structures
- Limits acute distention of cardiac chambers
- Limits direct spread of infection

Hemodynamic Effects of the Pericardium

- Diastolic coupling and ventricular interdependence
- Due to the finite space within the fibrous pericardial sac, the cardiac chambers are coupled during diastolic filling; filling of one ventricle may alter filling of the other
- Healthy pericardium (which is not maximally distended) with small amount of pericardial fluid, allows for the inspiratory increase in RV volume without impacting LV filling
- When the pericardium is maximally constrained (e.g. pericardial tamponade or constrictive pericarditis), increasing RV filling compromises LV filling; there is no room for the heart to expand further, the septum pushes into the LV, compromising LV filling ➔ ventricular interdependence.
- Intrapericardial pressure is coupled with the respiratory cycle
  - Normal pericardium transmits changes in intra-thoracic pressure to intra-pericardial pressure
  - Inspiration ➔ negative intrathoracic pressure ➔ decrease in intra-pericardial pressure

13.2 Acute Pericarditis (AP)

AP is a clinical syndrome of pericardial inflammation that is usually self-limited, lasting < 3 months (>3 months ➔ chronic pericarditis).

13.2.1 Etiology

Etiologies of acute pericarditis and pericardial effusion

Idiopathic	Number 1 cause of both AP and PEff (~50% of cases)
Viral infections	Enterovirus (coxsackie), Adenovirus, Herpesvirus, HIV (10% of HIV patients affected), HBV/HCV
Autoimmune systemic illnesses	SLE, RA, Sjogren, scleroderma Vasculitides (eosinophilic, churg-strauss, Takayasu, Behcet); Sarcoidosis, FMF, IBD, Still's disease
Malignancy	Almost exclusively metastatic disease—lung, breast, Hodgkin's lymphoma; Accounts for 6% of AP, and 15–20% of moderate to large PEff
Bacterial infections	Tuberculosis common in 3rd world countries; Otherwise: staph, pneumococcus, streptococcus
Post-MI	(Not including free wall rupture): Acute—acute inflammation due to the infarction Chronic—weeks to months later, immune reaction to the infarction (Dressler's Syndrome)
Post-pericardiotomy syndrome	(Not including acute hemorrhagic effusion post-surgery) 15% of post cardiac surgery patients
Radiation	Post thoracic XRT (e.g. for lymphoma)
Parasitic disease	Chagas disease
Hypothyroidism	Myxedema
Infiltrative diseases	Amyloidosis, sarcoidosis primary pericardial/cardiac malignancy

Note:

- Majority of cases of both AP and PEff are idiopathic
- There is considerable overlap in the etiologies for both conditions
- However, pericardial effusion can present without AP, AP can present without pericardial effusion

13.2.2 Clinical Manifestations and Diagnosis

Signs and symptoms can be present due to underlying etiology or systemic disease

- The common causes of AP (idiopathic, viral) in areas with low TB prevalence often have a relatively benign course, and often do not require extensive investigation (unless high risk features)
  - High-risk features include: Fevers, subacute course, large effusion, failure to improve within 7 days of treatment, myopericarditis, immunosuppression, oral anticoagulant use, trauma, signs and symptoms suggestive of an underlying etiology

The clinical diagnosis is made with ECG, echo, and with ≥2 of the following criteria:

1. Pericarditic chest pain
   Pleuritic and positional, worse when supine, better when sitting and leaning forward (>85–90% of cases)
2. ECG changes
   Widespread concave ST elevations, in multiple coronary territories; PR depression (more specific)/PR elevation in avR (~60% of cases)
3. Pericardial effusion
   New or worsening, (~60% of cases); AP can present without PEff ("dry pericarditis")
4. Friction rub (<35% of cases)
   Scratching/grating sound, best heard at the left sternal border with patient leaning forward. Three audible components that correspond to (1) atrial systole (2) ventricular systole and (3) ventricular diastole

- Additional supporting features:
  - Elevated inflammatory markers (WBC, ESR, CRP)—can be helpful for monitoring disease activity and therapeutic response
  - Elevation in CK-MB/troponin suggests concomitant myocardial injury and myopericarditis
- Advanced imaging:
  - CT imaging
    Can identify pericardial thickening and contrast enhancement of serous pericardium during active inflammation. Calcified pericardial thickening suggests chronic inflammation.
    Signal attenuation level in the effusion can help distinguish exudative vs. transudative
  - MRI
    Identifies pericardial thickening, pericardial enhancement from inflammation, and effusion characteristics
    Can also assess motion and loss of normal slippage of parietal pericardium

over epicardial surface during cardiac cycle, which suggests inflammation and pericardial adhesions

13.2.3 Management

- Physical activity restriction—limit to only activities of daily living
  - Non-athletes—until symptom resolution; athletes—3 months from onset of symptoms and repeat assessment prior to resuming rigorous activity
- Aspirin vs NSAIDs—individualized choice according to patient's specific pros and cons
- Colchicine—weight adjusted dosing, decreases recurrence, improves treatment
- Steroids—reserved for cases resistant to ASA/NSAIDs, contraindications to ASA/NSAIDs, or when there is increased chance for recurrent pericarditis
  - Lower doses preferred, tapering once symptoms resolve, or near normalization of CRP

13.2.4 Recurrent Pericarditis

A repeat episode of AP after a symptom free interval of at least 4–6 weeks from the first episode of AP

- Occurs in up to 15–30% of cases of AP, and up to 50% in those treated without colchicine
- Therapy is with prolonged medication courses and tapers of ASA, NSAIDS, or steroids
  - If those fail ➔ immune modulators and pericardiectomy are third and fourth line options

13.3 Pericardial Effusion (PEff)

13.3.1 Etiology

In addition to the causes of AP, other causes of PEff are:

High right atrial pressure states	PEff occurs from compromised epicardial venous drainage: ESRD/HD, pulmonary hypertension, CHF
Iatrogenic	Post procedures: e.g. PPM, central venous access, coronary dissection.
Hemorrhagic PEff	Conversion of AP on AC/antiplatelets, aortic dissection, malignancy, TB

13.3.2 Echocardiographic Assessment

Anatomic Assessment

- Size/Grade
  - There is always a physiologic amount of fluid (<50 cc) in the pericardial space—can be seen as echo-free space between epicardium and parietal pericardium during systole
  - Separation between epicardium and parietal pericardium that is present both in systole and diastole signifies >50 cc of effusion
  - Measurements should be of the largest separation achieved in any standard view, *during diastole*
  - A small PEff is less than 1 cm, which usually correlates to <100 cc. A large effusion is greater than 2 cm and correlates to greater than 500 cc; and a moderate PEff is in between

Grade	Amount	Echo size (cm)
Small	50–100 cc	<1
Moderate	100–500 cc	1–2
Large	>500 cc	>2

  Note: PEff size alone has poor correlation with hemodynamic effect and compromise; may provide clue to chronicity and etiology
- Distribution of effusion—circumferential vs. loculated
  - Loculated effusion can cause focal compression and tamponade physiology; if clinical suspicion high (e.g. post cardiac surgery)—localized effusion should be searched for, from multiple windows and views
- Rate of accumulation (if prior studies available)

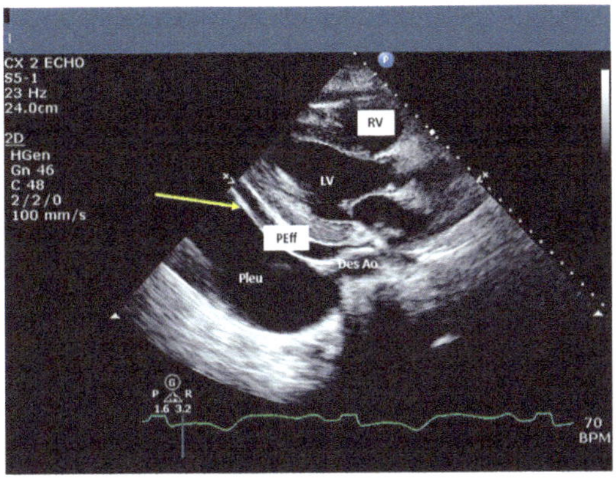

Fig. 13.2 **Differentiating pericardial effusion and pleural effusion**. Parasternal long axis image showing both a pericardial effusion and a pleural effusion. The descending thoracic aorta is an extra-pericardial, intrapleural structure. Thus, pericardial effusion is anterior to the descending aorta and does NOT include the descending aorta. However, the descending aorta can be visualized within the pleural effusion. *Desc Ao descending aorta, LV left ventricle, PEff pericardial effusion, Pleu pleural effusion, RV right ventricle*

- Left pleural effusion may mimic pericardial effusion—PLAX view and relation of effusion to descending aorta can help discern between the two (Fig. 13.2, Video 13.1)
- Epicardial fat vs. pericardial effusion
  - Adipose tissue can accumulate between myocardium and epicardium and may be confused with pericardial fluid
  - Epicardial fat—usually most prominent anterior to the RV, brighter than myocardium, moves with the heart; vs. transudative effusion—generally echo-lucent and does not move
- Other parameters to pay attention to:
  - Increased pericardial brightness
  - Wall motion abnormalities (for myopericarditis)
  - Chamber collapse (see cardiac tamponade section)

13.3.3 Management

- Medical treatment for underlying condition
- Pericardiocentesis/surgical pericardial biopsy/pericardial window
  - Can be performed for diagnostic studies (cultures, PCR) and/or management of significant PEff and clinical cardiac tamponade
- Fluid composition analysis—important for diagnostic purposes
  - Appearance—color, blood, fibrinous material, pus—should all be noted
  - Chemistry studies, microbiology studies and cytology should be done in the appropriate clinical settings

13.4 Cardiac Tamponade

Life threatening condition resulting from pericardial fluid accumulation causing increased pressure within the pericardial space that compromises venous return and impairs cardiac output.

The rise in pericardial pressure depends on the chronicity of effusion size

- A chronic effusion:
  - Increases slowly in size ➔ allows enough time for the pericardium to increase compliance ➔ less dramatic rise in pressure per change in volume ➔ less hemodynamic compromise
  - Hemodynamic stability can be maintained for longer time and much larger effusion size
  - Ultimately maximal pericardial constraint is reached and pericardial pressure increases, rising above ventricular cavity pressure ➔ tamponade. The steep pressure rise after the point of maximal constraint is the "last drop" phenomenon behind cardiac tamponade with chronic effusion
- An acute rapidly growing effusion:
  - Rapid rise in pericardial pressure can lead to tamponade at a much smaller effusion size
- Example: Acute aortic dissection or PPM lead perforation; tamponade occurs at much smaller effusion sizes (even as small as 100 cc) than, for example, a large effusion in a patient with ESRD on HD or chronic idiopathic peri-

carditis (where PEff as large as 1 L can be hemodynamically tolerated)

The resultant hypotension seen in tamponade occurs due to two main hemodynamic effects:

- Decreased left heart venous return/decreased preload
- Exaggerated ventricular interdependence—inability of the pericardium to accommodate the increased venous return to the RV during inspiration, causes the septum to bow into the LV and compromises LV filling

13.4.1 Clinical Manifestations

- Cardiac tamponade is a clinical syndrome characterized by: hypotension (or relative hypotension), tachycardia, increased JVD, and muffled hearts sounds (Beck's triad—JVD, muffled heart sounds, hypotension)
- ECG: low amplitude QRS, electrical alternans (changing of QRS axis due to movement of the heart)
- Pulsus paradoxus—inspiratory drop in systolic blood pressure > 10 mmHg

13.4.2 Echocardiographic Assessment (Fig. 13.3, Videos 13.2A and 13.2B)

Anatomic Assessment

- Reduced left ventricular volumes (EDV and ESV), LV "pseudo" hypertrophy
- IVC plethora—dilated IVC with minimal respiratory variation
- Diastolic chamber collapse
  - RA collapse—the right atrium is most commonly the lowest pressure chamber ➔ collapses first
  - RA collapse is least specific for tamponade (especially if isolated to systole, when RA pressure lowest and pericardial pressure highest)

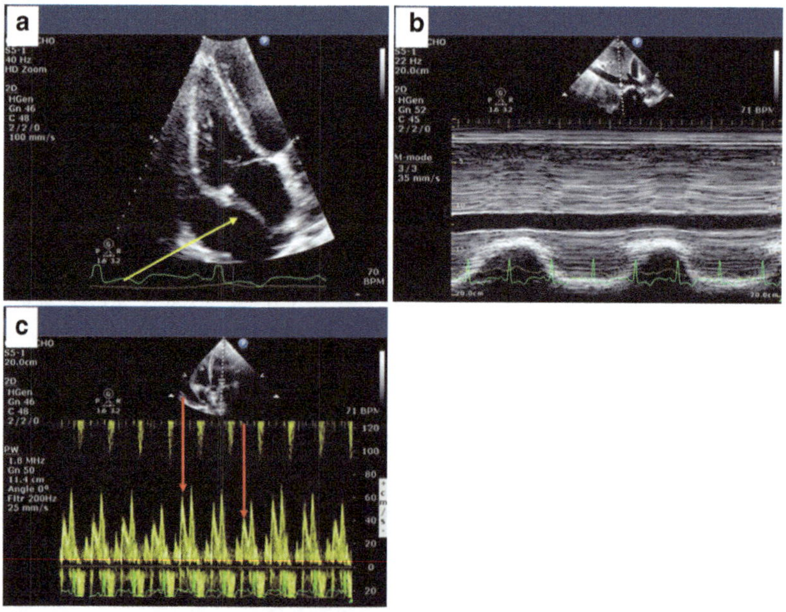

Fig. 13.3 **Echocardiographic findings in cardiac tamponade**. (**a**) Right heart zoomed apical view showing right atrial free wall compression (yellow arrow). (**b**) Subcostal m-mode showing dilated and plethoric inferior vena cava. (**c**) Spectral Doppler at the mitral valve tips showing significant (>25%) inspiratory decrease in mitral E velocity (red arrows)

- RA diastolic inversion lasting more >1/3 cardiac cycle ➔ specificity for tamponade higher
- RV collapse—more specific than RA collapse, less sensitive
- M-Mode can be used to visualize and time RA/RV collapse
- RV or RA collapse may not occur with pulmonary HTN/elevated right sided pressures

- Ventricular interdependence—abnormal IVS movement and change in ventricular chamber size with the respiratory cycle (not beat to beat variation)
  - Inspiration ➔ decrease in intrathoracic pressure ➔ increased venous return to right side ➔ RV increases in size more than LV
  - Expiration ➔ increase intrathoracic pressure ➔ increased return of blood to the left side ➔ LV larger than RV

Doppler Assessment

- Reduced stroke volume and cardiac output (calculated by LVOT area and VTI)
- Respiratory mitral and tricuspid inflow variation
  - MV—inspiratory decrease in MV E velocity > 25%
  - TV—Expiratory decrease in TV E velocity > 30%
  - Respirometer should be used to correlate inflow variation with the respiratory cycle
- Hepatic vein flow—expiratory decrease in forward flow and increase in diastolic flow reversal
- SVC flow—expiratory increase in flow reversal
- PV flow—expiratory increase in systolic flow and decrease or loss of diastolic flow

13.4.3 Special Situations

Localized/Regional Tamponade

- Loculated/focal effusion can cause localized chamber compression. Echocardiographic signs on standard views may be absent (20–25% not seen in TTE)
  - Can be seen post operatively (post pericardiotomy), dependent patients, post infarction
- May require TEE for diagnosis

Low-Pressure Tamponade

- Hypovolemic patients may have impaired filling of the heart even when intra-pericardial pressure is relatively low, if the intra-cardiac pressures are lower
- RA/RV collapse seen; signs of elevated filling pressures (IVC plethora) may be missing
- Initial treatment—increase intra-cardiac (RV) pressure (IV fluids)

Tamponade Without Respiratory Variation in Inflow Velocities

- Positive pressure ventilation
- Shallow breathing with minimal inspiratory drop in intra-thoracic pressure (e.g. chest wall trauma, post cardiac surgery patients, muscle weakness, muscle paralysis)
- Atrial septal defect with a significant shunt
  - Inspiratory changes in venous return are counter-balanced by changes in amount of inter-atrial shunting (same mechanism causing the classis fixed splitting of S2)
- Aortic insufficiency/volume overload— If left atrial pressure is high enough, changes in inspiratory pressure may not cause a significant change the PV-LA gradient

13.4.4 Management

- Temporizing measures: fluids, vasopressors, invasive hemodynamic monitoring—arterial line
- Echo guided pericardiocentesis (Fig. 13.4, Videos 13.3A, 13.3B, and 13.3C)
  - Blind pericardiocentesis has a high rate of complications (pneumothorax, cardiac wall puncture, death)
  - Echo is used to determine the location with largest fluid collection, confirm puncture/drainage of the pericardial space and monitor adequate drainage and procedural success
  - Common locations for needle puncture are: subcostal and apical.
  - After needle puncture, echo is used to determine proper placement with agitated saline injection and visualization of bub-

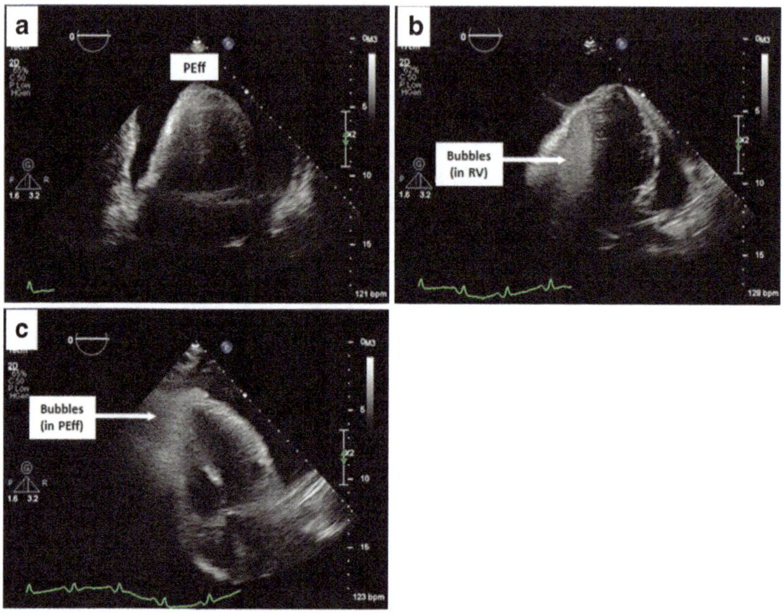

Fig. 13.4 **Echocardiographic guidance for pericardiocentesis.** (**a**) Apical 4 chamber view showing a large pericardial effusion prior to drainage procedure. (**b**) Agitated saline injection showing opacification of the right ventricle ➔ the needle was immediately withdrawn. (**c**) Agitated saline injection showing opacification of the pericardial space confirming proper puncture location. *Peff pericardial effusion, RV right ventricle*

bles within the pericardial space (and not the RV or LV cavity)

- Due to tomographic nature of echocardiographic imaging, needle/drain may not be directly visualized in the pericardial space.
- After confirmation of proper location with echo, fluoroscopy can be used to visualize guidewire advancement and ensure it is maintained within the pericardial space.
- Pigtail catheter or drainage catheter is advanced over the wire into the pericardial space and is used to complete the drainage.

  Note: If tamponade is due to aortic dissection—pericardiocentesis is relatively contraindicated; may worsen hemodynamic state; must be done while patient already in operating room.

13.5 Constrictive Pericarditis (CP)

CP is due to thickened, calcific, and adherent pericardium that limits diastolic filling.

13.5.1 Etiologies

CP can occur after any pericardial inflammatory process:

- Post cardiac surgery (30%)
- Idiopathic CP (25%)
- AP (15%)
  - The risk of CP from AP is low, <1% for idiopathic or presumed viral causes
  - Intermediate 2–5% for autoimmune and malignant etiologies
  - High >20% for bacterial causes, especially in purulent pericarditis or TB

- Effusive Constrictive Pericarditis
  - Can occurs after drainage of certain effusions ➔ two pericardial layers gradually thicken and stick together ➔ constrictive physiology.
  - One series, 8% of post pericardiocentesis patients developed CP
- Radiation (10%)—latent presentation, can present 20 years after initial radiation therapy
- Other causes—trauma, drug induced, asbestosis, sarcoidosis, uremic pericarditis, and rarely following recurrent pericarditis

13.5.2 Clinical Manifestations

CP classically presents with signs and symptoms of right heart failure (fatigue, SOB/DOE, abdominal swelling, peripheral edema).

- Physical exam findings: increased JVP, rapid "Y" descent, Kussmauls's sign (increased JVD with inspiration), pericardial knock (diastolic gallop after S2), ascites, and peripheral edema.
- Patients usually have clear lungs but can develop pleural effusions and congestion.
- Commonly misdiagnosed as HFpEF; BNP levels typically normal or lower than expected with HF
- Diagnosis: clinical signs and symptoms with evidence of impaired diastolic function due to pericardial constraint (by echo, CT, MR, or cardiac catheterization).

13.5.3 Echocardiographic Assessment (Fig. 13.5, Videos 13.4A and 13.4B)

Anatomic Assessment

1. M-Mode
   - Separation of the visceral and parietal pericardium by an echo-free space

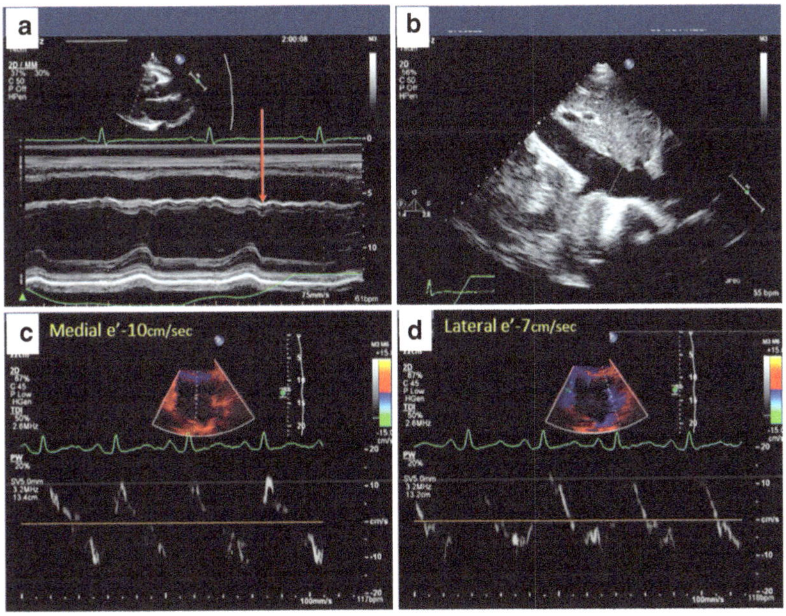

Fig. 13.5 **Constrictive pericarditis**. (**a**) M mode at the basal LV level showing early diastolic septal bounce (red arrow). (**b**) Subcostal view showing dilated and plethoric inferior vena cava. (**c**) Tissue Doppler imaging (TDI) at the medial mitral annulus with e' velocity of 10 cm/s. (**d**) TDI at the lateral mitral annulus with e' velocity of 7 cm/s (consistent with annulus reversus)

- Parallel motion of the visceral and parietal pericardium
- Premature opening of the pulmonic valve—due to atrial kick increasing RVEDP above PA diastolic pressure
- Septal bounce and septal shift

2. 2D imaging
   - Preserved LV and RV size and function; deformed heart shape may be seen
   - Moderate bi-atrial enlargement (vs. RCM with severe bi-atrial enlargement)
   - Plethoric IVC and hepatic veins (minimal or diminished respiratory variation)
   - Thickened pericardium
     - Often not seen with TTE (sensitivity—50%); TEE strongly correlates with CT evaluation of pericardial thickness (sensitivity and specificity—90%).
     - Note ~18–20% of CP have normal pericardial thickness ($\leq$2 mm)
   - Calcific pericardium (often requires CT imaging to appreciate, seen on CXR in ~20%)
   - Septal bounce—early diastolic shutter that occurs with each heart beat (represents rapid Y descent seen on cath)
   - Septal shift—movement of the IVS with each respiratory cycle (representative of ventricular interdependence due to pericardial tethering)

Doppler Assessment

1. MV inflow pattern—restrictive filling pattern (E:A 2:1, E DT <160)
2. Respiratory variations in Doppler patterns:
   - MV E velocity drop >25% with inspiration;
   - TV E velocity drop >40% with expiration
   - LVOT VTI/SV variation—inspiratory decrease in SV, LVOT VTI, and blood pressure
3. Isovolumic relaxation time (IVRT)—Inspiratory increase and expiratory decrease in IVRT (vs. no change in RCM)
4. Hepatic vein flow—Increased diastolic flow reversal during expiration (most specific if $\geq$0.7)
5. Tissue Doppler Imaging
   - Annulus reversus—medial e' > lateral e'
     - Lateral mitral annulus tethering to the thickened pericardium ➔ Normal or higher than normal medial e' velocities
   - Annulus paradoxus –E/e' values correlate inversely with increasing LAP
     - Medial e' velocity increases as constriction worsens

Strain imaging

1. pericardial restraint limits LV expansion, reduces twist/torsion
2. Reduced circumferential strain, reduced twist/torsion
3. Longitudinal strain is relatively preserved (regional reductions in longitudinal strain may be seen).

13.5.4 Other Imaging Modalities

CT imaging	MRI
• Highly accurate method for evaluating pericardial thickness and calcification. • Can also indirectly assess impaired diastolic filling with evaluation of chamber size/deformation, IVC/hepatic vein dilatation	• Gated MRI is the best imaging modality for assessing CP; tissue assessment for inflammation, pericardial adherence, and LGE

13.5.5 Cath Hemodynamic Assessment

- Equalization of cardiac chamber pressures (LVEDP ≅ RVEDP, $\leq$ 5 mmHg difference)
- Dip and plateau sign—sharp Y descent—on right atrial pressure tracings
- Mild-moderate pulmonary hypertension, RVSP generally $\leq$50 mmHg, RVEDP: RVSP $\geq$1:3
- Discordant LV/RV pressures with respiratory cycle
  - Inspiration ➔ increase in RVSP and decrease in LVSP

- Expiration ➔ increase in LVSP and decrease in RVSP
- In restriction ➔ concordant simultaneous LV and RV pressure tracings with both LVSP and RVSP increase with inspiration

- Ejection times vary with respiratory cycle

13.5.6 Constriction vs. Restriction

	Constriction	Restriction
MV filling pattern	Restrictive	Restrictive
Dip and plateau sign	Yes	Yes
Pressure tracings	Discordant	Concordant
Chamber pressures	LVEDP ≅ RVEDP, ≤ 5 mmHg difference	LVEDP > > RVEDP
TDI E' velocities	Medial e' preserved/ elevated Medial e' > lateral e'	Both medial and lateral e' reduced Lateral e' > medial e'
Septal Bounce Rapid 'Y' descent	Yes	No
Ventricular Interdependence	Yes: (+) septal shift, (+) MV/ TV inflow variation	No: (−) septal shift, (−) MV/ TV inflow variation
Pulsus Paradoxus	Yes	No
Bi-atrial enlargement	Moderate	Severe
PaHTN	Mild-moderate	Moderate-severe

13.5.7 Management

- Conservative management: 2–3 months of medical management ➔ assess for resolution
- Effusive constrictive pericarditis often resolves (common post-surgery, 50% are transient): trial of medical management before pericardiectomy
- Pericardiectomy—for chronic CP that failed medical therapy

13.6 Congenital Absence of the Pericardium

- Absence of the pericardium can be: complete—entire pericardium, complete left or right, or partial
- Most common variant—complete absence of the left pericardium (still very rare)

13.6.1 Clinical Manifestations

- Asymptomatic, incidentally found (by imaging or thoracic surgery)
- Symptoms may occur and include: chest pain, palpitations, dyspnea (median age at presentation—21)
- Laterally displaced apical impulse; the entire heart may be shifted leftward within the chest cavity

13.6.2 Echocardiographic Assessment

Anatomic Assessment

1. Unusual echo windows
2. RV appears enlarged in PSAX view; in apical view appears in the center of the image
3. Abnormal septal motion, exaggerated motion of the posterior wall (LV appears hyperdynamic)
4. "Tear drop" shape on apical windows
5. Associated congenital anomalies

Doppler Assessment

1. Absent pericardium ➔ reduction in negative intra-pericardial pressure during systole
   - Reduction of systolic to diastolic ratio in pulmonary vein flow
   - Reduction in SVC systolic flow
2. Severe TR may be seen

13.6.3 Management

1. Asymptomatic—generally no treatment required
2. Partial absence of left pericardium ➔ risk of compression, herniation or strangulation (of cardiac chambers, great vessels, coronaries). In these patients—surgical repair

13.7 Pericardial Cyst

- Most are congenital and detected as incidental finding, commonly between age 20–40
- Enclosed space, no communication with pericardial space, appear as round echo-lucent area
- Most common location—right cardiophrenic angle or near AV groove
- Management: for asymptomatic patients—conservative, with imaging follow up
- Rupture and hemorrhage can cause tamponade—very rare ➔ aspiration or surgical excision.

13.8 Pericardial Malignancy

13.8.1 Primary

Overall primary pericardial tumors are very rare
- Benign primary tumors more common than malignant
- – Include: lipoma, fibroma, hemangioma, lymphangioma, teratoma.
- – Found incidentally or due to palpitations/arrhythmias
- – Can grow to large size before causing compression
- – Appearance: discrete masses, sessile or pedunculated
- – Treatment—surgical excision (diagnostic & therapeutic)
- Malignant tumors—exceedingly rare
- – Most common—mesothelioma, followed by angiosarcoma
- – Non-specific symptoms: chest pain, shortness of breath, cough
- – Can cause effusion, myocardial invasion, constriction
- – Diagnosis requires pericardial biopsy (low yield of pericardial fluid cytology)
- – Treatment options limited; often non resectable, limited benefit of chemotherapy or radiation therapy

13.8.2 Secondary

- Tumor spread to pericardium—direct local invasion or metastatic spread
- Most frequent: lymphoma, melanoma, lung carcinoma, breast carcinoma
- Symptoms of pericarditis or effusion
- Diagnostic yield of fluid cytology variable (high for primary solid tumors, low for hematologic malignancies)
- Treatment guided by overall prognosis and clinical status

Further Reading

Ha JW, Ommen SR, Tajik AJ, et al. Differentiation of constrictive pericarditis from restrictive cardiomyopathy using mitral annular velocity by tissue Doppler echocardiography. Am J Cardiol. 2004;94(3):316–9. https://doi.org/10.1016/j.amjcard.2004.04.026.

Klein AL, Abbara S, Agler DA, et al. American Society of Echocardiography clinical recommendations for multimodality cardiovascular imaging of patients with pericardial disease: endorsed by the Society for Cardiovascular Magnetic Resonance and Society of Cardiovascular Computed Tomography. J Am Soc Echocardiogr. 2013;26(9):965–1012.e15. https://doi.org/10.1016/j.echo.2013.06.023.

Spodick DH. Acute cardiac tamponade. N Engl J Med. 2003;349(7):684–90. https://doi.org/10.1056/NEJMra022643.

Welch TD, Ling LH, Espinosa RE, et al. Echocardiographic diagnosis of constrictive pericarditis: Mayo Clinic criteria. Circ Cardiovasc Imaging. 2014;7(3):526–34. https://doi.org/10.1161/CIRCIMAGING.113.001613.

Aortic Disease

14

Learning Objectives

- To learn the causes, evaluation, and management of aortic atherosclerotic disease
- To learn the causes, evaluation, and management of aortic aneurysm
- To learn the causes, evaluation, and management of acute aortic syndromes

14.1 General Characteristics of the Aorta (Ao)

- The aortic wall is made up of three layers:
  - Intima—thin inner endothelium layer; delicate and easily damaged
  - Media—composed of smooth muscle and elastic fibers; bound by the elastic laminae; provides strength and elasticity
  - Adventitia—composed of collagen; contains vasa vasorum and nerves; vasa vasorum can reach the outer third of the media
- The elasticity of the media layer allows the aorta to accept systolic pressure and volume while maintaining continuous diastolic forward flow.
- With aging, the media undergoes degenerative changes → loss of elasticity → increase in pulse pressure seen in elderly patients; can lead to aortic dilatation.
- The aorta is divided into the thoracic aorta and abdominal aorta.
- This chapter will concentrate on the thoracic aorta.

14.2 Anatomy of the Thoracic Aorta (Fig. 14.1)

The thoracic aorta consists of:

- Aortic root
- Ascending aorta
- Aortic arch
- Descending aorta
- Note: nearly the entire thoracic aorta can be imaged with TEE however there is a "blind spot" at distal ascending aorta/proximal arch due to air in trachea and main bronchi.

The aortic root consists of (Fig. 14.2):

- Aortic annulus
- Sinuses of Valsalva (SOV)
- Sino-tubular junction

Electronic Supplementary Material The online version of this chapter (https://doi.org/10.1007/978-3-030-47041-8_14) contains supplementary material, which is available to authorized users.

T. Rambhatla, G. Perk, *The Echocardiography Companion*,
https://doi.org/10.1007/978-3-030-47041-8_14

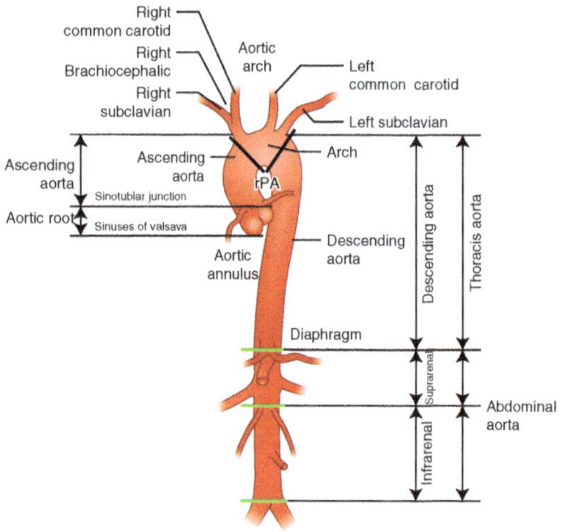

Fig. 14.1 **Thoracic aorta anatomy**. The thoracic aorta extends from the aortic annuls to the abdominal aorta which starts below the diaphragm. The thoracic aorta is divided into the aortic root (which consists of the aortic annulus, sinuses of Valsalva, and sinotubular junction), the ascending aorta, the aortic arch (which starts at the innominate artery and ends at the left subclavian artery), and the descending aorta

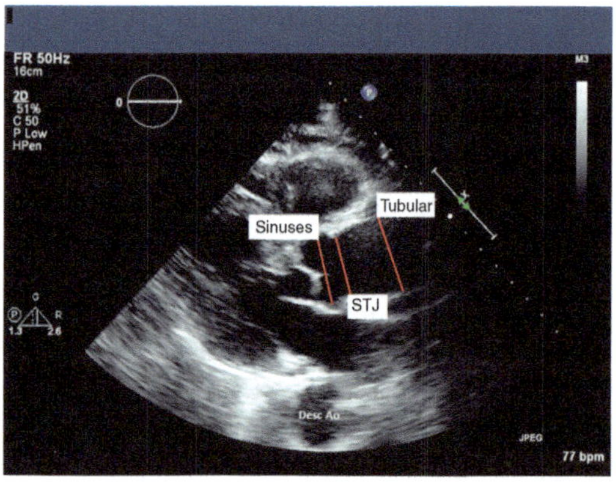

Fig. 14.2 Aortic root anatomy. Parasternal long axis view of the aortic root and the tubular ascending aorta. *Desc Ao descending aorta, STJ sinotubular junction*

- Aortic root measurements on TTE are performed in the PLAX view
  - Aortic Annulus:

    Measured at the hinge point of the aortic valve leaflets

    At mid systole

    Inner edge to inner edge

    Reference values (cm): Male: 2.6 ± 0.3, Female: 2.3 ± 0.2

    Indexed values (cm/m^2): Male: 1.3 ± 0.1, Female: 1.3 ± 0.1
  - Other root measurements

    Measured at end diastole

    Leading edge to leading edge

	Absolute (cm)	Indexed (cm/m^2)
Sinus of Valsalva	M: 3.4 ± 0.3 F: 3.0 ± 0.3	M: 1.7 ± 0.2 F: 1.8 ± 0.2
Sino-tubular junction	M: 2.9 ± 0.3 F: 2.6 ± 0.3	M: 1.5 ± 0.2 F: 1.5 ± 0.2
Tubular ascending aorta	M: 3.0 ± 0.4 F: 2.7 ± 0.4	M: 1.5 ± 0.2 F: 1.6 ± 0.2

14.3 Aortic Atherosclerosis

- In general, atherosclerotic plaque (atheroma) in the aorta increases in severity as the distance from aortic valve increases
- Prevalence in ascending aorta 8.4% < arch 31% < descending aorta 45%
- Identification of aortic atheroma has prognostic implications with increasing incidence of CAD, embolic phenomena, spontaneous CVA, and post bypass/cardiac catheterization CVA

Echocardiographic Assessment

- Although TTE can occasionally identify aortic atheroma from suprasternal view, it is not a reliable method.
- TEE (Fig. 14.3 and Videos 14.1A and 14.1B) can obtain high resolution views of the aortic intimal surface, mobile plaque, calcifications
- The aortic wall appears echocardiographically as two lines—adventitial-medial border and intima-lumen interface—separated by a hypoechoic space which represents the intimal-medial thickness (IMT).

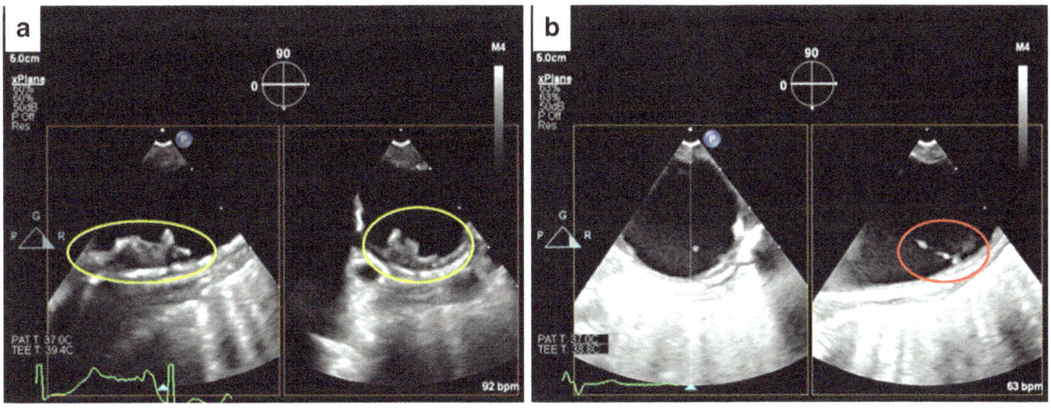

Fig. 14.3 **Aortic atherosclerosis**. (**a**) Transesophageal biplane view of the distal aortic arch showing very severe, complex atherosclerotic plaque (yellow circles). (**b**) Transesophageal biplane view of the descending aorta showing an elongated mobile component (clot) on the surface of atherosclerotic plaque (red circle)

- IMT—normally ≤ 1 mm.
- The aortic wall is normally smooth, continuous, and < 2 mm in thickness.
- There are different classification schemes to grade aortic atheroma
- For example - ASE consensus classification for aortic atheroma (Modified FAP criteria/ Savage classification

Grade	Atheroma severity	Atheroma thickness
1	Normal	<2 mm
2	Mild	2–3 mm
3	Moderate	3–5 mm
4	Severe	>5 mm
5	Complex	Grade 2,3, or 4 + mobile or ulcerated components

Clinical Manifestations

- Aortic atheroma is a manifestation of systemic atherosclerosis
- Increased incidence of co-existing CAD and PVD can be seen, as well as aortic aneurysm, renal artery stenosis, aortic valve stenosis, and mitral annular calcification
- Aortic atheroma is independently associated with advanced age, diabetes, smoking, hyperlipidemia and hypertension.
- Increased risk of CVA/embolization is seen with atheroma ≥4 mm, mobile atheroma, ulceration or thrombus, noncalcified plaques, and location in ascending aorta or aortic arch.
- The mainstay of treatment is statin therapy ± aspirin and aggressive risk factor modification.

14.4 Aortic Aneurysm

- Dilatation of any aortic segment beyond the normal range of reference values should prompt evaluation of the entire aorta.
- An aortic aneurysm results from stretching of all three of the aortic wall layers (intima, media, adventitia) and can involve more than one aortic segment
  - 60% involve the aortic root and/or ascending aorta
  - 10% involve the arch
  - 40% involve the descending aorta

- Aortic dilation is a nonspecific term that refers to both ectasia (enlargement beyond the reference value of the affected segment) and aneurysm (>1.5 × the normal measurement of that segment).

Etiology

- Primary aortic diseases that cause weakening of the wall of the aorta (connective tissue disease, Marfan's, inflammatory)
- Secondary/degenerative disease of the aorta (e.g. hypertension, AI/volume overload, AS) that lead to progressive dilation

Disease	Typical findings
Marfan's Syndrome	'Pear shaped' dilation localized to the annulus and SOV Caused by mutation in FBN1 fibrillin gene; 25% of mutations are sporadic Diagnosis—Ghent criteria
Bicuspid aortic valve	50% of patients with bicuspid aortic valve have aortic dilation Most common—tubular ascending aorta, less common—arch or root Caused by associated genetic abnormalities of connective tissue Screening of all first degree relatives recommended
Other connective tissue diseases	Ehlers-Danlos syndrome type IV; Loeys-Dietz syndrome;
Inflammatory/ infectious aortitis	Giant cell arteritis, Takayasu arteritis, mycotic syndromes, syphilis, Bechet's, ankylosing spondylitis
Degenerative/ secondary	HTN, volume overload, trauma, AS, subaortic membrane (post-stenotic dilatation)
Other	Idiopathic; familial thoracic aortic aneurysm syndrome

Morphologic Classification:

- Fusiform aneurysm
  - More common than saccular aneurysm
  - Caused by diffuse/circumferential weakening of the aortic wall
  - Appears as spindle shaped enlargement with tapered ends
- Saccular aneurysm
  - Less common
  - Focal weakening of the aortic wall
  - Appears as balloon-shaped outpouching

Echocardiographic and Multi-Modality Imaging Assessment

Aortic diameter is the principle predictor of aortic rupture making accurate measurement of the maximum aortic diameter of critical importance

- CT with contrast—first line
  - Very accurate and reproducible measurement
  - Considered superior to echo
  - Can accurately visualize all segments of the aorta and branch vessels
- TTE—second line (Fig. 14.4)
  - In most cases, aortic root dilatation can be serially assessed by TTE
  - However, dilatation beyond the sino-tubular junction is not adequately assessed with TTE.
  - TTE is very useful for family screening, assessing associated AI and LV function, and for disease limited to aortic root
- TEE—third line
  - Adequate for evaluation of aortic root and most of the ascending aorta
  - Has limitations in assessing the aortic arch and beyond

    Note: commonly there is a "blind spot' at the distal ascending aorta/proximal aortic arch due to air in the trachea or left main bronchus
  - TEE is considered third line modality because of its semi-invasive nature, limited

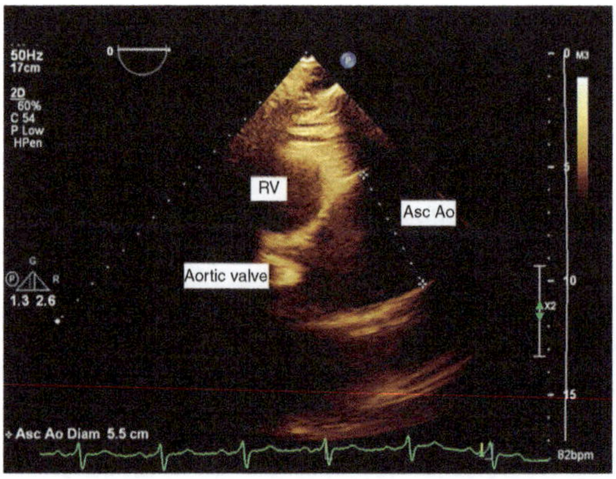

Fig. 14.4 **Aortic root aneurysm**. Parasternal long axis view showing large ascending aorta aneurysm, measuring up to 5.5 cm in diameter. *Asc Ao ascending aorta, RV right ventricle*

distal ascending aorta visualization, and inability to visualize arch vessels
- MRI—second line
  - Can accurately image entire aorta and avoids ionizing radiation
  - Preferred for follow-up of young patients

Management

- Medical treatment
  - Aggressive risk factor control
  - Target low systolic blood pressure, low LDL
  - Family screening when appropriate
- Surgical indications
  - Surgical intervention on the aortic root is undertaken when the estimated risk of complications (e.g. aortic dissection) outweighs the estimated surgical risk
  - Variables to consider when assessing risk for complications include aortic size, rate of change in aortic diameter, underlying pathology (for example, at a given aortic root diameter, risk of patients with Marfan's disease is higher as compared to other pathologies like HTN)
  - Variables to consider regarding risk of surgery include patient's age, comorbidities etc.

14.5 Sinus of Valsalva Aneurysm (SOVA)

Occasionally a localized aneurysm of one of the sinuses of Valsalva can be seen. Most common location—right coronary cusp (RCC).

Etiology

- Congenital—most common
  - Associated with bicuspid aortic valve, VSD
  - Can have a "wind sock" appearance
- Infectious—second most common cause
  - Infective endocarditis, syphilis
  - Generally appear with thickening of the aortic wall and abscess
- Trauma

Echocardiographic Assessment

- TTE (Fig. 14.5, Videos 14.2A and 14.2B)
  - Best seen on parasternal windows—PLAX or basal SAX
  - Contrast echo assists in diagnosis
- TEE
  - Best seen on a short axis view of the aortic valve
    Note: on TEE, the posterior aspect of the sinuses is better visualized as compared to the anterior aspect

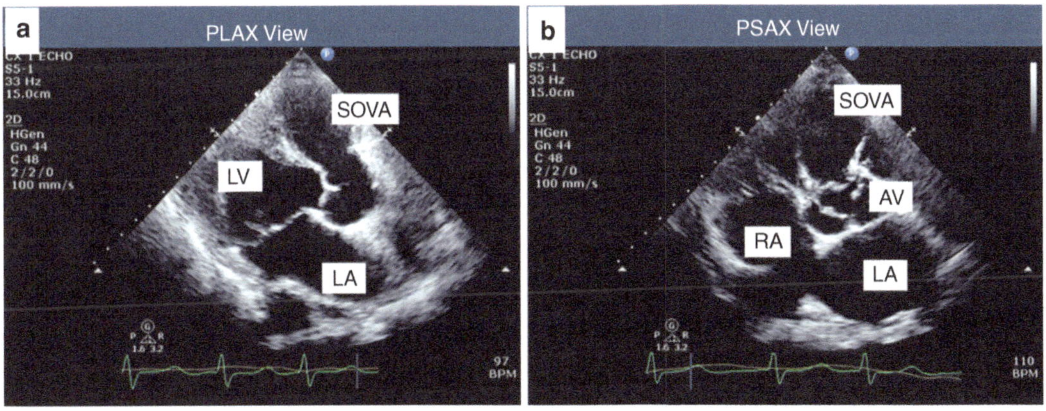

Fig. 14.5 **Sinus of Valsalva aneurysm.** (**a**) Parasternal long axis view showing a large sinus of Valsalva aneurysm (SOVA), of the right coronary sinus. (**b**) Parasternal short axis view showing the large right SOVA. *AV aortic valve, LA left atrium, LV left ventricle, RA right atrium, SOVA sinus of Valsalva aneurysm*

Clinical Manifestations

- May be asymptomatic and found incidentally on imaging studies
- Rupture of the aneurysm can occur into various cardiac chambers
  - Typically:
    RCC → RV or RA
    NCC → LA
    LCC → RV outflow
- Malcoaptation of aortic valve cusps → aortic regurgitation
- Thrombosis of aneurysm and thromboembolic complications

Management

If required, surgical correction is the treatment of choice.

14.6 Acute Aortic Syndromes (AAS)

AAS refers to a group of aortic pathologies that have common manifestations:

- Clinical presentation of acute "aortic pain"
- Damage to the aortic wall
- Risk of aortic rupture, necessitating timely diagnosis and treatment

AAS include:

- Aortic dissection
- Intramural hematoma
- Penetrating aortic ulcer
- Aortic aneurysm rupture

14.6.1 Aortic Dissection (AD)

AD results from a tear of the intima creating intimo-medial flap that allows blood to pulse into the media creating a false lumen and further propagation of the dissection.

Etiology

- The ultimate etiology for AD is the occurrence of linear tear in the intima that leads to the dissection flap
- Risk factors for intimal tear are:
  - HTN, atherosclerosis, smoking, cocaine
  - Bicuspid aortic valve, connective tissue disease (Marfan's, cystic medial necrosis), pre-existing aortic aneurysm
  - Inflammatory arteritis
  - Pregnancy, prolonged steroid use, trauma, iatrogenic (any instrumentation of the aorta—catheterization, surgery, cardiopulmonary bypass)

AD Classification

There are two main classification systems for AD: Stanford and DeBakey (Fig. 14.6).

- Stanford classification is based on whether or not the ascending aorta is involved.
- It is the more widely used classification.
- Most treatment algorithms rely on the Stanford classification
  - Stanford Type A
    Any dissection involving the ascending aorta
    More common (60% of AD) and caries a much higher mortality than type B
  - Stanford Type B
    Involves only the descending aorta (distal to left subclavian artery)
    Less common and has a lower mortality rate
- The DeBakey classification takes into account the site of the intimal tear
  - Type 1—starts at ascending aorta and propagates at least to the arch
  - Type 2—starts at the ascending aorta and limited to the ascending aorta only
  - Type 3—starts at the descending aorta and propagates distally or proximally (but not proximal to the left subclavian artery)

Echocardiographic and Multimodality Assessment (Fig. 14.7, Videos 14.3A and 14.3B)

- TTE
  - Low sensitivity for diagnosing AD
  - PLAX & suprasternal notch view
    Sometimes dissection flap can be visualized as a linear density that moves independent of the cardiac cycle (vs.

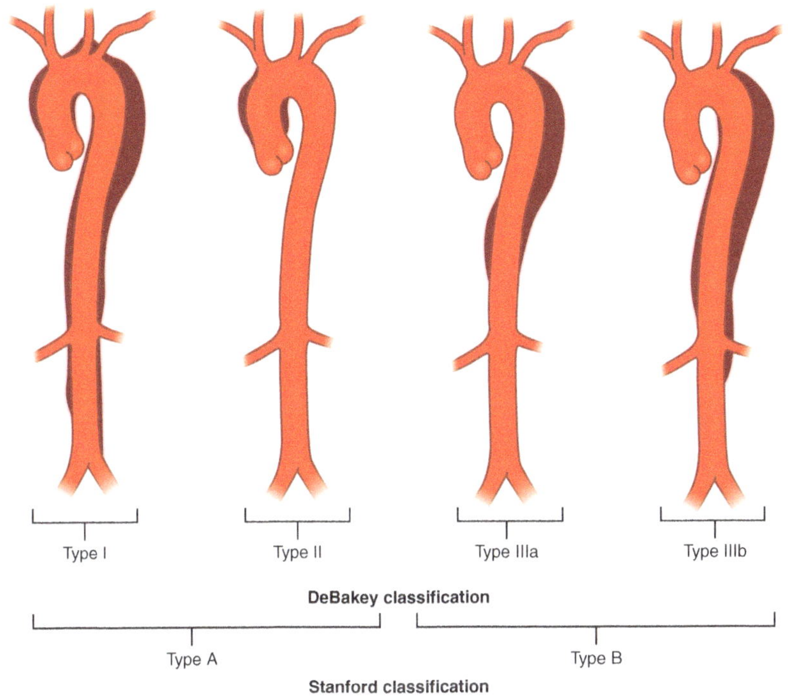

Fig. 14.6 Aortic dissection classification. The two most widely used classifications for aortic dissection are the DeBakey and the Stanford classifications. The Stanford classification is based on ascending aorta involvement (type A) or no ascending aorta involvement (type B), regardless of how far the dissection extends. The DeBakey classification takes into account the extent of the propagation of the dissection

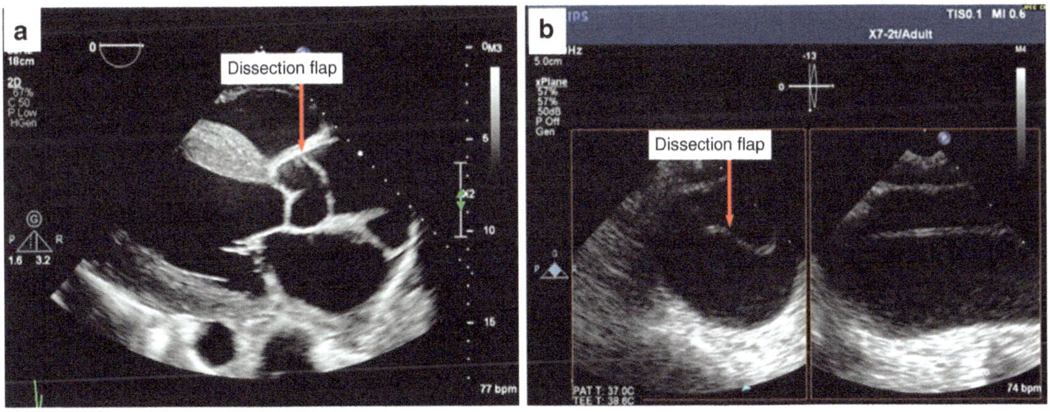

Fig. 14.7 Aortic dissection. (**a**) Parasternal long axis view showing a proximal ascending aorta dissection. (**b**) Transesophageal bi-plane view of descending thoracic aorta showing very extensive dissection (near circumferential) of the descending aorta

aortic wall artifact that moves with cardiac cycle)

Note: negative TTE does not rule out aortic dissection

  - TTE is very helpful in assessing complication of AD such as aortic regurgitation, pericardial effusion and tamponade, or wall motion abnormalities with ischemic cardiac injury due to dissection propagation into coronary ostium (most commonly—RCA).
- TEE
  - High sensitivity and specificity for diagnosing AD (98–99%)

    Note: important to remember there is a "blind spot" due to air in the trachea where TEE cannot visualize the distal ascending aorta-proximal aortic arch
  - As in TTE, important to differentiate between aortic wall reverberation artifact and intimal flap
  - Major benefits of TEE: rapid, portable, does not require contrast

    Note: if clinical suspicion is high and TEE negative → consider further imaging (sensitivity of TEE is very high but not 100%)
- Doppler assessment
  - Helpful in differentiating true and false lumen
  - Can help differentiating linear artifact from dissection flap
- Several echocardiographic characteristics can be used to differentiate the false lumen from the true lumen

	True lumen	False lumen
Anatomic assessment	Systolic Expansion Thicker wall (+)Atherosclerotic plaque	No systolic expansion Thinner wall (−)Atherosclerotic plaque
Color Doppler assessment	Brisk systolic blood flow Entry point may be seen with turbulence	Slow flow Areas of swirling/sludge Partial/complete thrombosis

- CT angiography
  - Very high sensitivity and specificity for AD diagnosis
  - Full extent of the dissection can be seen
  - Generally very rapid and readily available.
  - Does not require patient to be NPO for a long time
  - Does require contrast injection and involves radiation.

Clinical Manifestations

- Chest and back pain—presenting symptom in 86%

  Note: 6.4% of dissections present as "painless dissection"
- Syncope—presenting symptom in 13%
- Pulse deficit, absent carotid pulse, unequal blood pressures in both arms
- Hypertension (50%), normotension (35%), hypotension (15%)
- Widened mediastinum on CXR
- Complications from type A dissection
  - Myocardial ischemia, cardiac tamponade, aortic regurgitation, stroke
- Complications from type B dissection
  - Abdominal pain, spinal cord ischemia/peripheral neuropathy, renal failure, lower extremity ischemia

Management

As a general rule—type A dissection requires surgical treatment, type B may be managed medically

- Type A dissection
  - Medical management—60% mortality
  - Surgical management—26% mortality

    Note: when type A dissection is complicated by pericardial tamponade—extreme caution needed regarding pericardiocentesis; relieving tamponade can increase cardiac output → worsen dissection propagation → increase mortality. Pericardiocentesis should only be performed in operating room, ready to go on cardiopulmonary bypass.

- Type B dissection
  - Medical management—11% mortality
  - Surgical management—31% mortality
  - Surgery indicated for severe pain or symptoms due to dissection propagation (renal failure, limb ischemia, neurogenic symptoms)
- Mainstay of medical management—BP control and beta blockade
  - Beta Blockers—decrease shear stress on aortic wall
  - Vasodilators (avoid pure vasodilators without adequate beta blockade) and other BP treatments
- Causes of death in aortic dissection: tamponade, visceral/cardiac ischemia, aortic rupture

14.6.2 Intramural Hematoma (IMH)

Hemorrhage into the aortic media (without an obvious intimal tear).

Etiology

- Most common cause—spontaneous rupture of vasa vasorum
- Other causes:
  - Pathologic neovascularization of aortic plaque with micro-blood vessels and spontaneous bleeding
  - Chest wall trauma
- Risk factors include: HTN, DM, prior cardiac surgery, bicuspid aortic valve

  Note: Marfan's syndrome is not a risk factor
- Type B (distal IMH) is more common (60%)

Echocardiographic Assessment and Multimodality Imaging

- TEE (Fig. 14.8, Video 14.4)
  - Localized thickening of the aorta with possible compression of the true lumen
  - Discrete circumferential or crescent shaped thickening of the aortic wall >5–7 mm

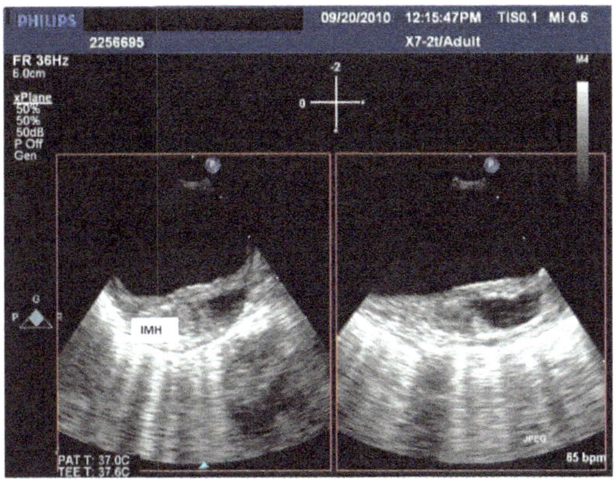

Fig. 14.8 **Intramural hematoma**. Transesophageal biplane view of the descending thoracic aorta showing an intramural hematoma. Notice the preserved intimal lining. *IMH intramural hematoma*

  - Intimal layer is smooth and continuous without intimal flap

    Displacement of intimal calcium into the lumen can be seen, however intima remains intact
- CT—Most common initial imaging modality
- MRI—superior for ruling out dissection flap and differentiating IMH from AD with a thrombosed false lumen

Clinical Manifestations and Management

- Accounts for 6 to 22–28% of AAS (different prevalence in western or eastern registries)
- Severe chest/back pain

  Note: acute MI, pulse deficit and visceral ischemia—unlikely
- IMH can progress to aneurysm, pseudoaneurysm, aortic rupture, and frank dissection
  - Predictors of progression: persistent pain, evidence of hypoperfusion, proximal root involvement (Type A) with aortic regurgitation, IMH > 1 cm
- Prognosis
  - Type A IMH—39% mortality rate; management is generally surgical
  - Type B IMH—8% mortality rate; management usually conservative: beta blockers, BP control

14.6.3 Penetrating Aortic Ulcer (PAU)

Focal area of atherosclerotic plaque that erodes/penetrates the internal elastic lamina into variable depth of the media.

Etiology

Risk factors: HTN, smoking, CAD, aortic aneurysm.

Echocardiographic Assessment and Multimodality Imaging

- Imaging modalities used for diagnosis: TEE, CT, MRI.
- Visualize:
  - Area of ulceration
  - Outpouching beyond expected aortic wall
  - Severe atherosclerotic plaque in the adjacent area

Clinical Manifestations

- PAU usually occur in the descending aorta
- Accounts for 2–11% of AAS
- Presents with back pain (75%), pleural effusion (30%)
- If PAU erodes deep into the media → rupture of vasa vasorum may occur → progression to IMH
- PAU can also progress to form a pseudoaneurysm, aneurysm, frank dissection or aortic rupture
- Treatment includes medical management, BP control, risk factor modification and surgical consideration

14.7 Coarcation of Aorta

Congenital narrowing of the descending aorta distal to the left subclavian artery.

- The type of coarctations is defined by its location relative to the ductus arteriosus (Fig. 14.9):
  - Post-ductal—most commonly seen in adults
  - Pre-ductal and Juxta-ductal coarctations—more commonly identified in infants and children
- 50% of patients with coarctation have a co-existent bicuspid aortic valve

  Note: 10% of patients with bicuspid aortic valve have aortic coarctation
- Other associated conditions:
  - Intracranial berry aneurysms—10%
  - Aortic aneurysm/dissection
  - Interrupted aorta

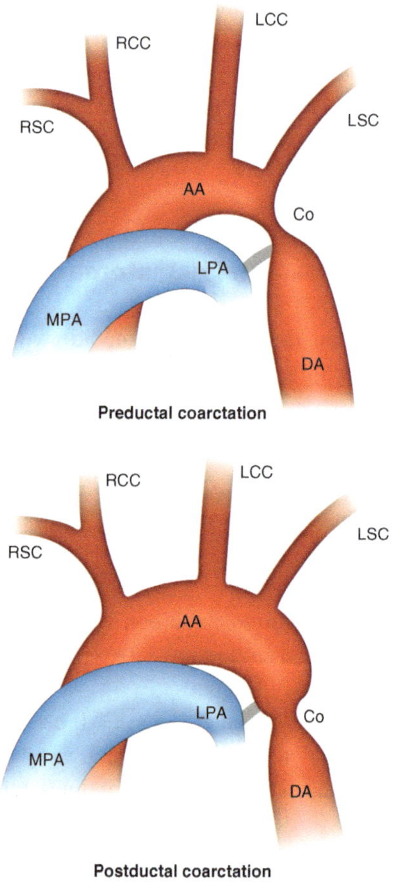

Fig. 14.9 **Aortic coarctation.** Anatomic types of aortic coarctation; pre-ductal—narrowing of the aorta just distal to the left subclavian artery; post-ductal—narrowing is distal to the ductus arteriosus (or ligamentum arteriosum)

– Membranous VSD
– Turner's syndrome (XO)
  10–20% have bicuspid aortic valve, 8% aortic coarctation; increased risk of dissection
– Shone complex

Echocardiographic Assessment

Anatomic Assessment

1. Discrete narrowing of the proximal portion of the descending aorta
   - TTE—suprasternal notch view
     Note: this view may not always visualize the narrowed segment which may be more distal/lower than visualized portion of the descending aorta
   - TEE—high esophageal views
2. LVH

Doppler Assessment

1. With hemodynamically significant coarctation (luminal narrowing ≥50%) → elevated peak systolic velocities across the coarctation segment (>2 m/s)
   Note: There can be low velocity/pressure gradient across the coarctation if there are well developed collateral vessels or PDA
2. Abdominal aorta spectral Doppler:
   - Delayed systolic upstroke (prolonged acceleration time) and prolonged deceleration time
   - Severe coarctation → continuous flow in diastole "pandiastolic antegrade flow"
     Note: Mild coarctation may not cause pandiastolic antergrade flow; loss of diastolic flow reversal is commonly noted

- Psuedocoarctation — increased gradient across descending aorta:
  – Redundant and tortuous distal aortic arch with kink just distal to the subclavian artery

Clinical Manifestations and Management

- Hypertension in children or young adults (measured on the arms)
- Blood pressure in lower extremities lower than upper extremities
- Rib notching from collateral circulation

Management (Adults)

- Treatment of HTN with beta blockers
- More prone to renal side effects from ACE inhibitors
- Indications for intervention:
  – Peak to peak gradient across coarctation > 20 mmHg
  – Peak to peak gradient < 20 mmHg with evidence of significant collateral flow, or in the setting of low forward stroke volume
- Surgical repair versus catheter-based angioplasty/stenting
  – Considerations for surgery vs. percutaneous repair include: patient's age, simple vs. complex anatomy, length of coarct segment, prior repair, concomitant disease and arch anatomy

14.8 Chest Trauma/Transection of Aorta

- Occurs due to rapid deceleration injury (MVA) and chest compression/blunt trauma (e.g. fall from significant height)
- Transection occurs at attachment points of the aorta to adjacent structures and leads to a perpendicular flap
  – Most feared complication is complete aortic rupture and mediastinal hemorrhage
- Most common site—aortic isthmus;
  – The isthmus is the transition zone between mobile ascending aorta / aortic arch and more fixed descending aorta → rapid deceleration may cause more stretching and trauma

 - Isthmus is likely weaker than other parts of the aorta
- Other rupture sites: gastro-esophageal junction at the diaphragm and sinuses of Valsalva

Further Reading

Berretta P, Patel HJ, Gleason TG, et al. IRAD experience on surgical type A acute dissection patients: results and predictors of mortality. Ann Cardiothorac Surg. 2016;5(4):346–51. https://doi.org/10.21037/acs.2016.05.10.

Erbel R, Aboyans V, Boileau C, et al. 2014 ESC Guidelines on the diagnosis and treatment of aortic diseases: Document covering acute and chronic aortic diseases of the thoracic and abdominal aorta of the adult. The Task Force for the Diagnosis and Treatment of Aortic Diseases of the European Society of Cardiology (ESC) [published correction appears in Eur Heart J. 2015 Nov 1;36(41):2779]. Eur Heart J. 2014;35(41):2873–926. https://doi.org/10.1093/eurheartj/ehu281.

Evangelista A, Isselbacher EM, Bossone E, et al. Insights From the International Registry of acute aortic dissection: a 20-year experience of collaborative clinical research. Circulation. 2018;137(17):1846–60. https://doi.org/10.1161/CIRCULATIONAHA.117.031264.

Goldstein SA, Evangelista A, Abbara S, et al. Multimodality imaging of diseases of the thoracic aorta in adults: from the American Society of Echocardiography and the European Association of Cardiovascular Imaging: endorsed by the Society of Cardiovascular Computed Tomography and Society for Cardiovascular Magnetic Resonance. J Am Soc Echocardiogr. 2015;28(2):119–82. https://doi.org/10.1016/j.echo.2014.11.015.

Hiratzka LF, Bakris GL, Beckman JA, et al. 2010 ACCF/AHA/AATS/ACR/ASA/SCA/SCAI/SIR/STS/SVM guidelines for the diagnosis and management of patients with Thoracic Aortic Disease: a report of the American College of Cardiology Foundation/American Heart Association Task Force on Practice Guidelines, American Association for Thoracic Surgery, American College of Radiology, American Stroke Association, Society of Cardiovascular Anesthesiologists, Society for Cardiovascular Angiography and Interventions, Society of Interventional Radiology, Society of Thoracic Surgeons, and Society for Vascular Medicine [published correction appears in Circulation. 2010 Jul 27;122(4):e410]. Circulation. 2010;121(13):e266–369. https://doi.org/10.1161/CIR.0b013e3181d4739e.

15 Congenital Heart Disease

Learning Objectives

- Understand the principles utilized for interpreting adult congenital heart disease (CHD) echocardiogram
- Learn the echocardiographic assessment and consequences of congenital heart diseases, as seen in the adult echocardiography laboratory

15.1 Atrial Septal Defects (ASD)

- ASD is the second most common congenital defect, and accounts for roughly 10% of all CHDs
- There is 2:1 female to male predominance
- Symptoms are often progressive; diagnosis delayed into adulthood.
- Anatomical types of ASDs:
  - Ostium secundum
  - Ostium primum
  - Sinus venosus ASD
  - Unroofed coronary sinus.

15.1.1 Interatrial Septum (IAS) Formation

The interatrial septum develops in several stages, starting at the 5th week gestation (Fig. 15.1)

- Septum primum, a crescent shaped tissue, grows in a cranial to caudal direction towards the endocardial cushions, separating the common atria
- The space between the leading edge of the septum primum and the endocardial cushion is called the ostium primum
- Before the septum primum seals off the ostium primum, fenestrations develop in the middle of it, which coalesce and form a second opening—the ostium secundum (OS)
- The ostium secundum allows blood to continue to flow from the right atrium to the left atrium once the septum primum has covered the ostium primum
- Failure of the septum primum to fuse with the endocardial cushions and seal off the ostium primum results in an ostium primum ASD
- Septum secundum develops on the right atrial side of the septum primum; it is an enfolding of the atrial wall which grows towards the ostium secundum, however not completely separating the atria
- The part of the septum primum that remains un-covered by the septum secundum is the fossa ovalis and is the only "true" interatrial septum in the adult

Electronic Supplementary Material The online version of this chapter (https://doi.org/10.1007/978-3-030-47041-8_15) contains supplementary material, which is available to authorized users.

T. Rambhatla, G. Perk, *The Echocardiography Companion*,
https://doi.org/10.1007/978-3-030-47041-8_15

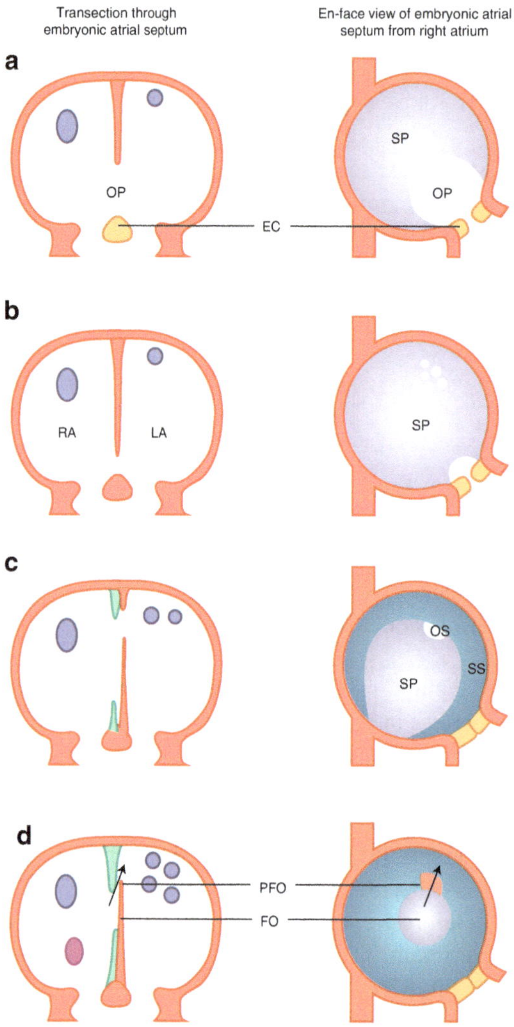

Fig. 15.1 **Embryologic development of the interatrial septum.** (**a**) Septum primum (SP) grows as a crescent shaped structure from the roof of the primordial common atria towards the endocardial cushions (EC); the space between the leading edge of the septum primum and the endocardial cushion is called the ostium primum (OP). (**b**) Before the septum primum seals off the ostium primum, fenestrations develop in the middle of it, which coalesce and form a second opening—the ostium secundum (OS). Septum primum then fuses with the endocardial cushions, closing ostium primum. (**c**) An enfolding of the atrial wall, the septum secundum (SS), develops on the right atrial side of septum primum and covers ostium secundum. (**d**) The septum secundum does not completely separate the atria; part of the septum primum remains uncovered by the septum secundum—the fossa ovalis (FO). The two septa only partially fuse; the septum primum acts as a flap valve (the "foramen ovale (FO)"), allowing the continued communication between the right and left atria (arrow)

- The septum secundum covers the ostium secundum, however the two septa only partially fuse; the septum primum acts as a flap valve (the "foramen ovale"), allowing the continued communication between the right and left atria
- Failure of septum secundum to completely overlap and cover the ostium secundum results in a secundum ASD. Most commonly, secundum ASD is due to a large ostium secundum (which is in fact a defect in the septum primum), that is too large for septum secundum to cover.
- After birth, when the lungs expand and pulmonary pressures drop, the septum primum and secundum fuse together closing the foramen ovale.
- Failure of fusion of the two septa occurs in roughly ¼ of the population creating Patent Foramen Ovale (PFO).

Classification of ASD

Based on size of the defect

- Small—<5 mm
- Medium—5–10 mm
- Large—10 mm

  Note: extent of shunt is subject to hemodynamic factors other than defect size alone (such as the competing forces of LV and RV compliance, pulmonary vascular resistance, valve disease, etc.)

15.1.2 Clinical Presentation

- Symptoms often manifest in adulthood
- Can present earlier depending on the size and extent of shunt
- Hemodynamically significant ASDs (Qp:Qs > 2:1) present with signs and symptoms of right sided volume overload—e.g. SOB, right heart failure, pulmonary hypertension

  Note: Patient presenting with unexplained dilation of right sided chambers should undergo a thorough evaluation for ASD. Typically, ASDs do not cause left sided overload or dilatation.
- Arrhythmias/palpitations
- Stroke/paradoxical embolus

  Note: Small ASD < 5 mm with no RV enlargement generally do not impact cardiac clinical course and remain asymptomatic. However, paradoxical embolus may still occur

Physical Exam

- Flow across the septal defect does not result in a murmur
- Increased flow across right sided valves (usually with Qp:Qs > 2:1) produces murmurs
  - Diastolic rumble across tricuspid valve
  - Ejection murmur across pulmonic valve
- Fixed split S2
  - No respiratory variation in the timing of aortic valve/pulmonic valve closure (A2 ➔ P2)

    Under normal circumstances

    Inspiration ➔ increase in right sided venous return ➔ increased flow through pulmonic valve ➔ delayed closure of PV ➔ wider separation between A2 and P2

    Expiration ➔ increase in left sided venous return from the pulmonary circulation ➔ AV closure moves closer to PV closure ➔ A2 and P2 occur simultaneously

    With an ASD, right and left sided chamber volumes are fixed during respiration

    Increase in venous return to the right side during inspiration results in less left to right shunting

    Increase in pulmonary venous return to the left side during expiration results in more left to right shunting

    Note: other conditions may cause wide split of S2 (e.g. RBBB, pulmonic stenosis) or paradoxical split of S2 (LBBB, aortic stenosis), however respiratory variations in the S2 split remain

15.1.3 Types of ASD

Ostium Secundum ASD

(Fig. 15.2, Videos 15.1A, 15.1B and 15.1C)

- The most common ASD, accounting for ~70%
- Usually an isolated defect

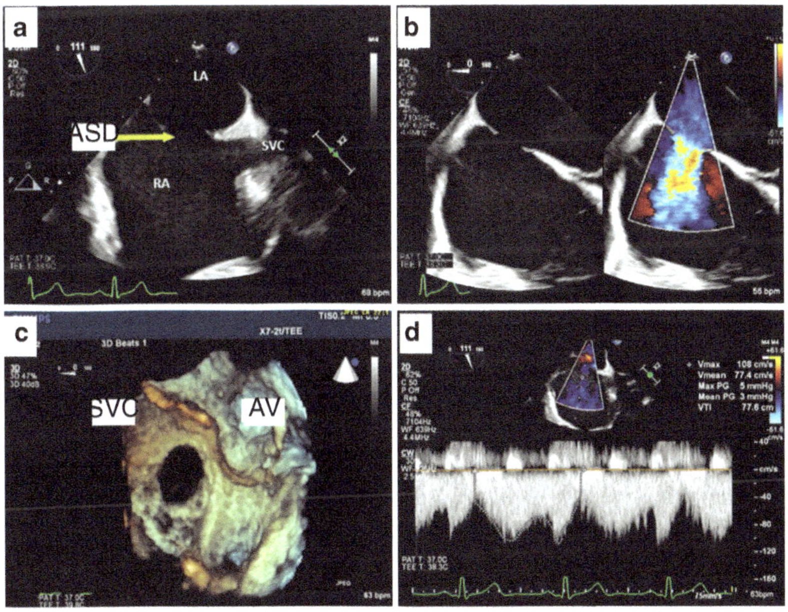

Fig. 15.2 **Secundum ASD.** (**a**) Mid-esophageal bicaval view showing a large secundum atrial septal defect. (**b**) Simultaneous color Doppler imaging shows significant left to right shunt. (**c**) Three-dimensional image from the right atrial perspective visualizing an oblong shaped secundum ASD. (**d**) Characteristic spectral Doppler tracing with continuous flow from left to right. *AV aortic valve, ASD atrial septal defect, LA left atrium, RA right atrium, SVC superior vena cava*

- Occasionally family history or specific genetic disorder is present
  - Holt-Oram syndrome: autosomal dominant disorder with hand and foot abnormalities and AV conduction defects
  - Others: Noonan syndrome, Treacher-Collins syndrome

Echocardiographic Evaluation

- Location—center of the IAS, typically in the superior region of the fossa ovalis (closer to the SVC, further away from IVC and TV)
- TTE has limited sensitivity for secundum ASDs (33% for small, 80% for medium, close to 100% for large secundum ASDs)
- TEE is often required to diagnose secundum ASDs—sensitivity close to 100%
- Secundum ASDs are often oblong or elliptical; significant variation in size can be seen during the cardiac cycle—to ensure measurement of the largest diameter multiple views are required
- Generally, TEE evaluation is required for proper assessment for suitability for percutaneous closure
  - Only secundum type ASDs are amenable to percutaneous closure
  - Requirements are:
    - ASD size: ≤40 mm (46 mm device is the largest available)
    - Surrounding rim tissue: ≥5 mm of rim tissue recommended to allow safe deployment of closure device
    - Note: Aortic rim can be smaller (generally > 3 mm acceptable)
  - Thorough assessment in multiple planes and with 3D imaging is necessary to accurately assess the size of the defect and the surrounding tissue
  - Contraindications to percutaneous closure include:
    - Cardiac thrombus
    - Contraindication to antiplatelet therapy
    - Inadequate rims
    - Non-isolated defect with associated abnormalities requiring surgical correction

Ostium Primum ASD (Partial AV Canal Defect) (Fig. 15.3, Video 15.2)

- Formed when the septum primum fails to fuse with the endocardial cushion; the ostium primum remains not fully covered; a form of AV cushion/AV canal defect
- Primum ASDs account for 10–20% of ASDs
- Primum ASDs can be seen in:
  - Down syndrome—35% of people with Down Syndrome have AV cushion defect
  - Ellis Van Creveld syndrome (consists of synpolydactyly, six fingers, splenic abnormalities)
- Associated abnormalities can include:
  - VSD—complete AV canal defect
  - Cleft anterior mitral valve and MR (Fig. 15.4, Videos 15.3A and 15.3B)
  - Double orifice MV
  - Single Papillary muscle MV (parachute MV)
  - Occasionally TV abnormalities
  - Conduction system abnormalities

Echocardiographic Evaluation

- Location—base of the heart, near AV valves
- TTE—100% sensitivity for primum ASDs, TEE often not required

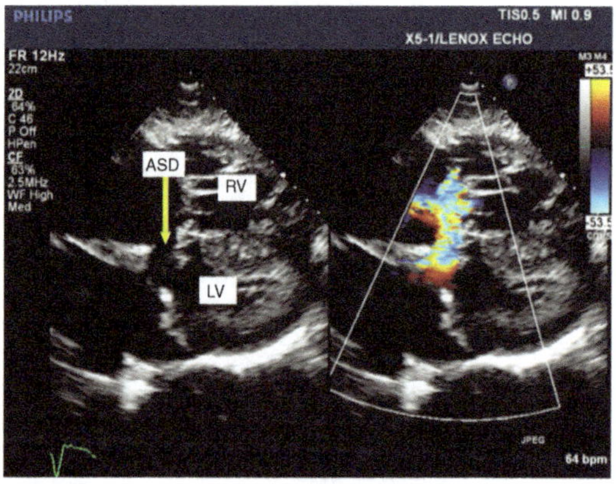

Fig. 15.3 Primum ASD. Subcostal, color compare image showing an ostium primum atrial septal defect (ASD). The defect is caused by failure of the septum primum to fuse with the endocardial cushions at the base atrium. Notice the mitral valve and tricuspid valve are at the same level, (no apical displacement of the tricuspid valve) which is seen with partial and complete endocardial cushion defects. *ASD atrial septal defect, LV left ventricle, RV right ventricle*

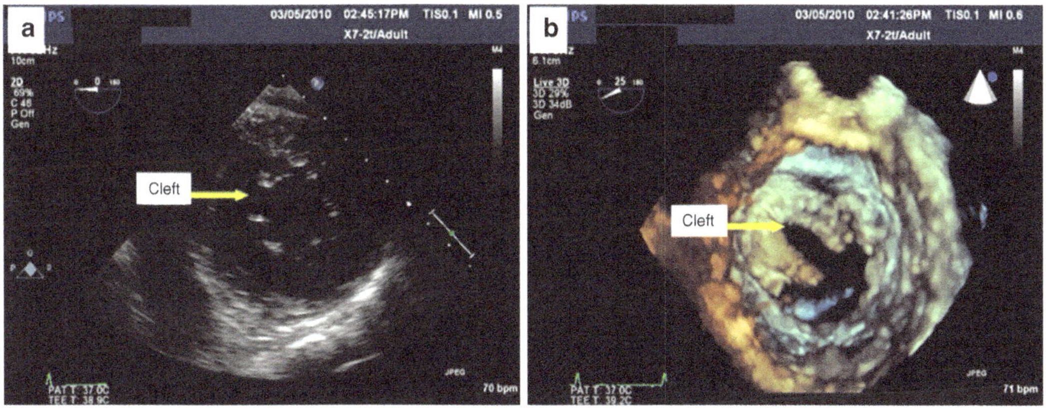

Fig. 15.4 Cleft mitral valve. (**a**) Parasternal short axis view showing a cleft anterior mitral valve. (**b**) Three dimensional image from the left ventricular perspective, showing the anterior leaflet cleft

- Common AV valve ➔ the MV and TV are at same level
  - Apical displacement of the tricuspid valve is lost
- Anterior displacement of the aorta ➔ aorto-mitral continuity is lost
  - Long narrow elongated LVOT ➔ "goose-neck" deformity

    Ratio of LVOT: LV inlet distance > 1.0

    LVOT obstruction can be seen; due to elongated LVOT and mitral valve abnormalities
- Cleft anterior MV (±mitral regurgitation)
- The cleft is best visualized on parasternal short axis view at the level of the leaflets
- TV disease with TR may be seen
- Primum ASD may be part of complete AV canal defect (ASD, inlet VSD, and common AV valve)

Sinus Venosus ASD

- Abnormal insertion of the vena cava (superior or inferior), overriding the interatrial septum
- Accounts for 5–10% of patients with ASDs

Echocardiographic Evaluation

- Location
  - SVC type—superior posterior aspect of the IAS ➔ "biatrial" insertion of the SVC
  - IVC type (less common)—at the IVC-RA junction
- Due to the posterior location of the ASD, TEE is almost always required for diagnosis

  Note: if clinical suspicion for ASD high (e.g. unexplained right heart dilatation) and no ASD seen on TTE, TEE is indicated to rule out sinus venosus ASD
- Almost always associated with partial anomalous pulmonary venous return of the right sided pulmonary veins

Unroofed Coronary Sinus

- Complete or partial absence of the wall between the coronary sinus and the left atrium
- Accounts for <1% of ASDs

Echocardiographic Evaluation

- Hardest ASD to visualized
- Associated congenital defects found in many patients
  - Common associations—persistent left SVC or anomalous pulmonary venous return
- Dilated coronary sinus can be seen on PLAX or apical four chamber view

  Note: prominent coronary sinus may be seen without a shunt (e.g. persistent left SVC, elevated right sided pressures).

15.1.4 Shunt Assessment with Echocardiography (Fig. 15.5)

- Spectral Doppler of the interatrial communication
  - Continuous flow (systole and diastole)
  - If size of ASD can be measured:

$$\text{Shunt flow} = \text{ASD Cross Sectional Area}(\text{CSA}) \times \text{ASD VTI}$$

- Shunt Calculation—Qp : Qs
  - Comparing pulmonary circulation flow (Qp) to systemic flow (Qs) allows assessment of the ratio between them
  - Qp—can be measured at the RVOT or the proximal PA

    $$\text{Qp} = \text{RVOT CSA} \times \text{RVOT PW VTI}$$

  - Qs—measured at the LVOT

    $$\text{QS} = \text{LVOT CSA} \times \text{LVOT PW VTI}$$

  - Significant shunt by echo: Qp:Qs > 1.5
- Important: decrease in shunt size or reversal of shunt occurs with long term complications:
  - Elevated right atrial pressures
  - Decreased RV compliance
  - Increased pulmonary pressure
  - Development of TR

15.1.5 Management

ASD Closure Indications

- For patients without significant pulmonary hypertension, ASD closure is considered / recommended based on the following parameters:
  - Significant net left to right shunt as evidenced by

    RA and/or RV enlargement

    Qp:Qs $\geq$ 1.5:1
  - No significant pulmonary HTN as evidenced by:

    PA pressure <50% systemic BP

    $\text{PVR} < \frac{1}{3}$ of systemic vascular resistance
  - No cyanosis (rest or exercise)

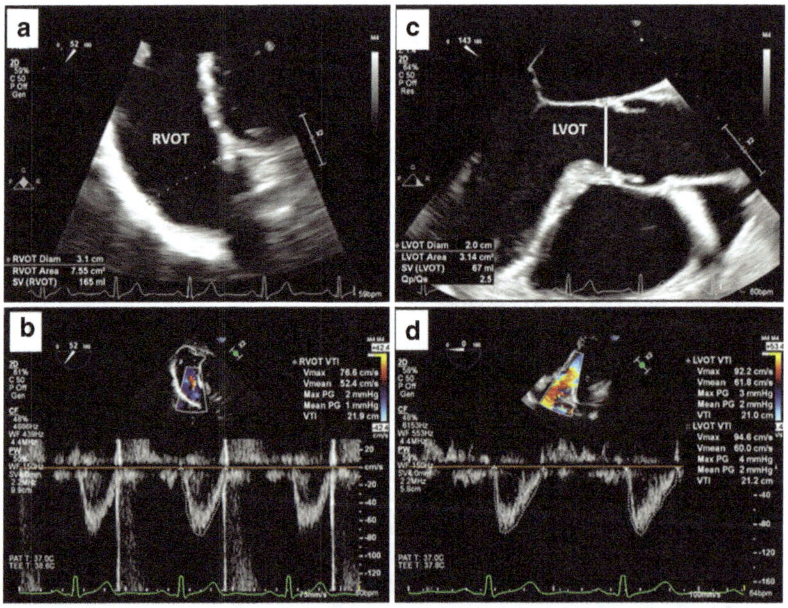

Fig. 15.5 **Shunt assessment.** Shunt magnitude is assessed by calculating the ratio between pulmonary blood flow and systemic blood flow (Qp:Qs). (**a, b**) Pulmonary blood flow is estimated by measuring the RVOT cross sectional area (CSA) and the RVOT VTI. Pulmonary stroke volume is then calculated by: $Qp = RVOT_{CSA} \times RVOT_{VTI}$ ($RVOT_{CSA} = \pi \times RVOT_r^2$); in this example RVOT stroke volume is 166 mL. (**c, d**) Systemic blood flow is estimated by measuring the LVOT cross sectional area and the LVOT VTI. Systemic stroke volume is then calculated by: $Qs = LVOT_{CSA} \times LVOT_{VTI}$; in this example LVOT stroke volume is 66 mL. Qp:Qs in this case = 2.5:1

- If above conditions & patient symptomatic (reduced functional capacity)—ASD closure recommended
- If above conditions & patient asymptomatic—ASD closure considered
- Other presenting symptoms—ASD closure considered
  - Paradoxical embolism (stroke)
  - Orthodeoxia-platypnea—dyspnea/deoxygenation when rising from recumbent to upright position
- For patients with pulmonary hypertension
  - If severe PHTN (systolic PA pressure > $\frac{2}{3}$ systemic systolic pressure and PVR greater than $\frac{2}{3}$ systemic and non-reversible) and net right to left shunt—ASD should not be closed
  - If moderate pulmonary HTN, net left to right shunt and pulmonary arterial pressures and PVR not meeting all above criteria—case by case decision regarding ASD closure
- Most secundum ASDs can be closed percutaneously
- Exceptions include:
  - Defect too large
  - Inadequate rims
  - Associated congenital anomalies (e.g. partial anomalous pulmonary venous return)
  - Significant tricuspid regurgitation (as it may persist after percutaneous closure)
- Non secundum ASDs always require surgical closure

15.2 Ventricular Septal Defects (VSD)

- The most common congenital defect in infants
- Often close spontaneously during childhood and early adulthood
- VSDs can occur anywhere in the interventricular septum (IVS)
- May be single or multiple
- May be associated with other cardiac malformations.

15.2.1 Anatomy of Interventricular Septum (IVS) (Fig. 15.6):

The IVS consists of several components

- Membranous
- Atrio-ventricular

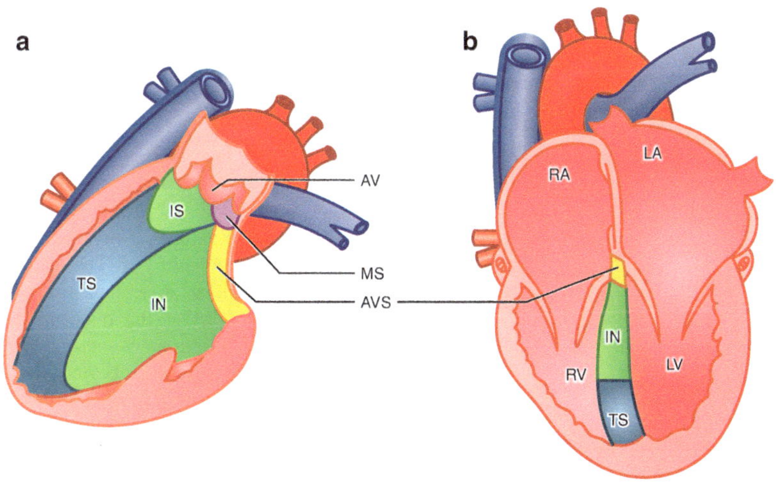

Fig. 15.6 **Anatomy of the interventricular septum.** The interventricular septum consists of four parts: the membranous septum, the trabecular or muscular septum, the infundibular or outlet septum, and the inlet septum. Note: due to the apical displacement of the tricuspid valve there is also an atrioventricular septum, separating the left ventricle and right atrium. *AV aortic valve, AVS atrioventricular septum, IN inlet septum, IS infundibular septum, LA left atrium, LV left ventricle, MS membranous septum, RA right atrium, RV right ventricle, TS trabecular septum*

- Trabecular
- Outlet (infundibular)
- Inlet

The main types of VSD correspond to the septal anatomy:

- Membranous defects
- Gerbode Defect
- Muscular defects
- Supracristal/Subpulmonic (outlet) defects
- AV canal (inlet) defects

15.2.2 Classification of VSDs

- The size of the defect and the PVR determine the physiologic effect of the VSD
- Small VSDs—can be asymptomatic; no cardiac compromise; loud systolic murmur (restrictive VSD). Larger VSDs—left sided volume overload; pulmonary hypertension
- Small VSD
  - Diameter ≤ 4 mm or ≤25% of the size of the aortic annulus
  - Small left to right shunt (generally Qp:Qs <1.5:1); no LV volume overload; normal PA pressure; normal PVR
  - Harsh systolic murmur heard
    Note: small VSDs still carry a risk of endocarditis or cerebral abscess
- Medium VSD
  - Diameter 4–6 mm or 25–75% of aortic annular diameter
  - Small to moderate left to right shunt (generally Qp:Qs 1.5–2.3:1); mild to moderate LV volume overload; usually no pulmonary hypertension
  - Patients may remain asymptomatic or develop mild CHF
- Large VSD ("unrestrictive")
  - Diameter > 6 mm or ≥75% aortic root diameter
  - Shunt size depends on the difference between systemic and pulmonary vascular resistance. When PVR drops after birth, there is moderate to large left to right shunt (generally Qp:Qs > 2.3); LV volume overload develops ➔ pulmonary venous pressure increases ➔ pulmonary hypertension develops
  - CHF symptoms manifest in infancy

15.2.3 Echocardiographic Assessment—General Principles (Fig. 15.7)

1. Septal anatomy
   - PLAX view—anteroseptum (which consists of the outlet or membranous septum and trabecular septum) is visualized
   - PSAX view
     - AV/basal level—membranous and outlet septum visualized
       Membranous septum towards 10 o'clock, outlet septum towards 2 o'clock
     - Mitral valve level—inlet and trabecular septum are visualized

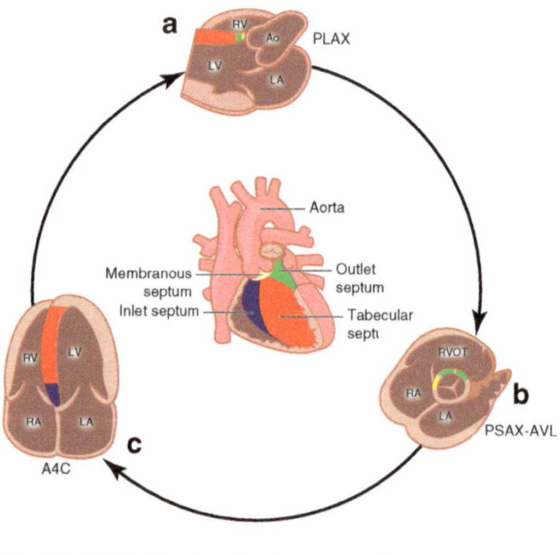

Fig. 15.7 Evaluating the interventricular septum on transthoracic echo. (**a**) The parasternal long axis view visualizes the anteroseptum which contains the muscular septum and either the outlet or membranous septum. Outlet and membranous septa are very close together and difficult to discern on this view. (**b**) The parasternal short axis view at the aortic valve level allows visualization of the membranous and outlet septa. The membranous septum is located at approximately 10 o'clock position and the outlet septum at 2 o'clock. (**c**) The apical four chamber view visualizes of the inlet septum; the five chamber view brings the more anterior membranous septum into view. *AO Aorta, LA left atrium, LV left ventricle, RA right atrium, RV right ventricle*

- Mid ventricular level—trabecular septum is visualized
- Apical view
  - Four chamber view—inlet and trabecular septum are visualized
  - Five chamber view—membranous and trabecular septum visualized
    Membranous and outlet septum are very close together and hard to distinguish in apical view; PSAX view utilized to separate them
2. 2D assessment—visualize a 'gap' in the surface of the IVS endocardial surface
   - Better to examine the LV side of the IVS; the RV surface of the IVS has trabeculations and breaks in the continuity of the endocardium ➔ may mimic VSD
3. Doppler assessment
   - Color Doppler—flow across the septum from left to right (as long as significant pulmonary hypertension has not developed and LV pressure is greater than RV pressure)
   - Small VSDs may not be visualized with 2D imaging and require Doppler imaging
   - Spectral Doppler is helpful to further evaluate color Doppler signal
     - Classic VSD spectral Doppler is high velocity systolic jet with minimal diastolic component (large pressure gradient between LV and RV during systole, diastolic LV and RV pressures are nearly equal)

15.2.4 Types of VSD

Membranous VSD
(Fig. 15.8)

- Most common type, accounts for 70–80% of VSDs
- The membranous septum is the thinnest potion of the IVS; located at the base of the heart, continuous with the inlet, outlet, and muscular septa.
- VSDs in this location typically extend into at least one of the other adjacent septa
- Close proximity to the aortic and tricuspid valves ➔ may lead to valvular insufficiency

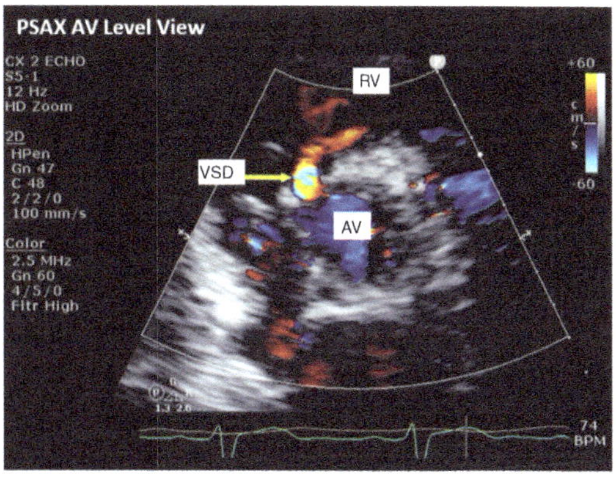

Fig. 15.8 **Membranous VSD**. Parasternal short axis transthoracic image at the aortic valve level showing left to right color flow at 10 o'clock position, consistent with a membranous ventricular septal defect. *AV aortic valve, RV right ventricle, VSD ventricular septal defect*

Echocardiographic Assessment

- Membranous VSD can best be distinguished from VSDs in adjacent septa on the PSAX view at the level of the aortic valve
- Typical location—10 o'clock position
- Due to the close proximity with the tricuspid valve, 20% of patients develop a membranous septum aneurysm ("windsock deformity")

Gerbode Defect
(Fig. 15.9)

- The most superior portion of the membranous IVS is called the atrioventicular septum
- This part of the septum is continuous with the inferior RA and superior LV
- The apical displacement of the tricuspid valve (relative to the mitral valve) creates a part of the IVS that separates LV from RA
  Note: An acquired Gerbode defect can occur (membranous VSD and acquired perforation of the TV leaflet, endocarditis, post-surgery) causing LV to RA shunt.

Muscular (Trabecular) VSD

- Accounts for ~10% of VSDs
- More common in children; often small and close spontaneously early in life

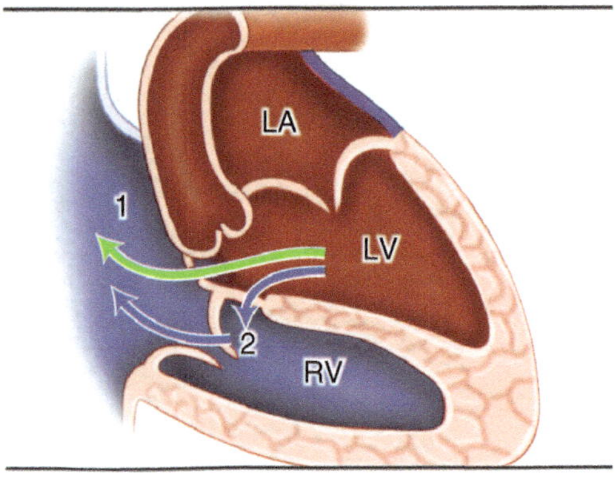

Fig. 15.9 **Gerbode defect**. A Gerbode defect is a left ventricle to right atrial shunt; can occur in several ways: a defect in the atrioventricular septum (green arrow) or a membranous ventricular septal defect with tricuspid septal leaflet pathology (blue arrow). *LA left atrium, LV left ventricle, RV right ventricle*

Echocardiographic Assessment

- Usually located in the distal apical portion of the IVS
- Often small; can be multiple ("Swiss cheese" septum)
- Defect completely surrounded by muscular tissue, no adjacent valves or other structures → typically no associated valve dysfunction

Outlet VSD (Supracristal/Subaortic/Infundibular) (Fig. 15.10)

- Rare defect, accounts for ~ 5% of VSDs
- More common in Asian patients

Echocardiographic Assessment

- Location: outlet septum, adjacent to both PV and the AV
- On PSAX view—typically located at 2 o'clock position
- Can be seen in the five chamber view, however hard to distinguish from membranous VSD
- Because of the close proximity to the aortic valve—progressive AI (due to aortic cusp prolapse) and/or sinus of Valsalva aneurysm (SOVA) can develop
  - Coronary cusp prolapse—75% - RCC

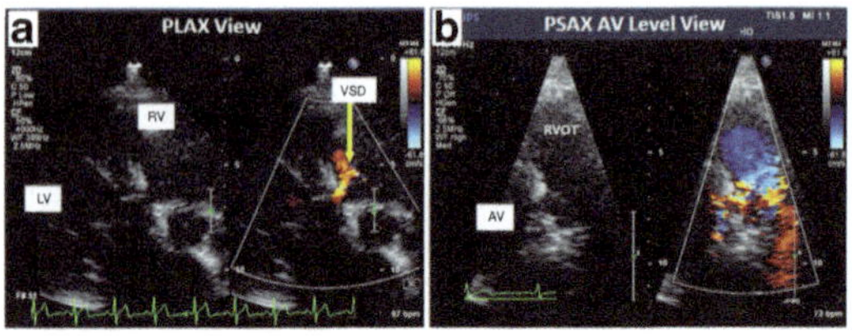

Fig. 15.10 **Supracristal (infundibular/outlet) VSD**. (**a**) Parasternal long axis image of the anteroseptum shows left to right shunt across the outlet septum. In this view it is difficult to distinguish between a membranous VSD and an outlet VSD. (**b**) Parasternal short axis view showing a VSD at a 2 o'clock position, confirming the diagnosis of a supracrital VSD. *AV aortic valve, LV left ventricle, RV right ventricle, RVOT right ventricular outflow tract, VSD ventricular septal defect*

  - SOVA—may be complicated by rupture (into the RV, RA or left side)
  - Presence of AI or SOVA should be taken into consideration when deciding about surgical correction and its timing

Inlet VSD (Complete AV Canal Defect/Endocardial Cushion Defect/AV Septal Defect)

- Accounts for ~5% of VSDs
- Failure of correct fusion of the endocardial cushions results in a range of defects of the atrioventricular septum, at the crux of the heart
- Components of the defect include:
  - Inlet VSD
  - Primum ASD
  - Anomalies of the AV valves (extreme - single AV valve which did not separate into TV and MV)
- Associated with Down's Syndrome
- Typically requires surgical repair early in infancy

Echocardiographic Assessment

- Location: inlet septum at the base of the heart
- Best seen in apical 4 chamber view (note: the 5 chamber view shows the anterior portion of the IVS, typically the membranous septum)
- Common AV valve can be seen
  - No apical displacement of the TV
  - Significant valvular insufficiency present

15.2.5 Management

VSD Closure Indications:

- Hemodynamically significant shunt (Qp:Qs ≥ 1.5:1) and signs of LV volume overload without pulmonary HTN or elevated PVR
- Note: If severe PHTN present (PASP > $\frac{2}{3}$ systemic pressure and PVR > $\frac{2}{3}$ systemic) – VSD closure should not be done
- If PA pressure and PVR elevated, however not to above cutoffs—individualized decision and consultation with adult CHD and PHTN specialists
- History of infective endocarditis (when no contraindications to closure)
- Significant or progressive aortic regurgitation
- Catheter based closure can be considered for isolated uncomplicated muscular VSDs and selected cases of membranous VSD.

15.3 Patent Ductus Arteriosus (PDA)

- The ductus arteriosus (DA) is an arterial connection between the aorta and the main pulmonary artery (PA) (typically—from the aorta, distal to the left subclavian artery to the junction between main PA and left PA)
- In fetal life, due to high pulmonary vascular resistance and low systemic (placental) resistance, flow in the DA is from the PA to the descending aorta (right to left)
- After delivery with onset of respirations:
  - Lungs expand ➔ systemic oxygen saturation rises ➔ pulmonary vascular resistance drops
  - Systemic vascular resistance increases
  - These changes cause reversal of flow in the DA; ultimately the DA constricts and obliterates (likely due to drop in prostaglandin E2 content); the ligamentum arteriosum is the remnant of the fetal DA.
- Failure of the DA to constrict and obliterate results in patent ductus arteriosus
- PDA sequela:
  - Left to right shunting
  - When large enough: pulmonary hypertension, left sided volume overload

    Note: degree of left to right shunt depends on the size and length of the PDA as well as the systemic and pulmonary vascular residence (small shunt—Qp:Qs < 1.5:1, large shunt—Qp:Qs > 2.2:1)
- Increased risk of endarteritis (regardless of size)
- Continuous machinery murmur is usually present at the left second intercostal space

Echocardiographic Assessment (Fig. 15.11, Video 15.4)

- Best views for imaging PDA—high PSAX view at the AV level and suprasternal notch view
- PDA itself may or may not be seen on 2D imaging (small size, usually within 0.9-11mm) however typical color Doppler flow can be picked up on above views
- Dilated PA, and signs of left sided volume overload can be seen with large PDA
- Doppler imaging:
  - Color—continuous flow (throughout systole and diastole); generally towards the transducer (when the shunt is left to right)
  - Spectral Doppler shows high velocity continuous flow with systolic accentuation
  - Shunt calculation (Qp:Qs):

    When measuring output at the LVOT and RVOT—note that Qp:Qs comes out reversed

    Since the shunt occurs <u>outside</u> the heart:

    Stroke volume calculated at the RVOT does NOT include the shunt volume

    Stroke volume calculated at the LVOT DOES include the shunt volume

    However, the pulmonary circulation sees the RVOT stroke volume + shunt volume (that is added at the level of the PA bifurcation); the systemic circulation sees the LVOT stroke volume – shunt volume (that is lost at the level of the DA)

Management

PDA Closure Indications:

- Significant PDA with net left to right shunt and signs of left side volume overload

  Note: as long as there is net left to right shunt, closure should be considered, even if there is pulmonary hypertension and elevated PVR

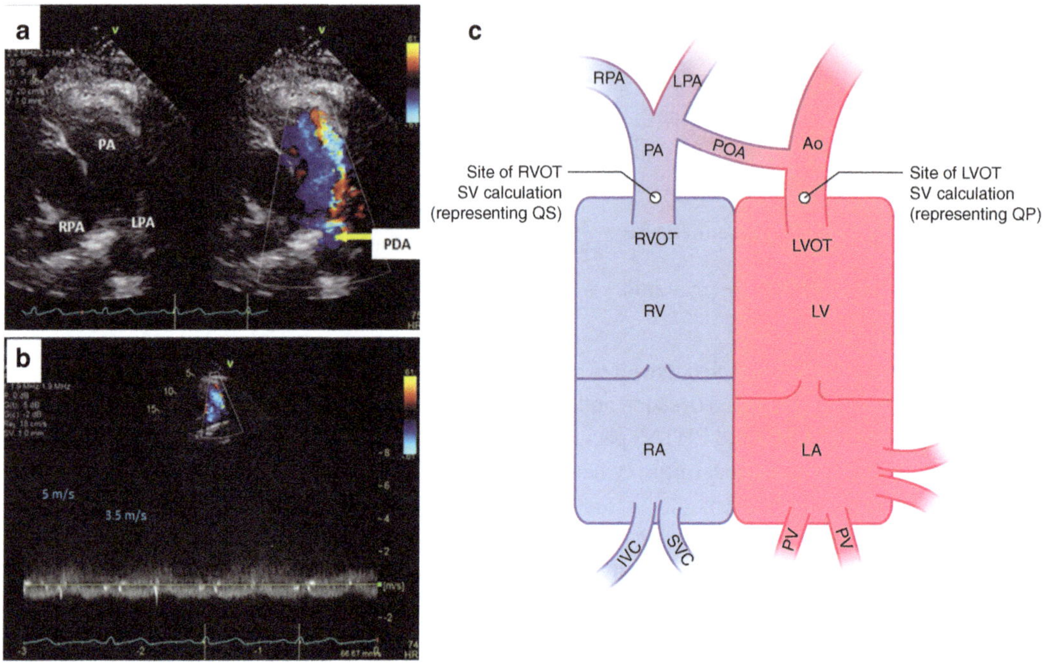

Fig. 15.11 **Patent ductus arteriosus.** (**a**) Parasternal short axis slightly superior to the aortic valve level showing a patent ductus arteriosus (PDA) with flow into the proximal left pulmonary artery (yellow arrow). (**b**) Continuous wave Doppler of ductal flow showing the classic continuous, high velocity, left to right flow, seen in PDA. Note: high velocities throughout systole and diastole (5 m/s and 3.5 m/s respectively) suggest normal pulmonary artery pressures: systolic aorta to pulmonary gradient—100 mmHg, diastolic gradient—49 mmHg. (**c**) Since PDA is an extra-cardiac shunt, Qp:Qs calculation is reversed; Qp is measured at the LVOT, and Qs is measured at the RVOT. *Ao aorta, LPA left pulmonary artery, LVOT left ventricular outflow tract, PA pulmonary artery, PDA patent ductus arteriosus, RPA right pulmonary artery, RVOT right ventricular outflow tract*

- Closure is contraindicated if there is irreversible PHTN and net right to left shunting (class III)
- Prior episode of endarteritis
- Small PDAs—closure may be considered (whether PDA is audible or non-audible) for reducing risk of endarteritis
- PDA may be closed percutaneously (coils or occluder device) or surgically ligated
- Anatomical considerations as well as patient's age and risk determine the procedure of choice

15.4 Tetrology of Fallot (TOF) (Fig. 15.12)

- The most common cyanotic congenital heart disease
- TOF is a combination of 4 abnormalities:

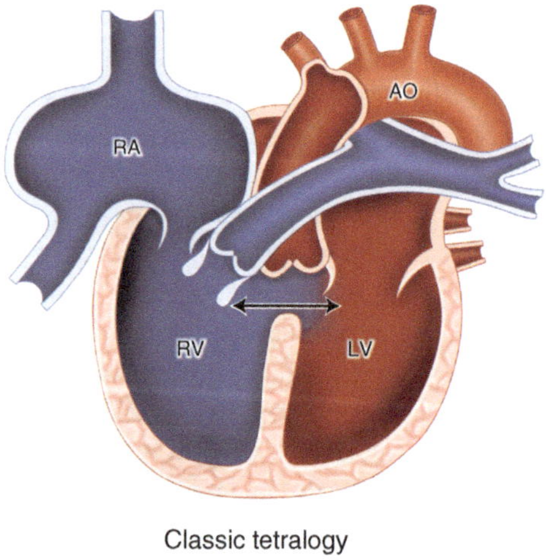

Fig. 15.12 **Tetralogy of Fallot.** Classic Tetralogy of Fallot is a combination of four abnormalities: large outlet VSD, overriding aorta, right ventricular outflow tract obstruction, and right ventricular hypertrophy. *Ao aorta, LV left ventricle, RA right atrium, RV right ventricle*

1. Large outlet (subaortic) VSD
   - The VSD is large and unrestrictive, causing equalization of LV and RV pressures
   - IVS is misaligned, anteriorly deviated and overrides the PA
2. RVOT obstruction
   - Can occur at subvalvular level, pulmonic valve annular level, pulmonic valve level or supra-valvular. Multiple level obstructions can also be seen
   - Hypertrophy of muscle bands in the infundibular septum further increases the outflow obstruction
   - If RVOT obstruction mild ➔ cyanosis may not be evident
3. Overriding aorta
   - Aorta displaced to the right, overriding the VSD
   - The extent of aortic override varies significantly (10–95% override)
   - Classic TOF override is usually ~50%
4. RVH
   - Severity is proportional to the extent of aortic override and RVOT obstruction ➔ influences the direction of shunt
   - Cyanosis manifests when RVSP > LVSP

Common Associated Anomalies:
- 25%—right aortic arch
- 10%—anomalous coronary artery (e.g. LAD arising from RCA)
- PDA, multiple VSDs, complete AV canal

Clinical Manifestations
- Degree of RVOT obstruction determines the clinical presentation
- Mild RVOT obstruction ➔ usually left to right shunt
- Significant RVOT obstruction ➔ RV pressure increases ➔ right to left shunting ➔ cyanosis
- Tet spells
  - Seen in infants and older children with uncorrected tetralogy
  - Hyperpnea, irritability and profound cyanosis,
  - Can be triggered by pain, hypovolemia, fever, vigorous exercise
  - Requires immediate management and referral for surgical correction
    Note: mainstays of medical management of Tet spells: supplemental oxygen, squatting position (increases SVR and promotes flow from RV into pulmonic circulation rather than systemic circulation), IV fluids, beta blocker therapy

Management
- Most patients with TOF undergo complete repair as their initial surgical procedure (patch closure of the VSD, RVOT enlargement, relief of RVOT obstruction)
- Very important to define coronary anatomy pre-operatively as TOF can be associated with anomalous origin of LAD with a path that traverses the RVOT
- Most common post-operative complication is pulmonic insufficiency

15.5 Transposition of the Great Arteries (TGA) (Fig. 15.13)

- Malformation of the truncus arteriosus resulting in abnormal communication between the great arteries and ventricles (LV connects with the PA and RV connects with the aorta)

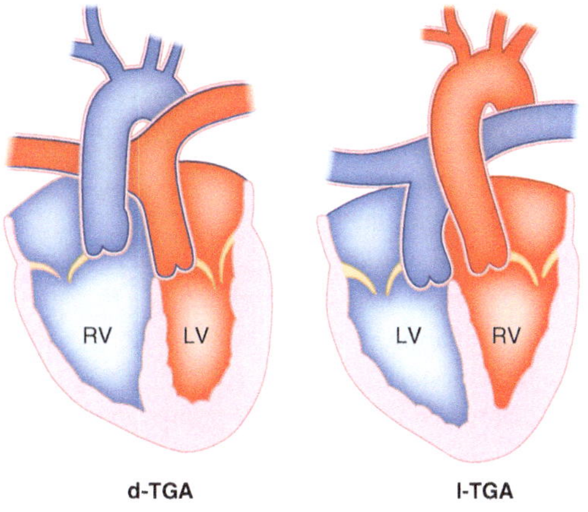

Fig. 15.13 **Transposition of the Great Arteries.** There are two types of transposition of the great arteries (TGA): D-TGA and L-TGA. In D-TGA, there is ventricular-arterial discordance with atrioventricular concordance. Two parallel circulations are created; immediate survival depends on the presence of a shunt. In L-TGA there is ventricular-arterial discordance AND atrioventricular discordance. A "corrected" circulation is created (however with the morphologic right ventricle functioning as the systemic ventricle). *Ao aorta, LV, left ventricle, PA pulmonary artery, RV right ventricle*

- Two Types of TGA: D-TGA and L-TGA
  - D stands for "dextro"—referring to the looping of the ventricles, such that the morphologic right ventricle is positioned to right of the morphologic left ventricle; the aorta is positioned anterior and slightly to the right of the pulmonary artery
  - L stands for "levo"—abnormal looping of the ventricles, such that the morphologic left ventricle is positioned to the right of the morphologic right ventricle; aorta is positioned anterior and to the left of the pulmonary artery
    Note: easy way to remember:
    D for "death"—in D-TGA there are two parallel circulations; incompatible with life without some type of shunt (ASD/VSD/PDA); typically requires immediate intervention
    L for "live"—circulation is overall preserved (hence also referred to as congenitally corrected transposition—"two wrongs make a right"); complications are in the long term (see below)

15.5.1 D-TGA

- Second most common cyanotic CHD—accounts for 5% of all CHD, 20% of cyanotic CHD
- Ventricular-arterial discordance with atrial-ventricular concordance resulting in two parallel circulations:
  - Venous return ➔ RA ➔ RV; RV pumps deoxygenated blood ➔ aorta ➔ systemic circulation ➔ returns to the RA
  - Pulmonary veins return oxygenated blood ➔ LA ➔ LV; LV pumps oxygenated blood ➔ PA ➔ pulmonary circulation ➔ return to LA via pulmonary veins
- Survival of the neonate before surgery depends on presence of left to right shunt
- Shunt can be at any level—ASD, VSD, PDA
- Shunting allows oxygenated blood from the left sided circulation into the right side, to be pumped into the systemic circulation

15.5.2 L-TGA (Congenitally Corrected TGA)

- Ventricular-arterial discordance with atrial-ventricular discordance (inversion of the ventricles plus transposition of the great vessels) - "two wrongs make a right"—one circulation, in series
  - Oxygenated blood from the pulmonary veins ➔ LA ➔ morphologic RV; RV pumps oxygenated blood ➔ aorta
  - Deoxygenated blood from systemic venous return ➔ RA ➔ morphologic LV; LV pumps deoxygenated blood ➔ PA
- Does not cause cyanosis

15.5.3 Echocardiographic Assessment (Fig. 15.14, Videos 15.5A, 15.5B, 15.5C and 15.5D)

1. Identifying the morphologic RV
   - RV is heavily trabeculated
   - Contains the moderator band
   - The valves always follow ventricles—identifying the TV identifies the morphologic RV
     - TV is apically displaced
     - TV has 3 leaflets (need TEE to identify)
2. Both great vessels run in parallel and do not cross
   - In normal anatomy—when viewing both great arteries—one always seen in short axis and the other in long axis (e.g. on PSAX view the aorta in seen in the center in cross section, PA is seen anterior and to the right in long axis—"hamburger and hotdog" appearance)
   - With TGA—both vessels run in parallel—on PSAX view both are seen in cross section
     Note: on CXR this is seen as a narrow mediastinum, because the great vessels are behind each other
3. The morphologic RV is the systemic ventricle; RV (systemic) failure develops as the RV cannot withstand the high systemic pressures over the long run

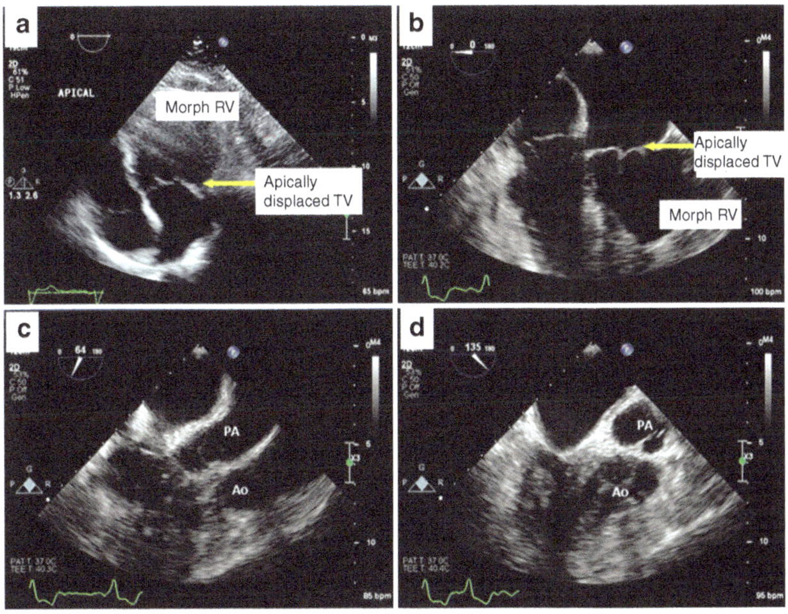

Fig. 15.14 Echocardiographic appearance of transposition of the Great Arteries. (**a**) Transthoracic apical four chamber view (**b**) transesophageal four chamber view; both showing the morphologic right ventricle in the left ventricle position. The morphologic right ventricle is identified by the apically displaced tricuspid valve. (**c**, **d**) Transesophageal images showing the great vessels running in parallel to each other; (**c**) long axis orientation, (**d**) short axis orientation. *Ao aorta, PA pulmonary artery*

  - RV dilatation, LA dilatation, heart failure signs and symptoms
  - If TR present—high velocity TR (systemic ventriculo-atrial regurgitation)
4. The morphologic LV is the pulmonary ventricle
   - If AI present—low velocity jet
5. Identifying the great vessels:
   - Pulmonary artery
     - Arises from the morphologic LV
     - Can be seen bifurcating into the right and left pulmonary arteries
   - Aorta
     - Arises from the morphologic RV
     - Coronary arteries can be seen at the semilunar cusps

Common Associated Anomalies

- 50% of patients with D-TGA have a VSD, 70–80% of L-TGA have a VSD
- 25% of patients with D-TGA have LVOT obstruction (which may be functional or anatomical), 30–60% of patients with L-TGA have LVOT obstruction
- Coronary artery anomalies are common with D-TGA
- TV anomalies are very common with L-TGA (up to 90% in L-TGA autopsy series); Ebstein like displacement of TV is seen in 20–50% of L-TGA
- Mitral valve anomalies are seen both in D and L TGA

15.6 Truncus Arteriosus

- Failure of the truncus arteriosus to divide into the PA and aorta
- Persistence of a single arterial trunk with single semilunar valve (truncal valve), that separates distally into the aortic and pulmonary arteries
- Large malalignment VSD that is straddled by the overriding single truncus (similar to TOF)
- Accounts for 0.7% of all CHD (4% of all critical CHD)

Echocardiographic Assessment

- Adult patients are seen post surgical repair
- Aortic root/RV conduit (stenosis/regurgitation) should be evaluated
- Suprasternal notch view to evaluate for coarctation of aorta
- Evaluate for post-surgical complications with incomplete VSD repair

Common Associated Anomalies

- 20–25% of patients with TA have DiGeorge syndrome (microdeletion of 22q11 associated with abnormal facies, thymic hypoplasia, and parathyroid gland abnormalities)
- Abnormalities of the truncal valve
- Abnormalities of the aorta (right aortic arch, interrupted aortic arch, hypoplastic arch ± coarctation)
- Coronary artery anomalies

Management

- Surgery required soon after birth with separation of PA and aorta, placement of a conduit from RV to PA, and VSD closure

15.7 Ebstein's Anomaly (Fig. 15.15, Videos 15.6A and 15.6B)

- Abnormal development of the RV myocardium, and failure of the tricuspid valve leaflets (most often the septal leaflet) to separate completely (delaminate) from the underlying myocardium

Echocardiographic Assessment

- Abnormal apical displacement of TV; defined as >8 mm/m^2 and measured from position of the anterior mitral leaflet (on apical four-chamber view)
- Typically the adherent leaflet is the septal leaflet; posterior leaflet may be tethered as well
- Anterior leaflet appears elongated, redundant, fenestrated ("sail" like); may float into RVOT
- The abnormal TV results in tricuspid regurgitation
  - The TR is typically low velocity (no pulmonary hypertension)

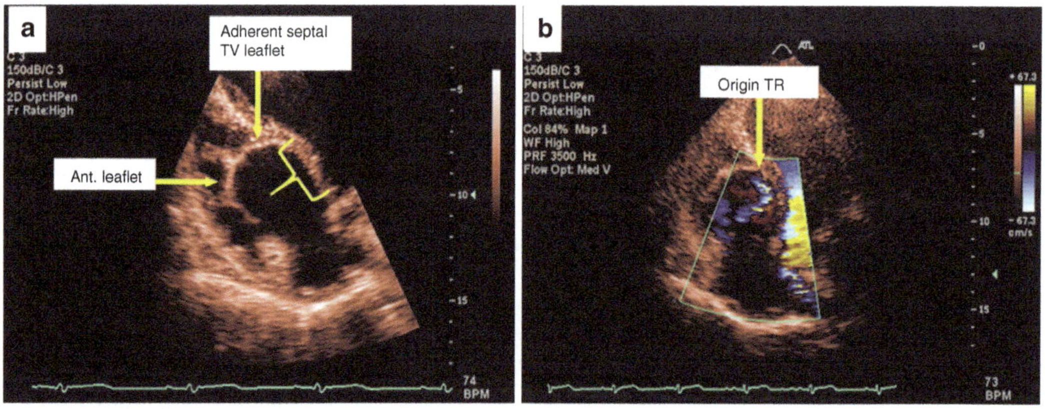

Fig. 15.15 **Ebstein's anomaly**. (**a**) RV focused, apical four chamber view showing exaggerated apical displacement of the adherent tricuspid valve septal leaflet (yellow bracket). In addition, the other leaflet (likely anterior) shows an elongated 'sail like' appearance. (**b**) The origin of tricuspid regurgitation is apical-anterior and can be difficult to visualize and quantify. *Ant anterior, TR tricuspid regurgitation, TV tricuspid valve*

- TR jet originates apically/anteriorly; may be missed
- Quantification is challenging
- The displaced TV divides the RV into two chambers
  - Proximal "atrialized" portion of the RV
  - Distal "functional" portion of the RV
  - The distal RV chamber may appear small on apical four chamber view, despite being enlarged (due to volume overload); this can be more accurately assessed by cardiac MRI
  - In some cases, the functional part of the RV may consist of only the RVOT
  - RV walls of the atrialized portion are thin and hypokinetic
- No pulmonary hypertension or pulmonic valve abnormalities
- ASD or PFO—seen in 50% of cases
  - Enlarged RA and often high RAP ➔ right to left shunt

    Note: Ebstein anomaly is a unique instance where right to left shunt can occur in the presence of normal PA pressure

Clinical Manifestations

- Degree of clinical manifestations depends on the severity of the anatomic abnormality
- Factors effecting clinical presentation:
  - Degree of TV displacement
  - Severity of TR
  - Severity of RV dilatation and dysfunction
  - Presence of ASD/PFO
- Symptoms include:
  - Right heart failure
  - Exertional hypoxemia
  - Right to left shunt with varying degrees of hypoxia/cyanosis
  - Cerebral abscesses
  - Arrhythmias—20–50% of patients have WPW
- EKG shows right atrial enlargement with "Himalayan p waves", atypical RBBB, and T wave inversions

Management

- Surgical TV repair is the treatment of choice - free septal leaflet from septum and placement of an annuloplasty ring
- Feasibility depends on degree of tethering of leaflets, size of RV, and mobility of the anterior leaflet; the smaller the functional RV is, the less likely repair is to be successful

15.8 COR-Triatriatum

Very rare congenital anomaly

- **Cor-Triatriatum Sinister**
  - Membrane bisecting the LA into two chambers –

    Upper chamber—contains the pulmonary veins

    Lower chamber—contains the inflow into the mitral valve
  - Hemodynamic consequences depend on level of obstruction at the membrane

    Clinical presentation resembles mitral stenosis; echocardiographic assessment demonstrates gradient above the MV
  - Often associated with other congenital defects
- **Cor-Triatriatum Dexter**
  - Membrane bisecting the right atrium
  - Less common than cor-triatriatum sinister
  - Can appear like a large Eustachian valve

15.9 Fontan Procedure/ Circulation

- Palliative surgical procedure for patients with single ventricle physiology (only one functional well-developed ventricle; other ventricle, if present, is less than 30% of its normal size)

- Conditions treated by Fontan procedure include (but not limited to):
  - Hypoplastic left heart
  - Tricuspid/pulmonic atresia
  - Double inlet RV
- With single ventricle physiology, there is only one functional ventricle, which needs to pump blood to the high resistance systemic circulation as well as the low resistance pulmonary circulation
- The Fontan procedure essentially diverts the systemic venous return into the pulmonary circulation, bypassing a pumping chamber
  - The single ventricle acts as a systemic ventricle
  - The pulmonary blood flow is passive, driven by central venous pressure and augmented by changes in intrathoracic pressures, as well as the relaxation of the systemic ventricle
- In order for the Fontan circulation to be effective the following conditions must be met:
  - Low PVR
  - Preserved systolic and diastolic function of the systemic ventricle
  - Pulmonary arteries large enough such that no mechanical obstruction is imposed
  - No or minimal atrio-ventricular valve regurgitation
- There are several forms of the Fontan procedure (Fig. 15.16), common ones are:
  - Atrio-pulmonary connection ("classic" Fontan)
    - The right atrial appendage is anastomosed to the main pulmonary artery
    - Blood from IVC and SVC drain into the RA which in turn connects to the pulmonary circulation
  - Cavo-pulmonary connection, utilizing either an intra-cardiac conduit or extra-cardiac conduit
    - The SVC is connected directly to the right pulmonary artery
    - A conduit connects the IVC to the pulmonary artery
    - An extra-cardiac conduit (in the pericardial space) is commonly used

Long Term Complications

- Atrial arrhythmias are very common
  - Probably less common following cavo-pulmonary connection than following atrio-pulmonary connection
  - High risk for thrombus, even on anticoagulation (can be seen in RA, conduit, left atrial appendage, PV orifices)

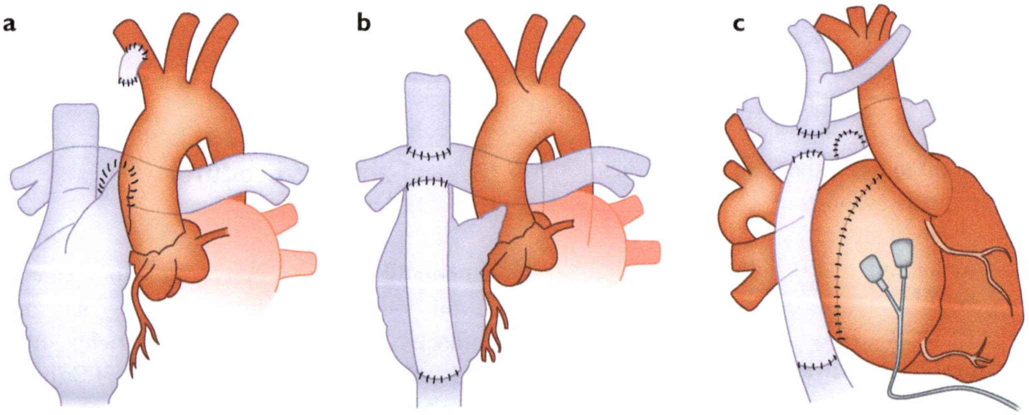

Fig. 15.16 Fontan connections. (**a**) Classic Fontan circulation; the right atrial appendage has been anastomosed to the pulmonary artery to direct venous blood directly from the right atrium into the pulmonary artery, bypassing the right ventricle. (**b**, **c**) Modifications of the original Fontan creating caval-pulmonary connection utilizing conduits, either intra-cardiac (**b**) or extra-cardiac (**c**)

- Cyanosis—from persistent right to left shunting (either via intentional fenestrations of the Fontan or from other unintentional communications between systemic venous return and pulmonary venous circulation
- Reduced exercise tolerance
- Ventricular dysfunction, low output state, dyspnea, fatigue and end organ dysfunction
- Atrio-ventricular valve regurgitation
- Kidney dysfunction, liver disease
- Thromboembolic events are seen in up to 33% of patients
  - Risk factors include:
    - Low flow in the Fontan conduit/Fontan obstruction
    - Atrio-pulmonary connection with right atrial dilatation
    - Low cardiac output
    - Atrial arrhythmias
  - Systemic events
    - Seen in patients with fenestrated Fontan
  - Pulmonary events
    - Can be complicated by low cardiac output due to increase in PVR
- Protein losing enteropathy
- Pulmonary disease (restrictive lung disease/plastic bronchitis)

Echocardiographic Assessment

Key points to remember when evaluating patients post Fontan

- Multiple variations of the Fontan procedure exist—important to review prior surgical data
- Fontan circulation is typically a low velocity system (venous flow)
- Often TTE views are limited; TEE (and often cardiac MRI) may be required for full assessment

15.10 Blalock-Taussig-Thomas Shunt

- Palliative surgical procedure used to augment pulmonary blood flow
- Can be used as early palliation for patients with TOF or single ventricle physiology (surgically simpler operation, that can be done even on newborns when required)
- Creates a direct connection between the subclavian artery and the pulmonary artery
  - Modified Blalock-Taussig shunt uses a Dacron graft to connect right subclavian artery to PA

Further Reading

Puchalski MD, Lui GK, Miller-Hance WC, et al. Guidelines for Performing a Comprehensive Transesophageal Echocardiographic: Examination in Children and All Patients with Congenital Heart Disease: Recommendations from the American Society of Echocardiography [published correction appears in J Am Soc Echocardiogr. 2019 May;32(5):681] [published correction appears in J Am Soc Echocardiogr. 2019 Oct;32(10):1373–1378]. J Am Soc Echocardiogr. 2019;3(2):173–215. https://doi.org/10.1016/j.echo.2018.08.016.

Silvestry FE, Cohen MS, Armsby LB, et al. Guidelines for the echocardiographic assessment of atrial septal defect and patent Foramen Ovale: From the American Society of Echocardiography and Society for Cardiac Angiography and Interventions. J Am Soc Echocardiogr. 2015;28(8):910–58. https://doi.org/10.1016/j.echo.2015.05.015.

Warnes CA, Williams RG, Bashore TM, et al. ACC/AHA 2008 guidelines for the management of adults with congenital heart disease: a report of the American College of Cardiology/American Heart Association Task Force on Practice Guidelines (Writing Committee to Develop Guidelines on the Management of Adults With Congenital Heart Disease). Developed in Collaboration With the American Society of Echocardiography, Heart Rhythm Society, International Society for Adult Congenital Heart Disease, Society for Cardiovascular Angiography and Interventions, and Society of Thoracic Surgeons. J Am Coll Cardiol. 2008;52(23):e143–263. https://doi.org/10.1016/j.jacc.2008.10.001.

Cardiac Masses

16

Learning Objectives

- Review the various intra-cardiac masses encountered in clinical echocardiography
- Learn the differential diagnosis of intra-cardiac masses
- Learn the characteristics that help differentiate abnormal masses from normal anatomic variants

16.1 Cardiac Tumors

- Most cardiac tumors are pathologically benign
- Significant consequences (embolization, arrhythmia, valve disease, and heart failure) can occur with benign or malignant tumors.

Tumor	Type	%
Myxoma	Benign	24.4
Lipoma	Benign	~8
Papillary fibroelastoma	Benign	~8
Angiosarcoma	Malignant	7.3
Rhabdomyoma	Benign	6.8
Rhabdomyosarcoma	Malignant	4.9
Mesothelioma	Malignant	3.6
Fibroma	Benign	3.2
Fibrosarcoma	Malignant	2.6
Lymphoma	Malignant	1.3
Leiomyosarcoma	Malignant	–

16.1.1 Benign Tumors

Myxoma
(Fig. 16.1, Videos 16.1A and 16.1B)

- The most common cardiac tumor, accounting for ~20–30% of all cardiac tumors.
- Location
  - 75%—in the left atrium, usually attached to the fossa ovalis
  - 15% occur in the RA
  - 10% in either LV or RV
- Characteristics
  - Usually a single pedunculated mass attached to the interatrial septum
  - Occasionally—cystic mass with grape like structure connected by a stalk to the septum
  - Vascular structure—takes up contrast either with contrast echo or angiography; has FDG uptake with PET imaging
  - CT cannot distinguish it from other structures based on attenuation or Houndsfields units

Electronic Supplementary Material The online version of this chapter (https://doi.org/10.1007/978-3-030-47041-8_16) contains supplementary material, which is available to authorized users.

T. Rambhatla, G. Perk, *The Echocardiography Companion*, https://doi.org/10.1007/978-3-030-47041-8_16

- Clinical manifestations
  - Systemic symptoms—fevers, chills, dyspnea
    Inflammatory markers—elevated ESR and IL-6 levels
  - Syncope—from dynamic mitral valve obstruction
    Rare—ventricular myxoma can obstruct the LVOT/RVOT
  - Stroke/embolism
    Thromboembolism occurs in up to 29% of patients
  - Tumor "plop"—from dynamic mitral valve (or tricuspic valve) obstruction
- Management
  - Surgery is usually indicated, even in asymptomatic patients, because of high risk of embolism or obstruction
  - Recurrence after surgery occurs in 2–5% of patients; higher rates in Careny Complex
    Note: Important to resect deeper than the stalk, to decrease risk of recurrence

Carney Complex

- Complex of pigmentation abnormalities (lentigines, blue nevi) and multiple tumors, including endocrine tumors, schwannoma, and myxomas
- Autosomal dominant inheritance
- Myxomas are often multiple and in unusual locations (not always attached to the fossa)

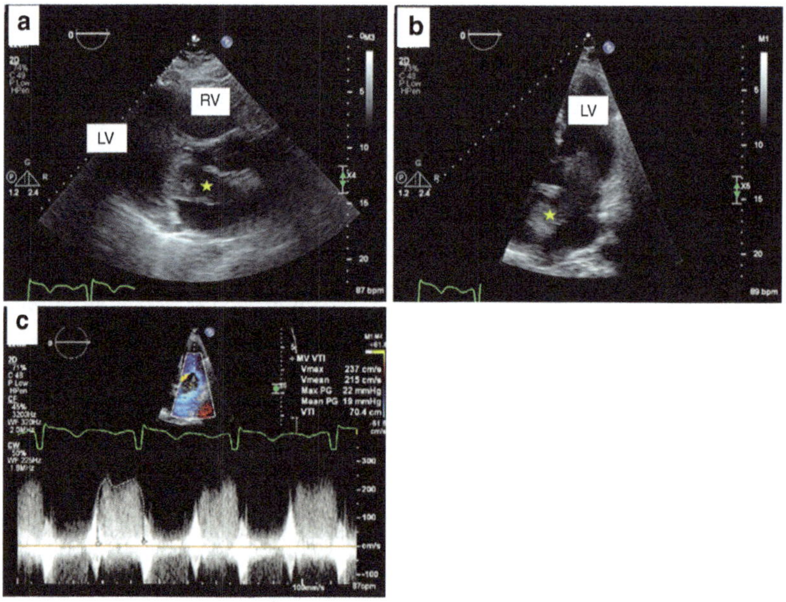

Fig. 16.1 **Myxoma.** (**a**) Parasternal long axis view showing a large myxoma (yellow asterisks) prolapsing into the mitral valve. (**b**) Apical four chamber view showing the myxoma attached to the inter-atrial septum and prolapsing through the mitral valve into the left ventricle. (**c**) Continuous wave Doppler across the mitral valve showing the myxoma causes functional mitral stenosis (mean inflow gradient—19 mmHg). *LV left ventricle, RV right ventricle*

Papillary Fibroelastoma
(Fig. 16.2, Video 16.2)

- Second most common primary cardiac tumor in adults
- Usually single, small (<1–1.5 cm), and arise from the endocardium
- Location
  - Typically—downstream aspect of a valve, on the leaflet tips
    - Account for 85% of valve associated tumors
  - More commonly left sided (>80%); aortic valve more than the mitral valve
- Characteristics
  - Highly mobile mass (dense elastin core coated by collagen) attached by a pedicle or stalk
  - Surface may have fingerlike projections
- Clinical Manifestations
  - CVA/TIA/embolic events—likely due to platelet/fibrin aggregates that embolize
  - Coronary occlusion can occur if fibroelastoma is located on a coronary cusp
  - Valve damage is rare
- Management
  - Symptomatic patients (prior embolic event or coronary occlusion)—surgical removal
  - Asymptomatic patients
    - Aspirin/anticoagulation—controversial
    - Surgical removal is considered for highly mobile and large fibroelastomas (>1 cm)

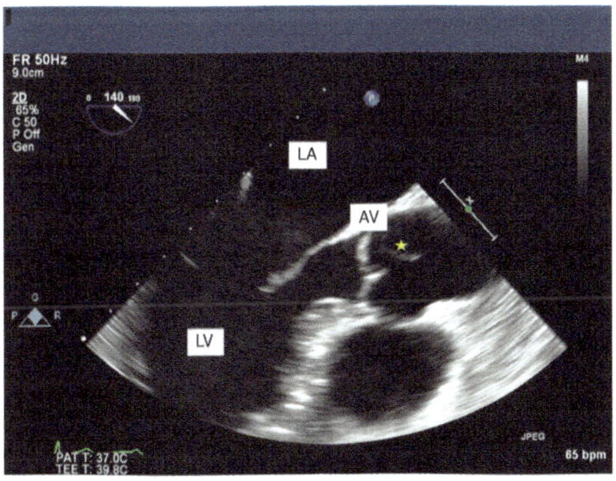

Fig. 16.2 **Fibroelastoma.** Transesophageal LVOT view showing a papillary fibroelastoma on the aortic side of the aortic valve (yellow asterisk). *AV aortic valve, LA left atrium, LV left ventricle*

Lipoma

- Second most common pediatric cardiac tumor; can also be seen in adults
- Can be located anywhere in the heart; right atrium—common location
- Typically, the lipoma is intra-myocardial (within the myocardial wall); classically asymptomatic and incidentally identified with imaging or at autopsy
- Does not embolize (vs. liposarcomas) and does not cause ventricular arrythmias (vs. fibromas)
- When located in the atrial septum—no sparing of the fossa ovalis (vs. lipomatous hypertrophy)

Rhabdomyoma

- Most common benign tumor in infants/children
- Typically small, multiple, and located in the wall of the ventricle or within the atrioventricular valves
- Often disappear in the first few years of life and generally do not require surgery
- 80% of children with rhabdomyomas have Tuberous Sclerosis
  - Autosomal dominant hamartoma syndrome with benign tumors in the brain and other organs associated with developmental delays and seizures

Fibroma

- Benign connective tissue tumor that arises from fibroblasts
- Generally seen in children less than 10 years old
- Location
  - Intramyocardial; usually the LV anterior wall, interventricular septum, or apex
- Characteristics
  - Can be large (2–5 cm); often calcified
  - MRI shows delayed hyper-enhancement
- Clinical Manifestations
  - Malignant arrhythmias—15% suffer SCD
  - Congestive heart failure
  - Conduction abnormalities
- Management—surgical resection (due to risk of SCD)

16.1.2 Malignant Tumors

- Malignant tumors can cause malignant pericardial effusions
- Generally, malignant tumors are not attached to the fossa ovalis

Angiosarcoma

- Most common primary malignant tumor
- 3:1 male predominance, generally presents at middle age
- Location
  - Usually in the right atrium with an associated pericardial effusion
- Characteristics
  - Generally large; may have already metastasized at time of diagnosis
  - Classic appearance: broad based RA mass near IVC (can mimic a clot in transit)
  - On CT imaging—"sun ray" pattern due to diffuse enhancement
- Clinical manifestations—fevers, right sided heart failure, tamponade
- Very poor prognosis; <6 month life expectancy

Rhabdomyosarcoma

- Accounts for ~20% of primary malignant tumors
- Location—within the myocardium, anywhere in the heart (atrial or ventricular walls)
- Clinical manifestations—depend on location of the tumor; may include chest pain, arrhythmias, conduction abnormalities, valve stenosis
  - By the time symptoms develop, the tumor usually has already metastasized
- Poor prognosis

Fibrosarcoma

- Can occur anywhere in the heart
- Often presents with nonspecific symptoms, delaying diagnosis
- Poor survival ~mean 11 months

Lymphoma (Fig. 16.3, Videos 16.3A and 16.3B)

- 80% are large B cell (a type of non-Hodgkin's lymphoma)
  - Seen in patients with AIDS—aggressive small noncleaved or immunoblastic type
- Location
  - Usually restricted to RA
  - 50% have an associated large pericardial effusion
- Clinical manifestations
  - Usually due to pericardial effusion or conduction abnormalities
  - 50% of patients have symptoms of right sided heart failure

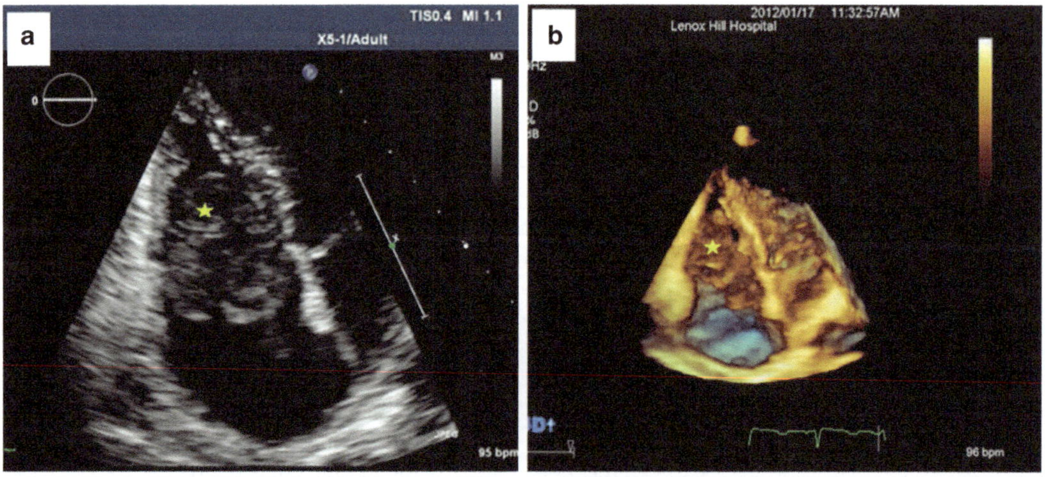

Fig. 16.3 **Cardiac lymphoma.** (**a**) Right heart- zoomed apical four chamber view showing a large lymphoma (yellow asterisk) originating in the right atrium and extending into the right ventricle. (**b**) Three-dimensional image showing the lymphoma across the tricuspid valve

- Diagnosis:
  Open biopsy is the gold standard
  Pericardial fluid cytology—14–60% sensitivity, endomyocardial biopsy—50% sensitivity
- Survival is <1 month without chemotherapy treatment

Leiomyosarcoma

- Develop from smooth muscle cells
- Location
  - Usually posterior wall of the left atrium, can come from the lining of the pulmonary veins
- Characteristics
  - Appearance is myxoid, similar to myxoma
- Management—radical surgical resection
- Poor prognosis, often <7 months after surgical excision

16.1.3 Cardiac Metastasis

- Cardiac metastases are more common than primary malignant cardiac tumors
- The most common tumors that metastasize to the heart are:
  - Renal Cell Carcinoma
    Metastasizes via direct extension through the IVC
    Can have the appearance of a thrombus
  - Lung carcinoma—direct extension from the lung to the heart
  - Breast Cancer—spreads to the heart via the blood stream, lymphatic systems, or pericardial extension
  - Melanoma—frequently metastasizes to the heart (myocardium/pericardium)—50% of metastatic cases involve the heart
    Metastases can occur years after treatment
    Can cause pericardial involvement—charcoal heart
  - Lymphoma—via lymphatic spread
  - Leiomyosarcomas—direct extension via the SVC

16.2 Non-tumor Massess

Blood Cyst
(Fig. 16.4, Video 16.4)

- Blood cysts are diverticula of cardiac valves, lined by endothelium and filled with blood
- They are generally sessile, broad based, and attached upstream on the cardiac valves
- Relatively common in newborns; disappear during infancy; rare in adults
- Generally incidentally found and cause no valve dysfunction
  - Rarely—large enough in size to cause valvular insufficiency or stenosis

Vegetations
(Fig. 16.5, Videos 16.5A and 16.5B)

- Irregular shape; highly mobile; oscillating mases
  Note: independent motion of the mass (i.e. motion unrelated to normal cardiac contraction and valve opening/closing) is an important characteristic that helps differentiate a vegetation from other findings (thickening/calcification)
- Can be infectious (bacterial or fungal) or non-infectious (sterile thrombi due to trauma, immune complexes/vasculitis, or hypercoagulable states)

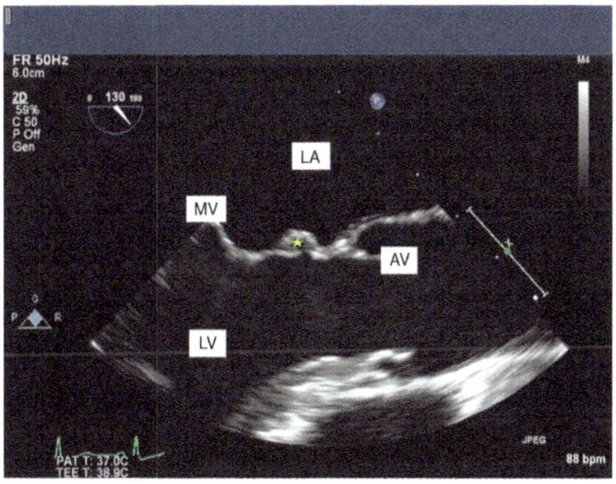

Fig. 16.4 **Mitral valve blood cyst.** Transesophageal LVOT view showing a small cystic mass on the atrial aspect of the anterior mitral valve leaflet (yellow asterisk). This finding is consistent with a mitral valve blood cyst. *AV aortic valve, LA left atrium, LV left ventricle, MV, mitral valve*

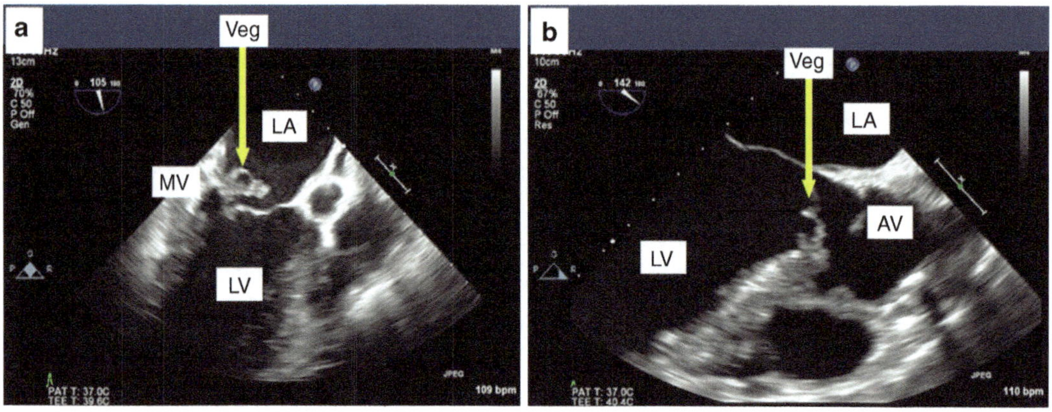

Fig. 16.5 **Infectious endocarditis.** (**a**) Transesophageal LVOT view showing large vegetation on the atrial aspect of the mitral valve. Note the extension of the infection into the mitral annulus with an irregular space, consistent with annular abscess. (**b**) Diastolic frame from a transesophageal LVOT view (different patient) showing large vegetation on the ventricular aspect of the aortic valve and completely torn/flail aortic valve; despite the diastolic frame, the valve is completely open with no coaptation of the cusps. *AV aortic valve, LA left atrium, LV left ventricle, MV mitral valve, Veg vegetation*

- Infectious vegetations are typically located on the upstream side of valves
- Libman-Sacks vegetations—associated with SLE, antiphospholipid antibodies—involve more basilar portions of the mitral or aortic valve (as opposed to leaflet tips), may be seen either on the upstream or downstream side of the valve, less mobile and may have less independent motion

Thrombus/Clot
(Fig. 16.6, Videos 16.6A, 16.6B, 16.6C, and 16.6D)

- Acute thrombus is often sessile, mobile, homogenous, echo-lucent, with irregular borders
- Chronic thrombus is often less mobile, can be laminated against the wall, and tends to be more echo-dense and calcified
- Echo contrast imaging shows a filling defect
- Thrombus in situ—occurs at sites of low flow
  - RAA, LAA in atrial fibrillation, LA in severe mitral stenosis, LV apex with severe apical hypokinesis/akinesis
- Intracardiac devices/wires/valves can be associated with in situ thrombosis
- Thrombus in transit –DVT that migrates to the RA/RV (possibly even to left heart though PFO/ASD)

16.3 Normal Variants

Eustachian Valve ("valve of the IVC")

- Embryologic remnant of the sinus venosus valve
  - In embryonic life, directed oxygenated blood towards the foramen ovale into the left heart
- Appears as a crescent shaped fold located at the IVC-RA junction at the inferior right atrium
- Can be of variable length and thickness
- Generally of no clinical significance; important to diagnose correctly and not confuse with pathological mass in the right atrium
  Note: Eustachian valve endocarditis has been described, albeit very rarely

Chiari Network
(Fig. 16.7, Video 16.7)

- Web like, fenestrated membrane arising near IVC and coronary sinus opening (from either the Eustachian valve or Thebesian valve)
- Appears as a filamentous, delicate, highly mobile structure
- 2–3% of the population have a prominent Chiari network
- Associated with interatrial septum aneurysm,

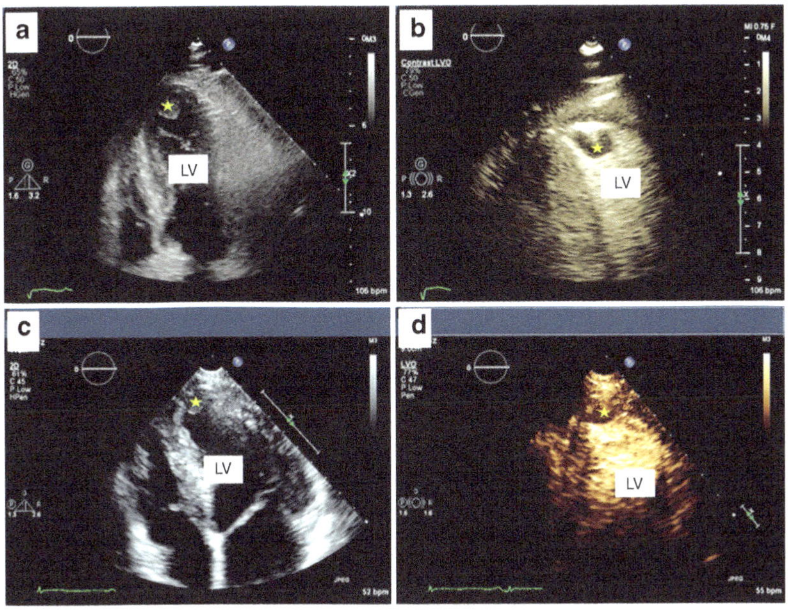

Fig. 16.6 **Left ventricular apical clot.** (**a**) Apical four chamber view showing a mobile sessile clot at the LV apex (yellow asterisk). (**b**) Contrast enhanced image from the same patient shows a clear apical filling defect. (**c**) Apical four chamber view showing a broad based, laminar apical clot (yellow asterisk). (**d**) Contrast enhanced image from the same patient shows the apical filling defect. *LV* left ventricle

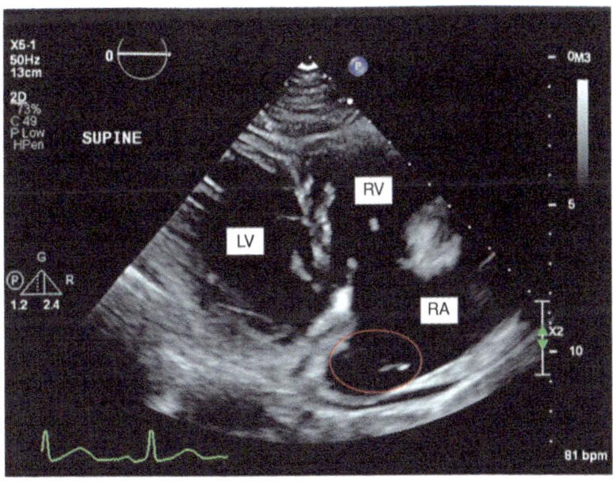

Fig. 16.7 **Prominent Eustachian valve/Chiari network.** Right ventricular inflow view showing a prominent Chiari network (red circle). The Chiari network appears as a highly mobile, thin filamentous structure at the junction of the inferior vena cava and the right atrium and can be of variable length and thickness. *LV* left ventricle, *RA* right atrium, *RV* right ventricle

PFO, and paradoxical embolism

- Generally of no clinical significance; important to diagnose correctly and not confuse with pathological mass in the right atrium
  - May cause difficulties during percutaneous procedures; entanglement or entrapment of right heart catheters has been rarely described

Crista Terminalis

- Ridge of myocardium that separates the trabeculated right atrial appendage from the smooth surfaced right atrium
- Extends from the SVC to IVC; when large enough can appear as RA mass
- The Crista Terminalis can be a source of atrial tachycardia and atrial fibrillation

Ligament of Marshall ("Coumadin Ridge") (Fig. 16.8, Video 16.8)

- A remnant of a fetal in-folding of the left atrial wall between the left superior pulmonary vein and the left atrial appendage
- Appears as a band like structure between the left superior pulmonary vein and the left atrial appendage
- Contains a nerve bundle, small atrial artery, and the remnant of the vein of Marshall

Lipomatous Hypertrophy of the interatrial septum

- Defined as >2 cm thickness of superior and inferior portions of the interatrial septum, with sparing of the fossa → "dumbbell shape"
- Contains un-encapsulated adipose (like hamartoma, not like a lipoma which is capsulated)
- More commonly observed in obese females
- Usually asymptomatic, but if large enough can cause SVC obstruction
  - Possible association with increased risk of atrial fibrillation and stroke

Moderator Band

- Muscular band located in the apical portion of the right ventricle that extends from the apical lateral wall to the interventricular septum
- One of the structures that helps identify the morphologic right ventricle in complex congenital heart disease
- Although it is located in the RV, it gets its blood supply from the LAD
  Note: RCA/acute marginal ischemia with preserved LAD/moderator band blood supply can lead to a "pseudo McConell's sign"—RV apical sparing due to preserved septal and moderator band contractility with RV free wall hypokinesis

LV Band ("LV tendon" or "false tendon") (Fig. 16.9, Video 16.9)

- Fibrous, fibromuscular, or muscular tendons in the apical or mid LV
- Typically connects the septum to the LV lateral/free wall; less commonly to a papillary muscle

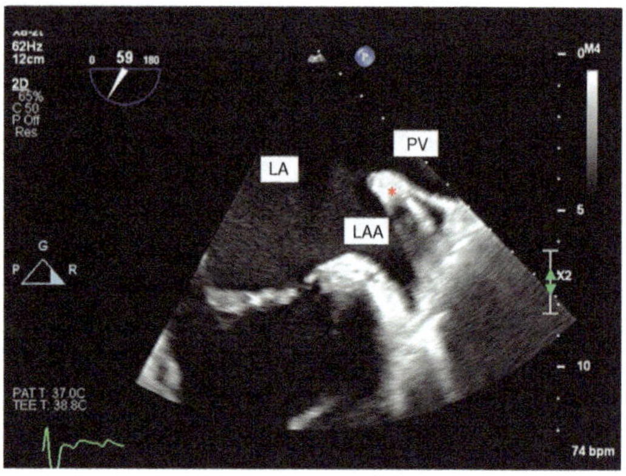

Fig. 16.8 **Coumadin Ridge**. Transesophageal image of the Ligament of Marshall/"coumadin ridge" (red star); appears as a band like structure between the left superior pulmonary vein and the left atrial appendage. It contains a nerve bundle, small atrial artery, and the remnant of the vein of Marshal. *LA left atrium, LAA left atrial appendage, PV pulmonary vein*

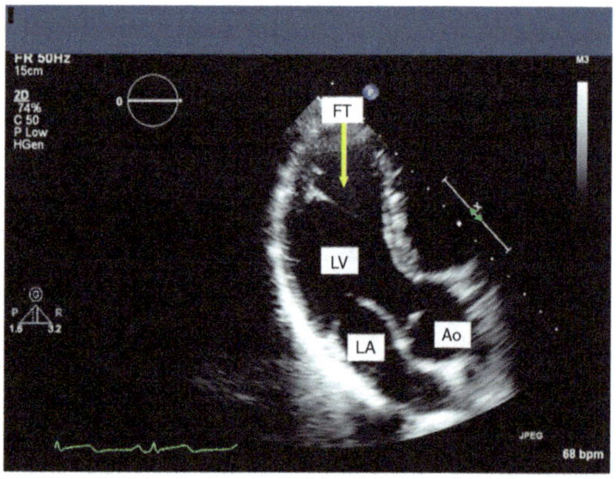

Fig. 16.9 **LV False tendon**. Apical three chamber view showing a left ventricular band (LV false tendon). It is a fibrous, fibromuscular, or muscular band that connects the septum to the LV lateral or free wall; no clinical significance but must not be confused with pathologic finding. *Ao aorta, FT false tendon, LV left ventricle, LA left atrium*

- Usually thin; can be thick and muscular, and can be calcified
- Usually asymptomatic, but has been linked to PVCs, thrombus, and thromboembolism

Lamble's Excrescences

- Thin, linear, filamentous fibrin strands that can develop at valve closure sites
- Appear as small (<1 cm), thread-like strands on the upstream surface of the aortic or mitral valves

- Occurs in older patients, >60 yrs of age
- Generally, asymptomatic, no embolic consequences and does not require treatment
  - If large and associated with embolism, a papillary fibroelastoma or vegetation should be considered

Arantius Nodules ("nodules of semilunar cusps")

- Normal leaflets of the aortic valve and pulmonic valve have a slight thickening or prominence located at the margin of each of the three cusps
- Hypertrophy and fibrosis of these nodules can cause valvular insufficiency

Further Reading

Klarich KW, Enriquez-Sarano M, Gura GM, Edwards WD, Tajik AJ, Seward JB. Papillary fibroelastoma: echocardiographic characteristics for diagnosis and pathologic correlation. J Am Coll Cardiol. 1997;30(3):784–90. https://doi.org/10.1016/s0735-1097(97)00211-8.

Lam KY, Dickens P, Chan AC. Tumors of the heart. A 20-year experience with a review of 12,485 consecutive autopsies. Arch Pathol Lab Med. 1993;117(10):1027–31.

Peters PJ, Reinhardt S. The echocardiographic evaluation of intracardiac masses: a review. J Am Soc Echocardiogr. 2006;19(2):230–40. https://doi.org/10.1016/j.echo.2005.10.015.

Reynen K. Cardiac myxomas. N Engl J Med. 1995;333(24):1610–7. https://doi.org/10.1056/NEJM199512143332407.

Interventional Echocardiography 17

Learning Objectives

- Become familiar with structural heart disease (SHD) interventions and the echocardiographer role
- Understand the major echocardiographic tasks for TAVR, mitral clip repair, mitral balloon valvuloplasty, and left atrial appendage occlusion

General Considerations

- Percutaneous interventions for various structural heart disease expanded dramatically over the course of the past decade
- Factors contributing to this rapid expansion include:
  - Improvements in imaging techniques, including real time 3-dimensional echocardiography
  - Improvements in catheter/device designs
  - Establishment of multidisciplinary heart-teams

17.1 Imaging for Structural Heart Disease Interventions

- Various modes of imaging are utilized for SHD interventions

Electronic Supplementary Material The online version of this chapter (https://doi.org/10.1007/978-3-030-47041-8_17) contains supplementary material, which is available to authorized users.

- Pre-procedure assessment often includes echo, CT and if needed cardiac MRI
- Intra-procedure guidance is done with fluoroscopy, echocardiography and occasionally fusion imaging, utilizing pre-procedure acquired CT images
- Echocardiography is the ideal modality for intra-procedure guidance;
  - Portable—can be done in real time at the procedure room
  - Superior spatial resolution as compared to fluoroscopy
  - Combining data from 2D, 3D and Doppler imaging can provide anatomic as well as hemodynamic information
  - Allows early identification of procedure success or complications

17.2 Real-Time 3 Dimensional Echocardiography

- Several important engineering advancements allowed the wide adoption of the technique into clinical medicine
  - Miniaturized matrix array transducer such that it fits in a regular sized TEE probe
  - Online display of the 3D rendered images
  - Ability to post-process the images.
- Full matrix array transducer (over 3000 elements) allows acquisition of large volume echocardiographic data sets (Fig. 17.1)

T. Rambhatla, G. Perk, *The Echocardiography Companion*,
https://doi.org/10.1007/978-3-030-47041-8_17

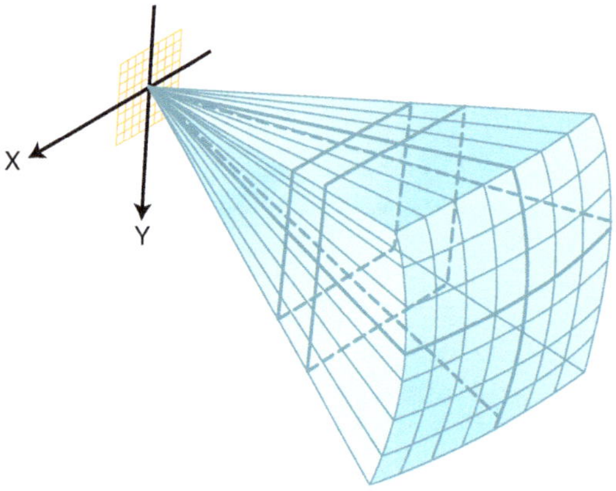

Fig. 17.1 **3D TEE Probe**. The full matrix array transducer has over 3000 elements and allows acquisition of large volume echocardiographic data sets. The beams are simultaneously steered in two orthogonal directions acquiring a series of 2D sectors along the elevation axis creating a pyramidal 3D data set

- The beams are simultaneously steered in two orthogonal directions acquiring a series of 2D sectors along the elevation axis creating a pyramidal 3D data set.
- Images can be obtained over 1 beat (presented in real-time) or gated over several beats
- 3D Color imaging also available
- Images can be processed and manipulated both in real-time and post-acquisition

17.3 SHD Interventions

- Currently a wide array of procedures can be performed percutaneously, obviating the need for open heart surgery
- A partial list of procedures includes:
  - Transcutaneous aortic valve replacement (TAVR)
  - Mitral valve clip repair
  - Atrial appendage exclusion
  - Mitral balloon valvuloplasty (BMV) for rheumatic mitral stenosis
  - Transcutaneous mitral valve replacement (TMVR) for selected indications
  - Prosthetic valve paravalvular leak (PVL) closure
  - Occlusion of intra-cardiac shunts (PFO, ASD, VSD)
  - Tricuspid valve clip repair
  - Alcohol septal ablation
  - Miscellaneous (pseudoaneurysm obliteration, intra-cardiac clot extraction and more)
- Echocardiographic evaluation:
  1. Pre-procedure testing
     - Comprehensive assessment including chamber quantification, LV wall motion and ejection fraction, valve function, presence of pericardial effusion
     - Defining the anatomy, pathology and hemodynamic consequences of the lesion in question
     - Verifying absence of contraindications for trans-catheter procedure (e.g. intra-cardiac clot) or findings that may alter the approach
  2. Intra-procedure monitoring and guiding
     - Quick assessment at the start of procedure to verify no new contraindications
     - Guidance during access to the left heart (see below)
     - Continuous visualization of all wires/guides/devices for improved accuracy and safety of the procedure
     - Real time assessment of all procedure stages
     - Immediate evaluation of success of the procedure
     - Rapid identification of complications and guidance of their treatment (e.g. pericardiocentesis)
  3. Post-procedure follow up
     - Often done by TTE (certain cases require TEE surveillance)
     - In the immediate post procedure period (hours/days)—assessment for procedure related complications
     - Long term—verifying correction of underlying pathology as well as cardiac response to the treatment (e.g. chamber size and function, pulmonary pressures)

17.4 Approach to the Left Heart

Several techniques can be utilized to approach the left heart during SHD interventions

1. Retrograde arterial approach
   - Most common access technique for TAVR procedures
   - Can be used also for aortic PVL procedures, occasional mitral PVL procedure (depending on PVL location), aortic/LVOT pseudoaneurysm occlusion
   - Can be done using femoral puncture or arterial cut down if required
   - Vessel size may be a limiting factor for utilizing retrograde arterial approach; assessed by pre-procedure contrast CT
   - Echocardiography is used once aortic valve is crossed; can verify course of wires in the left heart and avoidance of mitral valve apparatus
2. Central venous access and trans-septal puncture
   - Used for mitral clip procedure, atrial appendage occlusion, certain mitral PVLs, BMV, TMVR
   - Accurate location of the puncture site can be crucial for the success of the procedure
   - When specific puncture site is desired, TEE is essential for proper localization of the site
   - The fossa ovalis is imaged initially on the bivacal view
   - The trans-septal needle can be seen as it is pulled down from SVC towards the fossa
   - Tenting of the septum can be seen (Fig. 17.2, Video 17.1) as the interventionalist pushes the needle against the fossa
   - Biplane imaging is utilized to ascertain the location of the tenting both in the superior/inferior axis as well as the anteroposterior axis
   - The needle location can be adjusted according to the echocardiographic assessment
   - Once location has been optimized the puncture is performed either by further pressure on the needle or by applying radiofrequency energy through the needle.
   - Crossing of the septum can be directly seen by echo, as well as by the appearance of bubbles in the left sided chambers, immediately upon crossing
   - Once a wire is across the septum, further confirmation of the puncture site can be obtained by echocardiographic imaging of the point of crossing
3. Trans-apical puncture
   - Direct puncture of the left ventricular apex
   - Can be done percutaneously or utilizing mini thoracotomy and a cutdown
   - Used for certain mitral PVLs, TMVR, rarely for TAVR
   - Care must be taken to avoid lungs and coronary arteries
   - Echo can identify the intracardiac needle/wire once the puncture has been performed
   - Upon completion of the procedure, echo is used to verify closure of the site, lack of pericardial effusion or new wall motion abnormalities

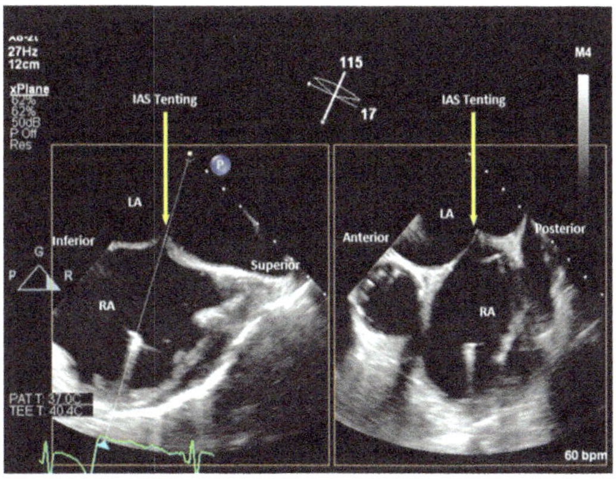

Fig. 17.2 **Tenting the interatrial septum**. TEE Biplane imaging from the bi-caval view as seen prior to trans-septal puncture. Accuracy in trans-septal puncture is key to the success of multiple procedures (as well as for avoiding complications). The biplane imaging is utilized to ascertain the tenting location both in the superior/inferior axis (left side of the image) as well as the anteroposterior axis (right side of the image). *IAS interatrial septum, LA left atrium, RA right atrium*

17.5 Specific Procedures

- As mentioned, numerous procedures can now be performed by catheter-based technique
- The echocardiographer must be familiar with the specific pathology to be addressed, devices to be used and possible complications of the procedure
- Several procedures will be reviewed in detail in the following sections, highlighting their unique echocardiographic requirements.
- For less common procedures, please refer to specific literature

17.5.1 TAVR

Indications:

- Symptomatic severe aortic stenosis in patients at extreme surgical risk, high surgical risk and intermediate surgical risk.
- Results from low risk trial were recently published, showing favorable TAVR outcomes
- TAVR is also approved for valve in valve procedure for failed bioprosthetic valve

Pre-procedure Imaging:

Goals of pre-procedure echocardiographic imaging:

- Establish the severity and subtype of aortic stenosis
- Evaluation of left ventricular function and ejection fraction
- Assess for presence and severity of other valvular disease
- Aid in TAVR valve sizing.

Pre-procedure study should include:

- Comprehensive TTE with detailed anatomic and hemodynamic evaluation of the aortic valve, chamber size and function, other valve disease, presence of pericardial effusion.
- Aortic root assessment:
- Most commonly, aortic root anatomy and dimensions are determined by CT imaging
- When echocardiographic assessment is required, TEE-3D based measurements are preferred
  - Aortic annulus is measured at the nadir of the valve leaflets attachments (virtual plane, there is no true aortic annulus) (Fig. 17.3)

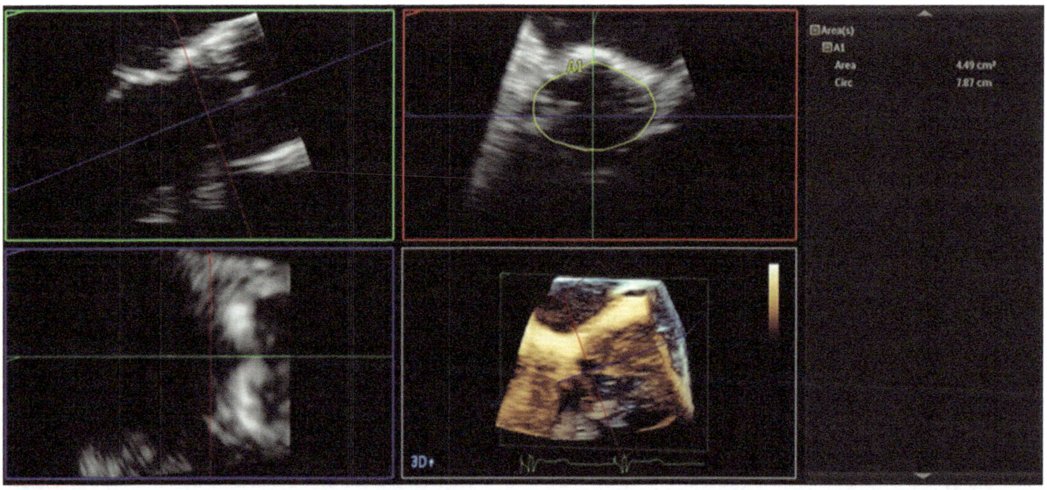

Fig. 17.3 **3D Aortic annulus planimetry.** A full volume data set is acquired from the LVOT view. The orthogonal planes are oriented (each separately) such that the annulus can be seen "en face". The annulus can be traced directly (no geometric assumptions regarding shape are required)

  - Left coronary artery height (i.e. distance of coronary ostium from the aortic annulus) can only be measured by 3D based multiplaner reconstruction
  - Diameters of the aortic sinuses, sino-tubular junction (STJ) and the tubular ascending aorta should be recorded
  - Severity and distribution of calcifications (in LVOT, aorto-mitral curtain, aortic root) should be noted

Intra-procedure Imaging:

Intra-procedure imaging can be done with TTE or TEE

TEE	TTE
Deeper anesthesia required	No need for anesthesia/ sedation
Continuous imaging	Intermittent imaging/ procedure delay during image acquisition
Probe may interfere with fluoroscopic images	Imaging windows may be in sterile field/ unapproachable
High resolution imaging (2D and 3D)	Image quality may be compromised (patient's position, body habitus etc.)
	Anterior structures/PVL might be better visualized
Shortening of LV/RV may limit chamber quantification and function assessment	Standard views to assess LV and EF
May help avoid complications/immediate diagnosis of complications	Possible delay in diagnosis of complications

- Pre-deployment aortic balloon valvuloplasty can be performed to facilitate valve delivery.
- Possible complications include:
  - Cardiac tamponade
  - Acute coronary occlusion
  - Severe aortic regurgitation
- If complication is suspected, echocardiography can help quickly make accurate diagnosis.

Currently, mainly two types of valves are in clinical use (Fig. 17.4):

- Self-expanding valve (Medtronic Core/ Evolut valves)
- Balloon expandable valve (Edwards Sapien valves)

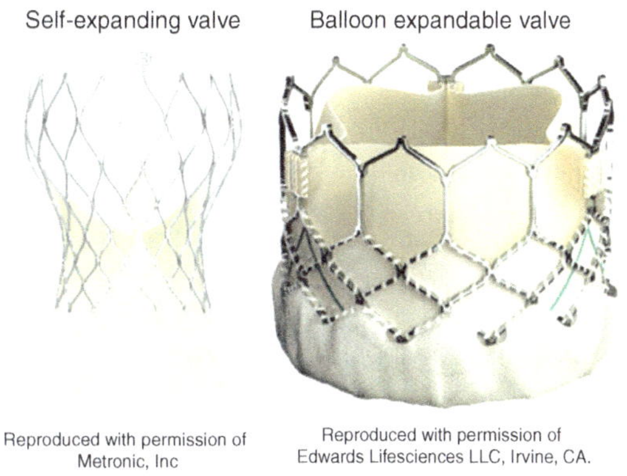

Fig. 17.4 **Current common TAVR valves in clinical use**. The two commonly used valves are the self-expanding, Medtronic valve and the balloon-expandable Sapien valve. Other designs are being developed and tested and will likely enter the market as well

- Other valves are being developed and tested and will likely become ready for clinical use in the near future

The TAVR valve must be positioned accurately, according to the valve-specific recommendations

- Most commonly, valve positioning is done based on fluoroscopy imaging; TEE can assist

Immediately following valve deployment, echocardiographic assessment is preformed.

Goals of Immediate Post-deployment Evaluation:

- Confirm valve positioning—although this is commonly done by fluoroscopy, echocardiography (in particular TEE) is useful for confirmation
- Assess valve function:
  - Leaflet motion
  - Hemodynamic assessment with measurements of velocities and gradients
  - Evaluation for presence and severity of paravalvular (and valvular) regurgitation
- If hemodynamic instability occurs, assessment for possible complications:
  - LV/RV function
  - Presence of pericardial effusion and signs of chamber collapse
  - Aortic root complications (e.g. dissection, hematoma)
  - Valve malfunction

Post-procedure Follow Up:

Comprehensive echocardiography at standard intervals (Fig. 17.5, Videos 17.2A and 17.2B). Studies should include:

- Full assessment of chambers size and function
- Other valves function, pulmonary pressures, diastolic function
- Detailed assessment of TAVR valve function –
  - Velocities
  - Gradients
  - Calculated valve area
  - Doppler velocity index
- Quantification of trans-valvular and paravalvular aortic regurgitation

17.5.2 Mitral Clip Repair

Indications:

- Severe mitral regurgitation due to primary/degenerative disease of the mitral valve in patients who are at prohibitive risk for surgery
- Patients with moderate to severe or severe mitral regurgitation due to left ventricular dysfunction (“functional/secondary” MR), who have heart failure symptoms despite optimal medical therapy

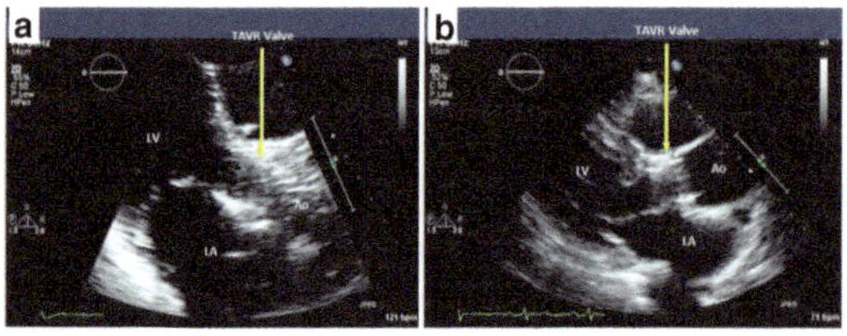

Fig. 17.5 **TAVR valve on transthoracic echo.** (**a**) Parasternal long axis view of a Medtronic self-expanding valve. Note the stent of the valve is longer as compared to the Sapien valve. Leaflets can be hard to image due to acoustic shadowing from the valve stent. (**b**) Parasternal long axis view of a Sapien balloon-expandable valve. The stent is shorter (however, side lobe artifacts make it appear longer than it is). Acoustic shadowing from the valve stent can obscure the valve leaflets. *Ao aorta, LA left atrium, LV left ventricle*

Pre-procedure Imaging:

Both TTE and TEE are required for appropriate planning of mitral clip procedure

Pre-procedure studies should include:

- Assessment of chambers size and function
- Quantification of the severity and definition of the mechanism of mitral regurgitation. TEE is essential for clarifying the origin of the MR jet and for detailed evaluation of leaflet anatomy (e.g. presence of clefts or calcifications at the grasping area)
- Measurement of pre-procedure mitral valve area (must be >4cm^2 to avoid post clip stenosis)
- Assessment for concomitant other valve disease
- Detailed anatomic assessment of the inter-atrial septum, including full visualization of the fossa ovalis and verification of adequate height for trans-septal puncture (Fig. 17.6)
- Exclusion of potential contra-indication (e.g. left atrial appendage clot)

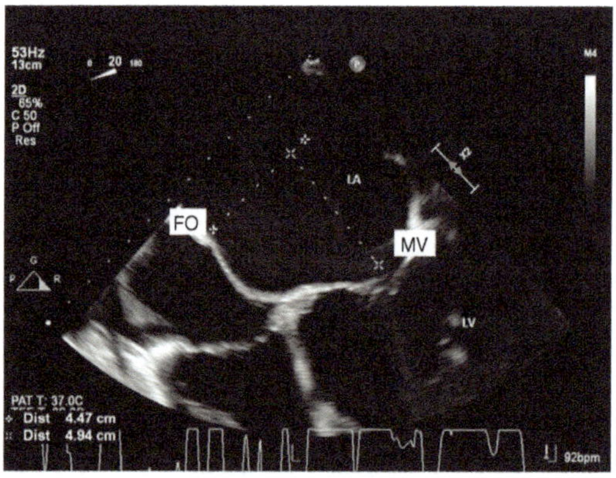

Fig. 17.6 **Optimizing trans-septal puncture height.** Mid-esophageal four chamber view showing the height of the fossa ovalis above the mitral valve. A minimum height is required for steering and advancing the clip delivery system. Pre procedure imaging should verify adequate height is available. *FO fossa ovalis, LA left atrium, LV left ventricle, MV mitral valve*

Intra-procedure Imaging:

TEE (2D and 3D) is the main imaging modality used during mitral clip procedures. Every step of the procedure relies heavily on echocardiographic guidance

- Trans-septal puncture:
  - Accurate location of the trans-septal puncture is crucial for the success of the procedure
  - Biplane visualization of the fossa ovalis at mid-esophageal view at aortic valve short axis with the orthogonal bicaval view is particularly useful for guiding the trans-septal puncture
  - Optimal location for the puncture—postero-superior aspect of the fossa ovalis (Fig. 17.7)
  - In addition, sufficient height above the mitral valve (generally > 4 cm) is important for facilitating steering and maneuvering of the clip delivery system
- Advancing delivery system into left atrium:
  - Initially, a steerable guide catheter is advanced into the left atrium
  - Tip is radio-opaque; can be easily identified by fluoroscopy and echocardiography
  - Guide must be advanced under continuous echocardiographic surveillance to avoid injury
  - Clip delivery system is then advanced through the catheter into the left atrium
  - The tip of the clip is visualized as it is advanced beyond the catheter, into the LA
  - The delivery system is deflected and advanced towards the mitral valve; the mid-esophageal LVOT view provides guidance regarding manipulations in the anterior-posterior axis, while the inter-commissural view provides guidance in the medial-lateral axis.
  - The clip is positioned above the origin of the mitral regurgitation jet
- Orienting the clip:
  - Clip arms are opened while the clip is in the left atrium
  - The clip is oriented such that the open arms are perpendicular to the mitral valve coaptation line
- Advancing into the left ventricle
  - Once the clip is oriented properly, arms are closed and clip advanced into the LV
  - Minimizing manipulation in the LV is important to avoid entangling of the cords/sub valvular apparatus
  - Correct orientation of the clip arms should be verified after advancement into the LV.
- Leaflet grasping:
  - Grasping is done under continuous echocardiographic surveillance
  - Optimal grasping view—2D, midesophageal, LVOT view (Fig. 17.8, Video 17.3)
  - The clip is pulled back until the mitral leaflets are captured; the grippers are than lowered
  - Clip arms are slowly closed under color Doppler surveillance; reduction in the MR jet can be assessed
  - If reduction in MR seems suboptimal, the clip arms can be opened and the clip re-positioned

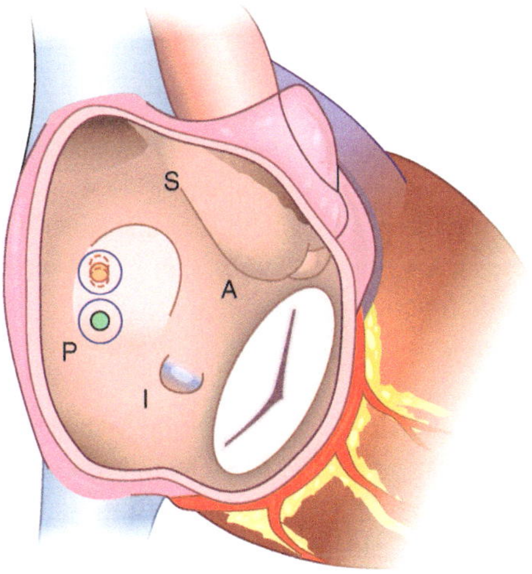

Fig. 17.7 **Optimal site for trans-septal puncture.** Diagram showing the preferred location (within the fossa ovalis) for optimal trans-septal puncture site for mitral clip procedure (orange location) and left atrial appendage occlusion procedure with a Watchman device (green location). *A anterior, I inferior, P posterior, S superior*

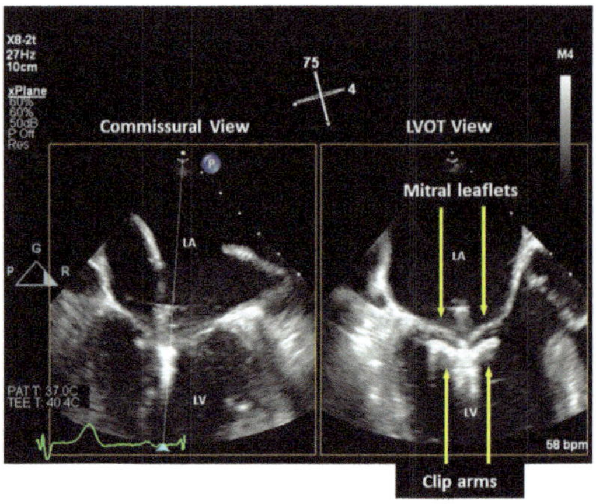

Fig. 17.8 **Mitral clip—leaflet grasping**. Biplane view utilized to guide leaflet grasping during mitral clip procedure. The starting view is the commissural view (on the left side of the screen). The orthogonal view is the LVOT view. The clip arms are oriented such that they are perpendicular to the mitral valve closure line. Note that on the commissural view, the arms are perpendicular to the screen. In the LVOT view the open clip arms can be seen, immediately below the valve leaflets. Once the leaflets are "caught" on the clip arms, the grippers are lowered and the leaflets are grasped. This should be performed under continuous echocardiographic surveillance to assure proper tissue grasp on the clip. *LA left atrium, LV left ventricle*

- Clip deployment:
  - After leaflet grasping and before deployment, echocardiographic evaluation should be performed

    Adequate leaflet grasping is assessed (to minimize risk of clip detachment)

    Sufficient reduction in mitral regurgitation needs to be achieved

    Gradient across the mitral valve should be measured to assure absence of mitral stenosis
  - If above evaluation is satisfactory, the clip is released
  - Repeat assessment of MR severity needs to be performed after clip release; tension exerted on the clip prior to deployment may have affected severity of the pre-release residual MR
  - If significant residual MR seen → additional clip/s can placed
- Retraction of delivery system:
  - Upon release of the clip, the delivery system should be pulled back into RA under echocardiographic surveillance, to minimize risk of injury

Immediately following device deployment, echocardiographic assessment is preformed.

Goals of Immediate Post-deployment Evaluation:

- Detailed quantification of residual mitral regurgitation
- Measurement of trans-mitral gradient
- Assessment of the size of the residual inter-atrial communication as well as direction of inter-atrial shunt. Most commonly, the shunt is only left to right and the puncture site heals spontaneously. If a very large defect is seen, torn tissue is present, or right to left shunting is identified, device closure of the defect should be considered.
- Exclusion of any complications should be carried out (e.g. pericardial effusion, device detachment)

Post-procedure Imaging:

Comprehensive echocardiography at standard intervals. Studies should include:

- Full assessment of chambers size and function
- Other valves function, pulmonary pressures, diastolic function
- Detailed assessment of mitral valve –
  - Clip/s stability
  - Residual MR severity—there may be multiple jets of residual MR (from both sides of the clip/s); multiple quantification parameters should be used to accurately estimate the severity of the residual MR
- Mitral inflow gradient

17.5.3 Mitral Balloon Valvuloplasty (BMV)

Indications:

- Symptomatic patients with severe rheumatic MS (MVA < 1.5 cm^2) and favorable valve morphology
- Asymptomatic patients with very severe MS (MVA < 1 cm^2) and favorable valve morphology
- Asymptomatic patients with severe MS, favorable anatomy and pre-pregnancy
- May be considered for asymptomatic patients with severe MS and favorable valve morphology
- May be considered for symptomatic patients with MVA > 1.5 cm^2 with evidence of hemodynamic significance (high pulmonary pressures, high mean mitral gradient)
- May be considered for severely symptomatic patients with severe MS and unfavorable valve morphology who are not surgical candidates
- May be considered for pregnant patients with severe MS who are symptomatic despite medical therapy (with favorable valve morphology)

Pre-procedure Imaging:

Both TTE and TEE are required for appropriate planning of mitral balloon valvuloplasty

Pre-procedure studies should include:

- Assessment of chambers size and function
- Detailed evaluation of the mitral valve:
  - Cause of mitral stenosis (rheumatic vs. other etiologies)
  - Severity of mitral stenosis
  - Valve anatomy as pertains to possible balloon valvuloplasty (Wilkins Score/other scoring schemes)
- Hemodynamic effects: transmitral gradient, pulmonary pressures
- Evaluation for concomitant valve disease with detailed quantification of associated mitral regurgitation (more than moderate MR precludes BMV as a treatment option)
- Exclusion of contra-indications (left atrial/appendage clot, severe/asymmetric commissural calcifications)

Intra-Procedure Imaging:

BMV can be performed under TTE or TEE guidance.

TEE provides more detailed imaging, such that each stage can be guided and monitored accurately, however generally requires general anesthesia.

Every step of the procedure can be imaged by echocardiography; imaging modality chosen determines the relative reliance on echocardiographic guidance vs. other (fluoroscopy)

- Trans-septal puncture:
  - Similar to mitral clip procedure, location of trans-septal puncture can be chosen based on TEE biplane visualization at mid-esophageal aortic valve/bicaval view
  - Optimal location for the puncture—postero-inferior aspect of the fossa ovalis
- Balloon positioning and inflation in mitral valve (Fig. 17.9, Videos 17.4A and 17.4B)
  - Following the trans-septal puncture, a wire is passed into the left ventricle
  - Inoue balloon is advanced over the wire into the left ventricle; echocardiographic assessment can confirm appropriate positioning of the balloon between mitral leaflets
  - Balloon inflation (from distal chamber to proximal chamber) is performed under echocardiographic surveillance

Immediately following balloon inflation, echocardiographic assessment is preformed.

Goals of Immediate Post-Inflation Evaluation:

- Evaluation for presence and severity of new mitral regurgitation
- Assessment of residual mitral stenosis

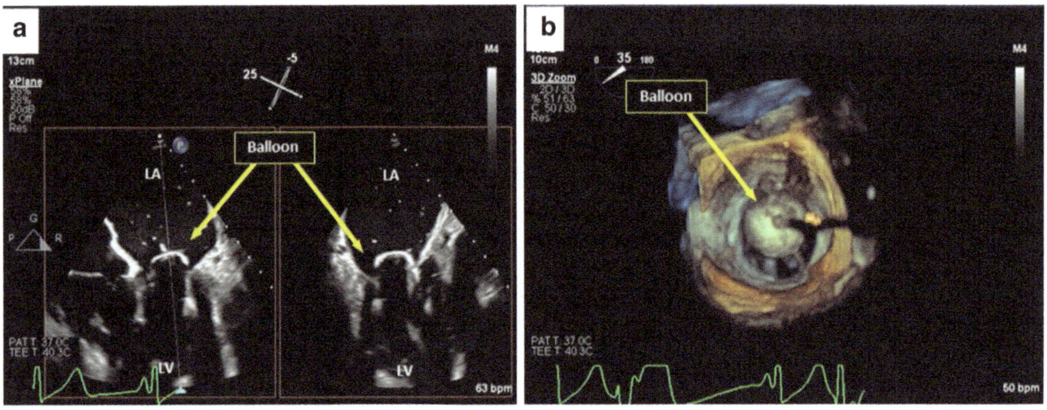

Fig. 17.9 **Mitral balloon valvuloplasty**. (**a**) Biplane view of balloon inflation during a mitral balloon valvuloplasty procedure. The balloon is inflated from distal chamber to proximal chamber under echocardiographic surveillance. (**b**) 3D view from atrial perspective showing the inflated balloon across the mitral valve. *LA left atrium, LV left ventricle*

  - Measurement of transmittal gradient
  - Planimetry of mitral valve area (if TEE utilized)
  - Commissural opening
  - Leaflet mobility
- If deemed necessary, repeat balloon inflations can be performed
- Assessment of the residual inter-atrial communication
- Exclusion of any complications

Post-Procedure Imaging:

Comprehensive echocardiography at standard intervals. Studies should include:

- Full assessment of chambers size and function
- Detailed assessment of mitral valve –
  - Mitral valve anatomy, commissural fusion, area by planimetry
  - Assessment of residual MR severity
  - Mitral inflow gradient
- Other valves function, pulmonary pressures

17.5.4 Left Atrial Appendage (LAA) Closure

Indications:
Patients with atrial fibrillation who cannot tolerate long term anticoagulation. Currently approved device - Watchman

- Important to note, post implantation, full anticoagulation with Warfarin is required for 45 days. Subsequently aspirin and Plavix are used for several months, followed by lifelong aspirin treatment.

Pre-procedure Imaging:

- TEE is required prior to Watchman procedure to rule out LAA clot
- Accurate measurements of LAA size are needed for optimal sizing of the Watchman device; the diameter of the LAA opening, as well as the depth of the LAA are measured at multiple angles from mid-esophageal view.

Intra-Procedure Imaging:

Watchman procedure is commonly done under TEE guidance. Intra-cardiac echocardiography can be used for guidance as well

TEE can help guide the various stages of the procedure:

- Trans-septal puncture
  - Biplane visualization (mid esophageal short axis aortic valve view and bicaval view) helps facilitate safe and accurate trans-septal puncture
- Manipulation of intra-cardiac wires and catheters

- Following trans-septal puncture, a wire, pigtail catheter and ultimately the Watchman device are introduced into the left atrium
- TEE surveillance with continuous visualization of all wires and catheters helps assure their safe manipulation
- Typically, prior to device placement, LAA angiogram is performed for further assessment of LAA anatomy

- Device positioning
  - Watchman device is introduced into LAA
  - Echocardiographic assessment includes
    - Measurement of device maximal diameter at multiple angles from mid-esophageal view to assure adequate compression of the device
    - Color Doppler interrogation to verify lack of residual flow around the device into the LAA
  - "Tag" test is performed by the interventionist to verify stability of the device in the LAA
  - Prior to deployment, if needed, the device can be recaptured and repositioned
  - Once all assessment is satisfactory, the device is deployed in the LAA

Immediately following device deployment, echocardiographic assessment is preformed.

Goals of Immediate Post-Deployment Evaluation
- Verify stable positioning of the device
- Confirm lack of residual communication between main left atrium and LAA
- Assessment of the residual inter-atrial communication
- Exclusion of any complications (mainly pericardial effusion)

Post-procedure Imaging

(Fig. 17.10, Videos 17.5A and 17.5B):

Typically, TEE is performed at standard intervals following Watchman procedure

Goals of the follow up TEE include:
- Verify good position of the Watchman device
- Confirm full clotting of LAA behind the device
- Evaluate (by color Doppler interrogation) for any residual communication between LAA and main left atrium
- Exclude any clot on the atrial surface of the device

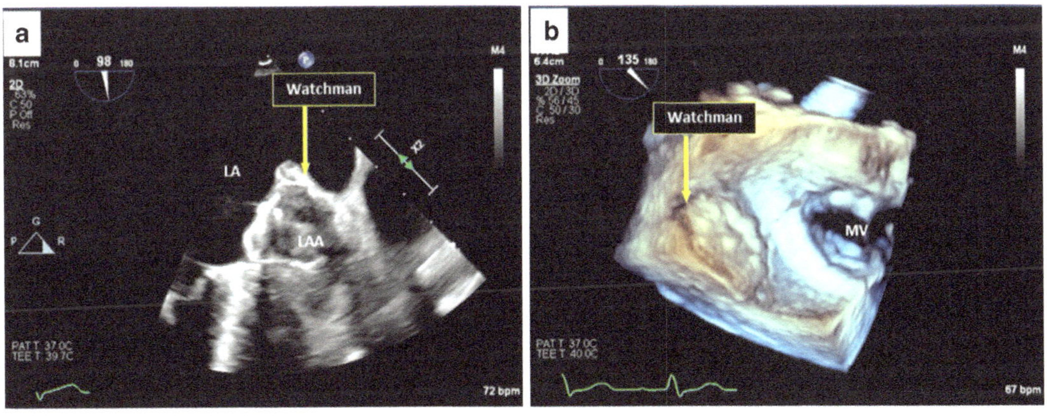

Fig. 17.10 **Post watchman device follow up**. (**a**) Two dimensional view of a Watchman device occluding the left atrial appendage. Good apposition of the device at the opening of the appendage is noted, as well as near complete clotting of the appendage cavity behind the device. No clot is seen on the atrial surface of the device. (**b**) 3D view from atrial perspective; the Watchman device is seen at 9 o'clock position, the mitral valve is seen deeper (partially cut on this image). *LA left atrium, LAA left atrial appendage, MV mitral valve*

Further Reading

Biner S, Perk G, Kar S, et al. Utility of combined two-dimensional and three-dimensional transesophageal imaging for catheter-based mitral valve clip repair of mitral regurgitation. J Am Soc Echocardiogr. 2011;24(6):611–7. https://doi.org/10.1016/j.echo.2011.02.005.

Hahn RT, Nicoara A, Kapadia S, Svensson L, Martin R. Echocardiographic imaging for transcatheter aortic valve replacement. J Am Soc Echocardiogr. 2018;31(4):405–33. https://doi.org/10.1016/j.echo.2017.10.022.

Hahn RT, Little SH, Monaghan MJ, et al. Recommendations for comprehensive intraprocedural echocardiographic imaging during TAVR. JACC Cardiovasc Imaging. 2015;8(3):261–87. https://doi.org/10.1016/j.jcmg.2014.12.014.

Pison L, Potpara TS, Chen J, et al. Left atrial appendage closure-indications, techniques, and outcomes: results of the European Heart Rhythm Association Survey. Europace. 2015;17(4):642–6. https://doi.org/10.1093/europace/euv069.

Perk G, Kronzon I. Interventional echocardiography in structural heart disease. Curr Cardiol Rep. 2013;15(3):338. https://doi.org/10.1007/s11886-012-0338-y.

Ruiz CE, Kliger C, Perk G, et al. Transcatheter therapies for the treatment of valvular and paravalvular regurgitation in acquired and congenital valvular heart disease [published correction appears in J Am Coll Cardiol. 2015 66(10):1207]. J Am Coll Cardiol. 2015;66(2):169–83. https://doi.org/10.1016/j.jacc.2015.05.034.

Wunderlich NC, Beigel R, Ho SY, et al. Imaging for mitral interventions: methods and efficacy. JACC Cardiovasc Imaging. 2018;11(6):872–901. https://doi.org/10.1016/j.jcmg.2018.02.024.

Index

T. Rambhatla, G. Perk, *The Echocardiography Companion*,
https://doi.org/10.1007/978-3-030-47041-8

B

C

D

E

R

S

T

GPSR Compliance

The European Union's (EU) General Product Safety Regulation (GPSR) is a set of rules that requires consumer products to be safe and our obligations to ensure this.

If you have any concerns about our products, you can contact us on ProductSafety@springernature.com

In case Publisher is established outside the EU, the EU authorized representative is:

Springer Nature Customer Service Center GmbH
Europaplatz 3
69115 Heidelberg, Germany

Batch number: 10732714

Printed by Printforce, the Netherlands